Evidence-Based
Treatment Approaches *for*
SUICIDAL ADOLESCENTS
Translating Science *Into* Practice

Evidence-Based
Treatment Approaches *for*
SUICIDAL ADOLESCENTS
Translating Science *Into* Practice

Edited by

Michele Berk, Ph.D.

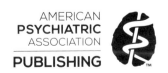

AMERICAN
PSYCHIATRIC
ASSOCIATION
PUBLISHING

If you wish to buy 50 or more copies of the same title, please go to www.appi.org/specialdiscounts for more information.

Copyright © 2019 American Psychiatric Association Publishing

ALL RIGHTS RESERVED

First Edition

Manufactured in the United States of America on acid-free paper
23 22 21 20 19   5 4 3 2 1

American Psychiatric Association Publishing
800 Maine Avenue SW Suite 900
Washington, DC 20024-2812
www.appi.org

Library of Congress Cataloging-in-Publication Data
Names: Berk, Michele, 1970– editor. | American Psychiatric Association
   Publishing, publisher.

Title: Evidence-based treatment approaches for suicidal adolescents :
   translating science into practice / edited by Michele Berk.

Description: First edition. | Washington, D.C. : American Psychiatric
   Association Publishing, [2019] | Includes bibliographical references and
   index.

Identifiers: LCCN 2018055779 (print) | LCCN 2018056530 (ebook) | ISBN
   9781615372515 (ebook) | ISBN 9781615371631 (pbk. : alk. paper)

Subjects: | MESH: Suicide—prevention & control | Suicide—psychology |
   Adolescent Behavior—psychology | Psychotherapy—methods | Risk Factors |
   Evidence-Based Practice

Classification: LCC RC569 (ebook) | LCC RC569 (print) | NLM WM 165 | DDC
   616.85/8445—dc23

LC record available at https://lccn.loc.gov/2018055779

British Library Cataloguing in Publication Data
A CIP record is available from the British Library.

Contents

PART I: Suicide Risk Assessment and Basic Safety Planning

PART II: Treatment Approaches

Contributors

Joan R. Asarnow, Ph.D.
Professor of Psychiatry and Biobehavioral Sciences, University of California, Los Angeles, David Geffen School of Medicine, and Semel Institute of Neuroscience and Behavior, Los Angeles, California

Kalina Babeva, Ph.D.
Clinical Instructor, University of California, Los Angeles, David Geffen School of Medicine, and Semel Institute of Neuroscience and Behavior, Los Angeles, California

Anthony Bateman, M.A., FRCPsych
Visiting Professor, University College London; Affiliate Professor in Psychotherapy, Copenhagen University; Consultant to the Anna Freud National Centre for Children and Families, London

Michele Berk, Ph.D.
Assistant Professor, Department of Psychiatry and Behavioral Sciences, Division of Child and Adolescent Psychiatry, Stanford University, Stanford, California

Chloe Campbell, Ph.D.
Deputy Director of the Psychoanalysis Unit, University College London

Stephanie Clarke, Ph.D.
Clinical Instructor, Department of Psychiatry and Behavioral Sciences, Division of Child and Adolescent Psychiatry, Stanford University, Stanford, California

Guy S. Diamond, Ph.D.
Associate Professor and Director of the Center for Family Intervention Science, Drexel University; Professor Emeritus, University of Pennsylvania School of Medicine, Philadelphia, Pennsylvania

Erika C. Esposito, B.A.
Graduate Student, Department of Clinical and Social Sciences in Psychology, University of Rochester, Rochester, New York

Christianne Esposito-Smythers, Ph.D.
Associate Professor and Director of Clinical Training, Department of Psychology, George Mason University, Fairfax, Virginia

Peter Fonagy, Ph.D., FBA, FMedSci, FAcSS
Professor of Contemporary Psychoanalysis and Developmental Science, University College; Chief Executive, Anna Freud National Centre for Children and Families, London

Catherine R. Glenn, Ph.D.
Assistant Professor, Department of Clinical and Social Sciences in Psychology, University of Rochester, Rochester, New York

Jennifer L. Hughes, Ph.D., M.P.H.
Assistant Professor of Psychiatry, University of Texas Southwestern Medical Center, Dallas, Texas

Quintin A. Hunt, Ph.D.
Assistant Professor of Counselor Education, University of Wisconsin-Superior, Superior, Wisconsin

Bora Jin, Ph.D.
Collaborating Researcher, Center for Family Intervention Science, Drexel University; Visiting Assistant Professor, Department of Child Development and Education, Myongji University, Seoul, Republic of Korea

Jaclyn C. Kearns, B.A.
Graduate Student, Department of Clinical and Social Sciences in Psychology, University of Rochester, Rochester, New York

Suzanne A. Levy, Ph.D.
Training Director, Attachment-Based Family Therapy Training Center, Center for Family Intervention Science, Drexel University, Philadelphia, Pennsylvania

Alec L. Miller, Psy.D.
Cofounder and Clinical Director of Cognitive Behavioral Consultants, LLP; Clinical Professor of Psychiatry and Behavioral Sciences, Montefiore Medical Center/Albert Einstein College of Medicine, New York, New York

Andrew C. Porter, M.Ed.
Graduate Student, Department of Clinical and Social Sciences in Psychology, University of Rochester, Rochester, New York

Jill H. Rathus, Ph.D.
Professor of Psychology, Department of Psychology, C.W. Post Campus of Long Island University, Brookville, New York

Trudie Rossouw, M.B.Ch.B, FFPsych, MRCPsych, M.D. (Res)
Consultant Child and Adolescent Psychiatrist and Honorary Senior Lecturer, University College London

Melisa D. Rowland, M.D.
Associate Professor, Department of Psychiatry and Behavioral Sciences, Medical University of South Carolina, Charleston

Manpreet K. Singh, M.D., M.S.
Assistant Professor, Department of Psychiatry and Behavioral Sciences, Stanford University School of Medicine, Stanford, California

Anthony Spirito, Ph.D., ABPP
Professor and Vice Chair, Department of Psychiatry and Human Behavior, Alpert Medical School of Brown University, Providence, Rhode Island

Amy S. Walker, Ph.D.
Associate Director of Training at Cognitive Behavioral Consultants, LLP, White Plains, New York

Jennifer Wolff, Ph.D.
Assistant Professor (Research), Department of Psychiatry and Human Behavior, Alpert Medical School of Brown University, Providence, Rhode Island

Isheeta Zalpuri, M.D.
Associate Clinical Professor, Department of Psychiatry and Behavioral Sciences, Stanford University School of Medicine, Stanford, California

Disclosure of Competing Interests

The following contributors to this book have indicated a financial interest in or other affiliation with a commercial supporter, a manufacturer of a commercial product, a provider of a commercial service, a nongovernmental organization, and /or a government agency, as listed below:

Peter Fonagy, Ph.D., FBA, FMedSci, FAcSS—*Chief Executive*: Anna Freud National Centre for Children and Families (AFNCCF); *Training*: clinicians in the UK and internationally in mentalization-based treatment. Revenues from these trainings go to the AFNCCF.

Alec L. Miller, Psy.D.—*Royalties*: Guilford Press book; *Consultant*: Behavioral Tech trainer fees; *Cofounder and Clinical Director*: CBC Treatment and Training Center

Jill H. Rathus, Ph.D.—*Trainer*: Behavioral Tech; *Author*: *Dialectical Behavior Therapy With Suicidal Adolescents*, *DBT Skills Manual for Adolescents*, and *DBT Skills in Schools*, all Guilford Press; *Codirector*: Cognitive Behavioral Associates, Great Neck, NY

Melisa D. Rowland, M.D.—*Stockholder*: MST Services, Inc., which has the exclusive licensing agreement through the Medical University of South Carolina for dissemination of MST technology and intellectual property.

Manpreet K. Singh, M.D., M.S.—*Research support*: From Stanford's Child Health Research Institute, National Institute of Mental Health, Office of Research on Women's Health, National Institute of Aging, Neuronetics, Johnson and Johnson, and Brain and Behavior Foundation. Dr. Singh has been on the advisory board for Sunovion.

The following contributors to this book have indicated no competing interests to disclose:

    Michele Berk, Ph.D.
    Guy S. Diamond, Ph.D.
    Christianne Esposito-Smythers, Ph.D.
    Catherine R. Glenn, Ph.D.
    Jennifer L. Hughes, Ph.D., M.P.H.
    Trudie Rossouw, M.B.Ch.B, FFPsych, MRCPsych, M.D. (Res)

Foreword

This volume brings together state of the art research and treatment development work with clinical descriptions of evidence-based and informed treatment strategies for adolescents presenting with suicidality and self-harm, a population at elevated risk for death by suicide and future suicidal and nonsuicidal self-harm. Clinicians and researchers alike will find the rich material in this volume to be a major resource in their efforts to prevent suicide, reduce suffering, and improve the lives of adolescents and their family members.

The loss of a patient to suicide is a heart-wrenching experience. Although there have been advances in knowledge and treatments, suicide is currently the second leading cause of death in adolescents and young adults. In contrast to other sources of mortality, tragically suicide death rates continue to increase in many of our communities and nations across the globe, and adolescents who self-harm are not only at risk for death by suicide but also for death by other unnatural causes as they mature and progress through adulthood. Research, clinical, and public health initiatives are needed to change these statistics and move us to a point where suicide rates decline, as we aspire toward the goal of "zero suicide" and making suicide a "never event" (see https://zerosuicide.sprc.org/). The material in this book provides important information on clinical treatment approaches that have shown promise in reducing the risk of suicide attempts and self-harm, an important component of our efforts to prevent the tragedy of premature deaths.

Following two chapters on risk assessment and safety plans, the book includes six chapters that present different approaches to psychosocial treatment. As would be expected, given that these different treatment approaches address common problems, some approaches are related and share common theoretical roots, and most share some common treatment foci and address similar targets and mechanisms (e.g., restricting access to dangerous self-harm methods, enhancing family support and functioning, strengthening emotion regulation). Yet, there are important differences between the approaches described in the various chapters, and the chapters offer clinicians different perspectives on how to best support safety and recovery in the adolescents and families for whom they provide care.

The volume also includes a chapter on pharmacological strategies for managing and treating suicidality. This combination of information on risk assessment and management, psychosocial treatment, and pharmacological treatment offers the needed information to consider both psychosocial and biologically based risk and protective factors. This perspective is increasingly recognized as crucial for improving physical and mental health and the outcomes for adolescents and their families. Not only has the field of psychiatry moved beyond the body and mind divide, but we have also learned that most adolescents presenting with suicidality and/or self-harm experience mental health disorders, and many of these young patients are treated with psychiatric medications. It is, therefore, crucial that clinicians caring for these patients understand the role, advantages, and potential harms associated with both psychosocial and pharmacological treatment strategies, as well as their combination.

Because we recognize the challenges in adopting new treatments, the book includes rich clinical descriptions and case examples as well as attention to the challenges of implementing treatments developed and evaluated in research laboratory settings in routine practice settings. These sections are sure to provide valuable information to clinicians and decision makers who wish to adopt these approaches in their settings.

Estimates suggest that one in five mental health professionals will lose a patient to suicide. As highlighted by Dr. Michele Berk in her introduction to this volume, as much as we want to, it is not possible to prevent every death. Yet, it is incumbent on us to do our very best to prevent these tragedies, and because most people who make fatal as well as nonfatal suicide attempts visit a health or mental health care provider in the months and sometimes weeks before their attempts, it is likely that opportunities will present to turn individuals toward building their lives and to prevent suicide attempts and deaths. The information provided in this book can be a valuable resource to support clinicians, policy makers, health and behavioral health system leaders, and researchers in developing knowledge, practices, and policies that can help us achieve the aims of alleviating suffering, improving lives of adolescents and families, and reducing the tragedies of suicide and premature deaths. We will never be able to prevent every death, yet this is a goal worth aspiring to, while recognizing that we can do our very best and still mental illness and/or other factors will overcome our best efforts. This volume offers critical strategies for helping us to do our very best for the adolescents and families who trust us to do this potentially life-saving work.

Joan R. Asarnow, Ph.D.
David Geffen School of Medicine,
Semel Institute of Neuroscience and Behavior,
University of California, Los Angeles

Acknowledgments

I would like to thank Tanya Llewellyn, Ph.D., and Stephanie Clarke, Ph.D., for their assistance in preparing this book. I would also like to thank the supervisors, mentors, and colleagues that I have worked with over the years who have taught me how to treat suicidal patients: Joan Asarnow, Ph.D., Aaron T. Beck, M.D., Gregory Brown, Ph.D., Christine Foertsch, Ph.D., and Marsha Linehan, Ph.D. Finally, I would like to thank my family: Talia Steidl, Samuel Steidl, Sheri Berk, Arthur Berk, and Stefanie Berk for supporting me in everything that I do.

Introduction

Michele Berk, Ph.D.

In this chapter, I provide the context for the book by reviewing the most recent statistics on the epidemiology of suicidal behavior in adolescents, as well as the literature on evidence-based treatment approaches. The literature review will include a brief review of the treatments to be described in the book, the data supporting each, and why each treatment was chosen for the book. It will also provide an overview of the goals and objectives of the book and briefly describe each chapter.

Suicide is the second leading cause of death among 10- to 24-year-olds in the United States (Centers for Disease Control and Prevention 2016). According to the Youth Risk Behavior Survey, a biannual national survey of high school students in the United States, just under 1 in 5 high school students reported seriously considering attempting suicide (17.7%), and just under 1 in 10 reported attempting suicide in the past year (8.6%; Kann et al. 2016). The prevalence of both suicidal ideation (SI) and suicide attempts (SAs) increases dramatically during adolescence (Nock et al. 2013). Suicide rates have continued to rise across age groups in the United States over the last 15 years, with females ages 10–14 years showing the greatest increase (200%; Curtin et al. 2016). In light of these alarming statistics, it is critical that mental health professionals who treat adolescents are familiar with evidence-based strategies for reducing suicide risk in youth.

Despite the magnitude of the problem, there are a surprisingly limited number of empirically supported treatments for decreasing suicidal behavior in adolescents. Randomized controlled trials (RCTs), in which subjects are randomly assigned to an experimental treatment group or to a control group (e.g., a different treatment approach, treatment as usual, wait list, etc.), are widely considered to be the gold standard approach for determining treatment efficacy in medical research, despite limitations (Bothwell et al. 2016). At present, there are only 16 RCTs of treatments for adolescents with histories of attempted suicide and/or nonsuicidal self-injury (NSSI) that target reduction in self-harm (SH) behavior as their primary outcome variable, including replication trials. Only eight of these trials yielded statistically significant results. Of these eight trials, only one has been replicated (dialectical behavior therapy, DBT; McCauley et al. 2016; Mehlum et al. 2014), and one failed two subsequent replication trials (developmental group therapy; Green et al. 2011; Hazell et al. 2009; Wood et al. 2001). A recent meta-analysis of 19 studies of therapeutic interventions for SH behavior (including studies focused on brief interventions conducted in emergency department [ED] settings that also focused on linkage to outpatient care as a primary outcome) found a significant advantage for therapeutic interventions versus control conditions for decreasing SH, with the strongest effect sizes for DBT, mentalization-based therapy (MBT), and cognitive-behavioral therapy (CBT) (Ougrin et al. 2015).

Although the results of extant research are promising, clinicians must make difficult decisions about how to most effectively treat adolescents at risk for suicide based on limited research findings. The relatively small amount of treatment research for adolescents at risk for suicide is likely due to the multiple challenges for investigators conducting research with this population (Berk et al. 2014; Iltis et al. 2013; Linehan 1997; Pearson et al. 2001). These challenges include 1) the significant anxiety associated with working with suicidal individuals; 2) managing liability if a subject is injured or dies during the trial; 3) the need for sufficient expertise and resources to monitor and treat suicidal subjects; and 4) the large sample sizes needed for sufficient statistical power to detect between-group differences in suicide-related outcomes (Pearson et al. 2001). These concerns have also resulted in the exclusion of suicidal individuals from research studies in general (Pearson et al. 2001). More research on effective treatments for youth at risk for suicide is urgently needed.

Working with suicidal patients is one of the greatest challenges faced by mental health professionals. The challenge is arguably even greater when working with adolescents because the death of a young person by suicide is uniquely tragic for all involved. As both a clinician and researcher working with this population, I have often felt anxious, ineffective, and helpless when working with teens and families who were desperate for help to prevent devastating outcomes and have struggled to find effective tools to help within the limits of our existing knowledge. The overarching goal of this book is to help clinicians navigate the difficulties of providing effective treatment to suicidal youth by bringing together in one volume the most current knowledge about treatments that have evidence for reducing the risk of suicide in youth in order to help clinicians provide the best possible evidence-based care to their patients. As somebody who has often been frustrated by *what we don't know* about how to help suicidal youth, my goal in this book is to provide clinicians with accurate, accessible, and comprehensive information about *what we do know*.

Overview of the Book

This book provides a practice-friendly review of six treatments that have been shown in RCTs (and which have not failed subsequent replication trials) to reduce suicidal and/or SH behavior in adolescents with prior histories of these behaviors, that is, in adolescents at highest risk of suicide. Each treatment approach is described in a chapter written by the treatment developer(s). The six treatments described in this book are 1) DBT for adolescents (DBT-A); 2) MBT for adolescents (MBT-A); 3) integrated CBT (I-CBT; which addresses co-occurring suicidal behavior and substance use); 4) multisystemic therapy (MST); 5) attachment-based family therapy (ABFT); and 6) the Safe Alternatives for Teens and Youths (SAFETY) program. In addition, Chapter 2, "Risk and Protective Factors for Suicidal Thoughts and Behaviors in Adolescents," provides an up-to-date, comprehensive review of research on risk factors for adolescent SAs and suicide deaths. Chapter 3, "Safety Planning and Risk Management," provides a review and guidelines for basic safety measures that should be taken with all youth at risk for suicide, regardless of treatment approach, and discusses hospitalization of suicidal youth. Chapter 10, "Pharmacological Approaches for Treating Suicidality in Adolescents," provides a review of the most recent research and clinical guidelines on medication management with suicidal youth.

In order to allow readers to easily find relevant information and to compare components of one treatment approach with another, each treatment approach–focused chapter follows a common structure, which includes the following: 1) an overview of the treatment approach; 2) theoretical model and proposed mechanisms of change; 3) review of current empirical evidence for the approach; 4) treatment components and primary intervention strategies; 5) a case example; 6) recommendations for how a clinician can implement the approach in his or her own practice; and 7) resources for obtaining training in the approach and suggested readings. The reader can also refer to Table 1–1 in this chapter for a quick guide to comparing the components of each treatment.

Because this book is geared toward a wide range of clinicians working across various practice settings, each treatment approach–focused chapter includes resources for obtaining training from the treatment developers in the fully adherent version of the treatment model (e.g., the version that has been tested in research) as well as recommendations for how to incorporate individual elements of the treatment when implementing the fully adherent model is not feasible. However, it is important to note that existing evidence for each treatment approach *supports only the fully adherent versions* of the treatment, exactly as conducted in the existing clinical trials. Hence, whereas using only parts of a treatment may make sense clinically, it is important to remember that there is no evidence to support the effectiveness of modified versions of the treatment protocol, and clinicians are essentially relying on *clinical judgment only* when choosing to do so. Further dismantling research is needed to provide empirical support and guidance regarding the effectiveness of using individual components of existing empirically supported treatments. Those clinicians who choose to adapt existing treatment approaches by using only components of the treatment instead of the full model are encouraged to collect outcome data for both clinical and research purposes to measure the effectiveness of the adaptation (Koerner et al. 2007).

TABLE 1-1. Summary of treatment approaches

Treatment approach	Treatment components	Treatment length	Number of clinicians required	Diagnostic focus	Primary mechanism of change	Strategies for enhancing commitment/adherence to treatment	Includes safety planning?	Includes parent and family sessions?	Outcome data on reductions in SA, NSSI, or SH
DBT	Individual therapy Multifamily skills group Telephone coaching Therapist consultation meeting	6 months	1 individual therapist 2 multifamily group leaders	Trans-diagnostic BPD	Increased use of DBT skills to regulate emotion	Pretreatment commitment phase Targeting therapy-interfering behavior in every session	Yes	Yes	SA, NSSI, SH
MBT-A	Individual MBT therapy MBT—family therapy	12 months	1 individual therapist and 1 family therapist	Trans-diagnostic BPD	Improved ability to mentalize	Treatment contract reviewed in initial phase of treatment	Yes	Yes	SH
I-CBT	Individual therapy for teen and parenting session for parent, provided concurrently with a joint family session at the end	12 months	1 teen therapist and 1 parent therapist	Trans-diagnostic AOD use disorders	Increased use of CBT coping skills	Motivational interviewing strategies used to enhance commitment	Yes	Yes	SA

TABLE 1-1.   Summary of treatment approaches *(continued)*

Treatment approach	Treatment components	Treatment length	Number of clinicians required	Diagnostic focus	Primary mechanism of change	Strategies for enhancing commitment/ adherence to treatment	Includes safety planning?	Includes parent and family sessions?	Outcome data on reductions in SA, NSSI, or SH
MST-Psychiatric	Home-based sessions with teens and families provided as needed by an MST team on call 24 hours a day	4–7 months	Team of 3–4 therapists plus a child psychiatrist, crisis caseworker, MST supervisor, expert MST consultant, and MST expert psychiatrist	Trans-diagnostic	Improved parent and family functioning	Session conducted in the home Focus on engagement with family in initial sessions	Yes	Yes	SA
ABFT	Family therapy	12–16 weeks	1 family therapist	Trans-diagnostic	Improved attachment security between adolescents and parents	Adolescent and parent alliance tasks	Yes	Yes	SA

TABLE 1-1. Summary of treatment approaches *(continued)*

Treatment approach	Treatment components	Treatment length	Number of clinicians required	Diagnostic focus	Primary mechanism of change	Strategies for enhancing commitment/ adherence to treatment	Includes safety planning?	Includes parent and family sessions?	Outcome data on reductions in SA, NSSI, or SH
SAFETY	Individual therapy for teen and parenting session for parent, provided concurrently with a joint family session at the end.	3 months	1 teen therapist and 1 parent therapist	Trans-diagnostic	Enhanced protective processes within youth, family, and social environments	Commitment to treatment/using safety plan Availability of home-based sessions	Yes	Yes	SA

Note. ABFT=attachment-based family therapy; AOD=alcohol/other drug; BPD=borderline personality disorder; CBT=cognitive-behavioral therapy; DBT=dialectical behavior therapy; I-CBT=integrated cognitive-behavioral therapy; MBT-A=mentalization-based therapy for adolescents; MST-Psychiatric=multisystemic therapy with psychiatric supports; NSSI=nonsuicidal self-injury; SA=suicide attempt; SAFETY= Safe Alternatives for Teens and Youths; SH=self-harm.

Definitions of Key Terms Used in This Book

One problem in suicide research has been the inconsistent use of terms across studies to describe SH outcomes, which has made it difficult to compare the results of one study with another (O'Carroll et al. 1996; Turecki and Brent 2016). In the United States, suicide attempt (SA) and NSSI behaviors are seen as distinct behaviors and differentiated on the basis of the presence or absence of intent to die versus other intended outcomes of the behavior, such as reducing negative emotion (Crosby et al. 2011; O'Carroll et al. 1996; Posner et al. 2007; Silverman et al. 2007). In contrast, in the United Kingdom and Europe these behaviors have typically been grouped together in a broader category of SH, which includes both SA and NSSI, regardless of intent (NICE 2004; Ougrin et al. 2012). Both SA and NSSI (Asarnow et al. 2011; Bridge et al. 2006; Wilkinson et al. 2011) have been shown to be robust risk factors for future SAs; hence, both approaches appear to have value. However, it is important to note that prior SAs are the strongest predictor of death by suicide (for a review, see Brent et al. 2013), are most proximally related to death by suicide, and are associated with greater risk of death/serious injury as a result of the behavior. Therefore, it is important to determine if a treatment specifically reduces SAs. The RCTs testing the treatments described in the book have used both SA and SH as study outcomes. To enable a precise understanding and comparison of the findings of each of these research studies, definitions of these terms are provided in Table 1–2 and a summary of the outcomes supported for each study are listed in Table 1–1.

Treatments With Randomized Controlled Trials That Are Not Reviewed in This Book

The focus of this book is on treatments targeting youth at highest risk of suicide. Hence, the book only includes treatments that were studied with samples of adolescents with prior SA or SH and that measure SA or SH as an outcome. Although the overall number of studies remains small when these inclusion criteria are broadened, there are a number of studies that have focused on interventions for lower-risk youth (e.g., youth with SI or other risk factors, not including SA or SH), primary prevention (e.g., youth who have never been suicidal), or engagement in follow-up care fol-

TABLE 1-2. Definitions of types of self-injurious behaviors

Suicide attempt (SA)	A potentially self-injurious behavior, associated with *some evidence of intent to die*
Nonsuicidal self-injury (NSSI)	Self-injurious behavior *not associated with intent to die* (e.g., intent may be to reduce negative emotion, to punish oneself)
Self-harm (SH)	Broader category including all intentional self-injury, with or without intent to die (i.e., SA and NSSI)

lowing an ED visit (for reviews, see Berk and Hughes 2016; Glenn et al. 2015; Ougrin et al. 2012, 2015).

There are two existing RCTs of treatments for youth with prior SA or SH that are not included in this book. The first is a brief, four-session parenting intervention conducted in Australia. Given the brevity of this approach, its psychoeducational focus, and its inclusion of parents only (i.e., no intervention was provided to teens), it deviates somewhat from the emphasis of this book on adolescent psychotherapy approaches. Moreover, the primary outcome measure used in the RCT was a summary score measuring severity of suicidality, which included SI as well as SA and SH, instead of measuring suicidal behavior as separate from suicidal thoughts. The second treatment is a group therapy approach that was studied in the United Kingdom and demonstrated significant reductions in SH in the initial RCT testing its efficacy (Wood et al. 2001); however, it failed to be replicated in two subsequent RCTs. For the sake of completeness, each of these treatments are described briefly below.

Resourceful Adolescent Parent Program

The Resourceful Adolescent Parent Program (RAP-P) is a four-session, parent-only, strengths-based psychoeducation intervention developed in Australia that focuses on building parents' strengths to foster resiliency in teens (Pineda and Dadds 2013). RAP was originally developed as a school-based universal prevention program for adolescent depression and includes adolescent (RAP-A), parent (RAP-P), and teacher components (RAP-T). Pineda and Dadds (2013) conducted an RCT comparing RAP-P as a stand-alone intervention plus routine care with routine care alone in a sample of 48 Australian adolescents with at least one episode of suicidality (including SI, SA, and NSSI) within the past 2 months. The parent intervention was delivered either in a mental health clinic or in the home and included an introductory session focused on education about adolescent suicidal behavior and practical strategies for decreasing SH (added to the original version of the RAP-P for this study), and three additional sessions focused on identifying parenting strengths, reducing parenting stress, providing information about normative adolescent development, and family conflict resolution strategies. Results showed that, compared with routine care alone, youth whose parents received routine care plus RAP-P reported significantly greater decreases in suicidality (based on a summary score including SI, SH, and SA) at 3- and 6-month follow-up assessments. These findings are noteworthy because family conflict is a key risk factor for adolescent suicidal behavior (Bridge et al. 2006), and an intervention for parents only may be easier to deliver and associated with greater treatment compliance than interventions that require regular teen participation. Readers who are interested in learning more about RAP-P are referred to the journal article describing this study (Pineda and Dadds 2013).

Developmental Group Therapy

Developmental group therapy was developed for use in the United Kingdom and tested in an RCT with 63 adolescents (ages 12–16 years) in the United Kingdom with a recent history of SH plus one additional instance of SH within the past year (Wood et al. 2001). Youth were randomly assigned to receive 6 months of either developmental group therapy or treatment as usual. At posttreatment follow-up, those in group therapy demonstrated a decreased likelihood of engaging in repeated (i.e., ≥ two) episodes of SH as well as a longer mean time until the first repetition of deliberate SH, compared with those in the treatment as usual group. The developmental group therapy utilized techniques from CBT, DBT, and psychodynamic therapy and was designed to be sensitive to the developmental needs of adolescents and to facilitate lessening of SH via "positive and corrective" therapeutic relationships. The intervention consisted of an initial assessment, six acute group sessions, and a long-term follow-up group. The acute portion of the group was structured around six themes related to SH in adolescents, which include relationships; school problems and peer relationships; family problems; anger management; depression and SH; and hopelessness and feelings about the future. The long-term portion of the group focused more on group process and had a psychodynamic orientation. On the basis of the positive outcomes of the original study, there were two subsequent replication trials conducted using developmental group therapy; however, neither study found significant between-group differences in SH outcomes, calling into question the effectiveness and transportability of the treatment (Green et al. 2011; Hazell et al. 2009).

Common Elements of Effective Treatments

As shown in Table 1–1, the treatments included in this book that have been shown to be effective at reducing SA and/or SH in adolescents share several common elements. First, all treatments include detailed safety planning with the adolescent and parent, which is essential for reducing risk of serious injury and/or death when working with youth at risk for suicide. Chapter 3 of this book provides a detailed review of evidence-based safety planning strategies, which are recommended for use with all suicidal youth, regardless of treatment approach.

Second, as shown in the recent meta-analysis of therapeutic interventions for SH in youth described above (Ougrin et al. 2015; see also Brent et al. 2013), family-based treatment components are associated with greater effect sizes for decreasing SH and are included in all of the treatments described in this book. Improving family functioning is a critical treatment target for suicidal youth (Brent et al. 2013). Family conflict has been identified as a key risk factor for adolescent suicide and suicidal behavior, and family cohesion has been identified as a protective factor (Bridge et al. 2006). Because parents play a critical role in maintaining youth safety, strengthening relationships between parents and teens is essential in enabling parents to implement safety strategies and to increase the likelihood that the adolescent will go to the parent for help in a suicidal crisis. All of the treatments discussed in this book include at least one or more of the following parent/family modalities: parent collateral sessions, family sessions, multifamily group sessions, and parent telephone coaching. Two of the treatment approaches are entirely family focused (ABFT and MST), two of the treatments conduct simultaneous teen and parent sessions plus a joint family session with both therapists at the end (I-CBT and SAFETY), one (DBT-A) includes parents in weekly multifamily group plus collateral and family sessions as needed, and one (MBT-A) includes monthly family sessions. As noted earlier, there is also one evidence-based treatment with evidence of efficacy in decreasing suicidality (RAP-P) that was not included in this book that is a parent-only intervention.

Third, all of the treatments focus specifically on reducing suicidal thoughts and behaviors across multiple psychiatric diagnoses and thus are predominately transdiagnostic in nature. Symptoms of psychiatric disorders that occur in conjunction with suicidality, such as depression, are typically targeted in their role as risk factors for suicidal behavior, rather than being the primary treatment target. In terms of each individual treatment approach, MST, ABFT, and SAFETY target suicidality across multiple diagnoses and are not diagnosis specific. I-CBT is designed for treatment of comorbid suicidality and substance use disorders. The original adult versions of DBT and MBT focused on the treatment of suicidality and comorbid borderline personality disorder (BPD); however, the adolescent adaptations of these treatments (DBT-A and MBT-A) have focused predominately on treatment of suicidality and SH and BPD traits as risk factors for suicidal behavior versus targeting the BPD diagnosis.

Fourth, the majority of the effective treatments discussed in this book are comprehensive programs consisting of multiple treatment modalities provided by multiple therapists. Hence, effective treatments for reducing suicidal and SH behavior in adolescents typically provide a higher "dose" of psychotherapy than is typically provided in standard outpatient care (e.g., once per week individual therapy sessions). In addition, in some of the treatments in the book, therapists are also available between sessions (typically 24/7) for phone contacts (DBT, MST, and SAFETY) and offer flexibility to provide additional sessions per week as needed in times of crisis. Treatments vary in length, ranging from a minimum of 3 months (SAFETY and ABFT) to a maximum of 1 year (I-CBT and MBT-A). The optimal treatment length and/or number of sessions for adolescents with histories of suicidal and SH behavior remains an empirical question; however, research has shown that more substantial treatment doses are associated with larger effect sizes for reducing SH (Ougrin et al. 2015).

Fifth, all treatments described in this book include interventions designed to enhance treatment compliance/adherence. Multiple studies have shown that suicidal adolescents have poor compliance with outpatient mental health treatment, with dropout rates as high as 77% (Burns et al. 2008; Piacentini et al. 1995; Spirito et al. 1992, 2011; Trautman et al. 1993). Hence, for treatment to be effective, specific strategies designed to improve compliance with treatment are essential. The treatments in this book use a variety of approaches to enhance compliance. DBT includes a "pretreatment commitment" phase, in which the teen is asked to commit to participating in all elements of the treatment for a period of time (typically, 6 months) and to working on reducing life-threatening behaviors. Multiple "commitment strategies" are used to obtain and strengthen commitment, enhance motivation to change, and problem-solve barriers to commitment. Parents are also asked to commit to participating in the family-based components of the treatment, to facilitate their teen's treatment attendance, and to implement the safety plan. Furthermore, "therapy-interfering" behaviors are a standard part of the individual session agenda in order to proactively address any issues that may result in treatment dropout. I-CBT, SAFETY, and MBT-A also include specific conversations about commitment to treatment participation, treatment goals, and safety plans. I-CBT uses motivational interviewing strategies to enhance commitment to reducing both suicidality and substance use. ABFT includes sessions focused on adolescent and parent alliance, in which treatment goals are reviewed and an agreement to work on them is obtained. Finally, MST addresses treatment compliance by delivering all sessions in the home or the community. SAFETY also conducts the first session in the home, with additional home-based sessions available as needed. It is important to note that strategies should address both teen and parent compliance, because parents play a critical role in facilitating their teen's participation in treatment.

Sixth, each treatment targets one or more known risk factors for adolescent SA and SH. The majority of the treatments target multiple risk factors in addition to offering flexibility within the manual to tailor interventions to match each adolescent's particular combination of risk factors. Chapter 2 provides a detailed review of modifiable risk factors for suicidal behavior in adolescents, and clinicians are encouraged to target risk factors in treatment, regardless of their treatment approach.

Conclusion

In summary, according to this review of the existing evidence-based treatments for decreasing SA and SH in adolescents, effective treatment strategies have included the following: detailed safety planning; parent and family-based interventions; decreasing suicidal and SH behaviors as the primary treatment target versus treating related diagnoses (e.g., depression) and assuming the suicidality will resolve as a result; a substantial dose of treatment (e.g., by providing multiple treatment modalities often involving multiple therapists and/or between-session availability of clinicians); and treatment compliance/adherence strategies. Recent reviews of the literature on treatment approaches for youth at risk for suicide have also identified these factors as common elements of efficacious treatments (Brent et al. 2013; Glenn et al. 2015; Ougrin et al. 2015).

Despite the existence of promising treatment approaches, there are challenges for clinicians attempting to implement these treatments in community practice. For example, the multiple visits, modalities, clinicians, and between-session contacts included in several of the treatments discussed may not be feasible in private practice or in clinics with limited resources. For this reason, each treatment approach–focused chapter includes a table at the end describing elements of the treatment that may be more easily utilized in practice when implementation of the full treatment package is not possible. Dismantling studies are needed to determine the essential elements of these treatment programs in order to reduce burden and increase feasibility of dissemination (Glenn et al. 2015). Although the focus of this book is on treatment strategies for youth who have already engaged in suicidal or SH behavior, it is important to also highlight prevention strategies for stopping these behaviors from occurring in the first place. Prevention efforts may include decreasing risk and increasing protective factors (e.g., interventions that enhance family functioning, decrease substance abuse and psychiatric illness, reduce traumatic experiences, and build coping and emotion regulation skills), increasing early identification efforts for youth at risk (e.g., via mental health awareness programs in schools and communities or screening for depression and suicide risk in primary care settings), reducing stigma associated with mental health treatment, and improving access to mental health services (Berk and Hughes 2016; Caldwell 2008; Nordentoft 2011; Turecki and Brent 2016). In addition, integration and collaboration across various systems that interact with suicidal youth, such as psychiatric inpatient units and EDs, community mental health providers, schools, and primary care providers, are important for identifying youth at risk, linking them to appropriate services, and increasing participation in treatment (Asarnow and Miranda 2014; Brent et al. 2013).

As noted, working with individuals at high risk for suicide can cause a range of intense emotions for clinicians (Hendin et al. 2000; Linehan 1993). As mental health practitioners, suicidality is one of the few issues we encounter in our work that involves life and death outcomes. As discussed at length in Chapter 2, although research has identified multiple risk factors for suicidal behavior, at present, there is no way to accurately predict which individuals at risk will actually attempt suicide or die by suicide at any given moment. As a result, it is important to note that as clinicians, *we do not have the power to completely prevent our patients from attempting suicide and/or dying by suicide.* As a postdoctoral fellow at the University of Pennsylvania first learning how to work with acutely suicidal patients, one of my supervisors, Dr. Gregory K. Brown, gave me the following piece of advice that has remained critical over the years in my ability to continue working with this patient population. He stated, "You cannot prevent patients from attempting suicide, you can only lower the risk." I have found this statement to be immensely helpful in managing the anxiety and sometimes overwhelming sense of responsibility that comes with working with this patient population, and I have made it my primary goal to utilize up-to-date research knowledge to "lower the risk" of suicidal behavior in my patients. The goal of this book is to help other clinicians familiarize themselves with the currently available evidence-based strategies for lowering the risk of suicide in their patients by providing an up-to-date review of evidence-based practices for suicide risk assessment, safety planning, psychopharmacology, and psychotherapy approaches for the treatment of suicidal adolescents.

References

Asarnow JR, Porta G, Spirito A, et al: Suicide attempts and nonsuicidal self-injury in the treatment of resistant depression in adolescents: findings from the TORDIA study. J Am Acad Child Adolesc Psychiatry 50(8):772–781, 2011 21784297

Asarnow JR, Miranda J: Improving care for depression and suicide risk in adolescents: innovative strategies for bringing treatments to community settings. Annu Rev Clin Psychol 10:275–303, 2014 24437432

Berk MS, Hughes J: Cognitive-behavioral approaches for treating suicidal behavior in adolescents. Curr Psychiatry Rev 12:4–13, 2016

Berk M, Adrian M, McCauley E, et al: Conducting research on adolescent suicide attempters: dilemmas and decisions. Behav Ther (N Y N Y) 37(3):65–69, 2014 24954969

Bothwell LE, Greene JA, Podolsky SH, Jones DS: Assessing the gold standard—lessons learned from the history of RCTs. N Engl J Med 374(22):2175–2181, 2016 27248626

Brent DA, McMakin DL, Kennard BD, et al: Protecting adolescents from self-harm: a critical review of intervention studies. J Am Acad Child Adolesc Psychiatry 52(12):1260–1271, 2013 24290459

Bridge JA, Goldstein TR, Brent DA: Adolescent suicide and suicidal behavior. J Child Psychol Psychiatry 47(3–4):372–394, 2006 16492264

Burns CD, Cortell R, Wagner BM: Treatment compliance in adolescents after attempted suicide: a 2-year follow-up study. J Am Acad Child Adolesc Psychiatry 47(8):948–957, 2008 18596554

Caldwell D: The suicide prevention continuum. Pimatisiwin 6(2):145–153, 2008 20835376

Centers for Disease Control and Prevention: 10 leading causes of death by age group, United States—2016, 2016. Available at: https://www.cdc.gov/injury/wisqars/pdf/leading_causes_of_death_by_age_group_2016-508.pdf. Accessed November 26, 2018.

Crosby AE, Ortega L, Melanson C: Self-directed Violence Surveillance: Uniform Definitions and Recommended Data Elements, Version 1.0. Atlanta, GA, Centers for Disease Control and Prevention, National Center for Injury Prevention and Control, 2011

Curtin SC, Warner M, Hedegaard H: Increase in Suicide in the United States, 1999–2014. NCHS Data Brief 241(241):1–8, 2016 27111185

Glenn CR, Franklin JC, Nock MK: Evidence-based psychosocial treatments for self-injurious thoughts and behaviors in youth. J Clin Child Adolesc Psychol 44(1):1–29, 2015 25256034

Green JM, Wood AJ, Kerfoot MJ, et al: Group therapy for adolescents with repeated self harm: randomised controlled trial with economic evaluation. BMJ 342:d682, 2011 21459975

Hazell PL, Martin G, McGill K, et al: Group therapy for repeated deliberate self-harm in adolescents: failure of replication of a randomized trial. J Am Acad Child Adolesc Psychiatry 48(6):662–670, 2009 19454922

Hendin H, Lipschitz A, Maltsberger JT, et al: Therapists' reactions to patients' suicides. Am J Psychiatry 157(12):2022–2027, 2000 11097970

Iltis AS, Misra S, Dunn LB, et al: Addressing risks to advance mental health research. JAMA Psychiatry 70(12):1363–1371, 2013 24173618

Kann L, McManus T, Harris WA, et al: Youth risk behavior surveillance—United States, 2015. MMWR Surveill Summ 65(6)(SS-6):1–174, 2016 27280474

Koerner K, Dimeff LA, Swenson CR: Adopt or adapt? Fidelity matters, in Dialectical Behavior Therapy in Clinical Practice: Applications Across Disorders and Settings. Edited by Dimeff LA, Koerner K. New York, Guilford, 2007, pp 19–36

Linehan M: Cognitive-Behavioral Treatment of Borderline Personality Disorder. New York, Guilford, 1993

Linehan MM: Behavioral treatments of suicidal behavior: definitional obfuscation and treatment outcomes, in The Neurobiology of Suicide: From the Bench to the Clinic. Edited by Stoff DM, Mann J. New York, New York Academy of Sciences, 1997, pp 302–328

McCauley E, Berk MS, Asarnow JR, et al: Collaborative adolescent research on emotions and suicide (CARES): a randomized controlled trial of DBT with highly suicidal adolescents, in New Outcome Data on Treatments for Suicidal Adolescents. Berk MS, Adrian M (Chairs). Symposium conducted at the meeting of the 50th Annual Convention of the Association for Behavioral and Cognitive Therapies (ABCT), New York, October 27–30, 2016

Mehlum L, Tørmoen AJ, Ramberg M, et al: Dialectical behavior therapy for adolescents with repeated suicidal and self-harming behavior: a randomized trial. J Am Acad Child Adolesc Psychiatry 53(10):1082–1091, 2014 25245352

NICE: Self-Harm: The Short Term Physical and Psychological Management and Secondary Prevention of Self-Harm in Primary and Secondary Care: Clinical Guideline 16. London, Gaskell & British Psychological Society, 2004

Nock MK, Green JG, Hwang I, et al: Prevalence, correlates, and treatment of lifetime suicidal behavior among adolescents: results from the National Comorbidity Survey Replication Adolescent Supplement. JAMA Psychiatry 70(3):300–310, 2013 23303463

Nordentoft M: Crucial elements in suicide prevention strategies. Prog Neuropsychopharmacol Biol Psychiatry 35(4):848–853, 2011 21130823

O'Carroll PW, Berman AL, Maris RW, et al: Beyond the Tower of Babel: a nomenclature for suicidology. Suicide Life Threat Behav 26(3):237–252, 1996 8897663

Ougrin D, Tranah T, Leigh E, et al: Practitioner review: Self-harm in adolescents. J Child Psychol Psychiatry 53(4):337–350, 2012 22329807

Ougrin D, Tranah T, Stahl D, et al: Therapeutic interventions for suicide attempts and self-harm in adolescents: systematic review and meta-analysis. J Am Acad Child Adolesc Psychiatry 54(2):97.e2–107.e2, 2015 25617250

Pearson JL, Stanley B, King CA, et al: Intervention research with persons at high risk for suicidality: safety and ethical considerations. J Clin Psychiatry 62(suppl 25):17–26, 2001 11765091

Piacentini J, Rotheram-Borus MJ, Gillis JR, et al: Demographic predictors of treatment attendance among adolescent suicide attempters. J Consult Clin Psychol 63(3):469–473, 1995 7608360

Pineda J, Dadds MR: Family intervention for adolescents with suicidal behavior: a randomized controlled trial and mediation analysis. J Am Acad Child Adolesc Psychiatry 52(8):851–862, 2013 23880495

Posner K, Oquendo MA, Gould M, et al: Columbia Classification Algorithm of Suicide Assessment (C-CASA): classification of suicidal events in the FDA's pediatric suicidal risk analysis of antidepressants. Am J Psychiatry 164(7):1035–1043, 2007 17606655

Silverman MM, Berman AL, Sanddal ND, et al: Rebuilding the tower of Babel: a revised nomenclature for the study of suicide and suicidal behaviors. Part 1: Background, rationale, and methodology. Suicide Life Threat Behav 37(3):248–263, 2007 17579538

Spirito A, Plummer B, Gispert M, et al: Adolescent suicide attempts: outcomes at follow-up. Am J Orthopsychiatry 62(3):464–468, 1992 1497112

Spirito A, Simon V, Cancilliere MK, et al: Outpatient psychotherapy practice with adolescents following psychiatric hospitalization for suicide ideation or a suicide attempt. Clin Child Psychol Psychiatry 16(1):53–64, 2011 20404070

Trautman PD, Stewart N, Morishima A: Are adolescent suicide attempters noncompliant with outpatient care? J Am Acad Child Adolesc Psychiatry 32(1):89–94, 1993 8428890

Turecki G, Brent DA: Suicide and suicidal behaviour. Lancet 387(10024):1227–1239, 2016 26385066

Wilkinson P, Kelvin R, Roberts C, et al: Clinical and psychosocial predictors of suicide attempts and nonsuicidal self-injury in the Adolescent Depression Antidepressants and Psychotherapy Trial (ADAPT). Am J Psychiatry 168(5):495–501, 2011 21285141

Wood A, Trainor G, Rothwell J, et al: Randomized trial of group therapy for repeated deliberate self-harm in adolescents. J Am Acad Child Adolesc Psychiatry 40(11):1246–1253, 2001 11699797

PART I

Suicide Risk Assessment and Basic Safety Planning

2

Risk and Protective Factors for Suicidal Thoughts and Behaviors in Adolescents

Andrew C. Porter, M.Ed.
Jaclyn C. Kearns, B.A.
Erika C. Esposito, B.A.
Catherine R. Glenn, Ph.D.

Introduction

Suicidal thoughts and behaviors (STBs) are relatively rare in childhood but increase drastically in prevalence during the transition to and throughout adolescence (Nock et al. 2008). Suicide is the second leading cause of death among youth 10–19 years old (Centers for Disease Control and Prevention [CDC] 2018). Lifetime prevalence rates of *suicide ideation* (SI; thoughts of killing oneself), suicide plans (making plans to kill oneself), and *suicide attempts* (SAs; direct and intentional self-harm with some intent to die) among youth are even higher at 12.1%, 4.0%, and 4.1%, respectively (Nock et al. 2013). Over the past decade, rates of suicide in youth have continued to rise (Centers for Disease Control and Prevention 2018) despite increased prevention and intervention efforts for this population (Glenn et al. 2015; Zalsman et al. 2016).

A primary reason for the lack of decline in STB rates is the poor understanding of the mechanisms that contribute to risk for STBs within the mental health community. Unfortunately, most existing research on STBs is focused on adult populations, and the adolescent-specific research that exists has largely been cross-sectional (i.e., examining relations between characteristics and STBs at a single point in time). There is a pressing need for longitudinal research that identifies *prospective* risk and protective factors for STBs that are specific to adolescents.

Risk and Protective Factors: Definitions

In this chapter, we broadly define *risk* and *protective factors* as characteristics of individuals and their experiences that are associated with and precede the occurrence of an STB (Kraemer et al. 1997). Risk factors indicate elevated risk for future STBs, or they weaken the positive effects of a protective factor. Protective factors indicate lower risk for future STBs or buffer against the effects of a risk factor (Kazdin et al. 1997; Rutter 1987). Risk and protective factors can be categorized in two ways. The first is by whether the factor is modifiable. *Fixed factors*, such as ethnicity or the death of a parent, represent characteristics that cannot be changed, neither on their own nor with intervention. *Variable factors*, such as depression severity or coping skills, represent characteristics that can be changed, either on their own or with intervention. Both types of factors are valuable. Fixed risk and protective factors are useful for identifying groups of people who, on average, have especially high or low risk for developing STBs or for whom a risk or protective factor may have strengthened or weakened effects. Variable risk and protective factors have malleable effects and, therefore, are optimal targets for intervention and prevention. A variable risk factor becomes *causal* if research can demonstrate that changing the factor results in a change in risk. Unfortunately, there is currently no evidence for causal risk factors for adolescent STBs (see section "Limitations"). As such, the evidence presented in this chapter focuses exclusively on fixed and variable (but not causal) risk and protective factors for adolescent STBs.[1]

---

[1]For a detailed discussion on the classification of risk and protective factors, see Kraemer et al. 1997 and Kazdin et al. 1997.

The second way risk and protective factors are categorized is by the amount of time that elapses between the occurrence of the factor and the occurrence of the STB. *Distal risk factors* predict STBs that occur distant in time from the risk factor (e.g., in the following months or years), whereas *proximal risk factors* have their effect on STBs that occur soon after the occurrence of the risk factor (e.g., in the following hours, days, or weeks). Because the occurrence of a distal risk factor indicates elevated risk of some future STB, these factors may be useful for identifying individuals who could benefit from selective preventions. Proximal risk factors, on the other hand, may be especially useful for risk assessment and short-term interventions because the occurrence of a proximal risk factor indicates elevated risk for STBs over the short term. Although there is no agreed-upon definition for determining how close "proximal" is, only six studies reviewed in this chapter measured the effect of risk factors on STBs with follow-up periods of 6 months or less (see section "Limitations"). We will highlight those studies at the end of this chapter.

Chapter Overview

In this chapter, we review existing research on risk and protective factors for adolescent STBs. We begin with a brief overview of prominent suicide theories that may provide an overarching framework for understanding risk for STBs in youth. We then focus the review on studies that examine specific categories of risk and protective factors that may be amenable to treatment (e.g., psychological and social factors) and briefly discuss risk factors that are not directly amenable to clinical intervention (e.g., family history of STBs), but they may be helpful in identifying high-risk groups of adolescents. Then, we review evidence for protective factors that may be bolstered in treatment. We conclude by highlighting fundamental gaps in current knowledge of STB risk during adolescence and suggest important directions for future research. Unless otherwise noted, we included studies only if they met the following three criteria:

1. In line with the definition of a risk factor (Kraemer et al. 1997), we focus exclusively on studies that used prospective designs in which the identified risk or protective factor was measured before the assessment of the STB. (Of note, we did not include studies that only examined demographic risk factors, such as gender, race/ethnicity, and socio-

economic status. In some sections, however, we do discuss demographic characteristics to highlight between-person differences in the effects of other risk or protective factors. Our rationale for this focus is that demographic characteristics [as distal and fixed factors] have limited utility as targets for intervention.)

2. To be consistent with the World Health Organization's definition of adolescence (World Health Organization [WHO] 2014), we only review studies in which at least one STB outcome was assessed in individuals ages 10–19 years.

3. Because this chapter is about *suicidal* thoughts and behaviors, we focus exclusively on studies in which a suicide outcome was distinguished from *nonsuicidal self-injury* (NSSI; i.e., the direct and intentional destruction of body tissue performed *without* intent to die; Nock 2009).

Theoretical Considerations

Theoretical models are useful for identifying potential risk and protective factors for clinical phenomena and provide a framework for testing how these factors work together to confer risk or protection. One of the earliest models or frameworks for understanding suicide was the sociological theory of Durkheim (1897), which posited that suicidal behavior resulted from disruptions in social factors. For instance, Durkheim theorized that a lack of social integration, or anomie, was a primary motivation for suicide. Notable psychological theories shared the central tenet that suicide was caused by extreme psychological distress or pain, with suicide providing the ultimate escape from this distress/pain (Baumeister 1990; Menninger 1938; Shneidman 1993). More rigorous empirical investigation of suicide theories began with the hopelessness theory of suicide (Abramson et al. 2000; Beck 1986), which provided testable hypotheses about the cognitive processes associated with suicidal acts (Wenzel and Beck 2008). These earlier theories helped to explain why an individual might desire suicide, but they did not provide a framework for understanding how an individual might move from thinking about suicide to acting on their suicidal thoughts—a transition that only occurs among approximately one-third of people who think about suicide (Nock et al. 2008, 2013). However, these initial theories did lay the foundation for more complex models of suicidal behavior that aim to explain this transition from suicidal thinking to suicidal action (e.g., three-step theory [Klonsky and May 2015], interpersonal theory of suicide [Joiner 2005], motivational-volitional model of suicidal behavior [O'Connor 2011]).

Currently, no theory of suicide has been developed specifically for adolescence, despite the significant social, emotional, and biological changes unique to this developmental period (Crone and Dahl 2012; Somerville et al. 2010; Steinberg 2005) that coincide with the drastic rise in STBs (Nock et al. 2008). The only suicide theory that has been directly tested in adolescents is the interpersonal theory of suicide (Joiner 2005; Van Orden et al. 2010)—one of the most prominent and empirically supported contemporary theories of suicide in adults (e.g., Ma et al. 2016). Therefore, we focus in the rest of this section on existing research testing the interpersonal theory in adolescents.

Interpersonal Theory of Suicide

The interpersonal theory posits that both a desire to die and the capability to do so must be present for potentially lethal self-injury to occur (Joiner 2005; Van Orden et al. 2010). Specifically, the theory suggests that active suicide desire results from a combination of thwarted belongingness (e.g., loneliness), perceived burdensomeness (e.g., liability to others), and feeling hopeless that these states will change (Joiner 2005; Van Orden et al. 2010). Potentially lethal suicidal behavior occurs when individuals have this desire for suicide and have acquired the capability to act on that desire. Acquired capability for suicide manifests in a reduced fear of death and an increased tolerance for physical pain (e.g., NSSI; Joiner 2005; Van Orden et al. 2010).

A recent review (Stewart et al. 2017) identified 17 studies that tested at least one component of the interpersonal theory among adolescents ages 12–17 years (compared with the over 66 studies of the interpersonal theory in adults; Ma et al. 2016). The review concluded that there is emerging empirical support for the interpersonal theory among adolescents, with the most reliable association between SAs and acquired capability (measured in five studies using proxy indexes such as intravenous drug use, NSSI, history of multiple SAs, and exposure to violence; Stewart et al. 2017). However, this review highlighted the need for further research, especially studies that address some notable limitations. The majority of the reviewed studies failed to explicitly test all three core interpersonal theory constructs (i.e., thwarted belongingness, perceived burden-someness, acquired capability), all used proxy indexes of the interpersonal theory constructs (e.g., low social support as a measure of thwarted belong-ingness), and only four studies utilized longitudinal designs (Stewart et al. 2017).

A study by Czyz et al. (2015) is the only prospective study that has tested all three interpersonal theory constructs in adolescents. Contrary to what the interpersonal theory would suggest, Czyz et al. did not find support for an interaction of the main interpersonal theory components (perceived burdensomeness, thwarted belongingness, and acquired capability) in predicting SAs over the subsequent 3 or 12 months among hospitalized youth. However, they found that males (but not females) with greater per-ceived burdensomeness and higher acquired capability (as indexed by the presence of multiple past suicide attempts) were more likely to attempt sui-cide 3 months after hospital discharge. Females with lower acquired capa-bility and greater thwarted belongingness were more likely to attempt suicide 3 months postdischarge. Across both genders, higher acquired capa-bility was the only construct to predict attempts over 12 months, con-trolling for baseline depressive symptoms.

Summary

Currently, no adolescent-specific theory of suicidal behavior exists. Some of the best evidence comes from testing the interpersonal theory in youth. Al-though components of the interpersonal theory have been examined in studies with adolescents, testing of the full model using a prospective design has been limited (Stewart et al. 2017). An adolescent-specific theoretical model of suicide would be useful for identifying developmentally relevant risk and protective factors and for helping conceptualize how these factors work together to confer risk during this unique developmental period.

Psychological Risk Factors

Although no adolescent-specific theories have been developed, the cur-rent body of evidence for adolescent risk factors offers a starting place for developing such theories. This section reviews existing psychological risk factors for adolescent STBs examined in prospective research. For the purposes of this section, we consider a risk factor "psychological" if it is related to psychopathology (e.g., psychiatric disorders and symptoms), a maladaptive behavior (e.g., NSSI, underage cigarette use), or a cognitive-affective process related to psychopathology (e.g., hopelessness, negative thinking). We begin this section by discussing research on psychiatric disorders because these have received the most attention as risk factors for adolescent STBs. Then, we dedicate the remainder of the section to discussing more time-varying psychological risk factors (e.g., depressive symptoms, hopelessness, NSSI). We conclude by reviewing past STBs as risk factors for future STBs.

Major Depressive Disorder

Suicidal thoughts and behaviors have long been considered phenomena that occur in the context of major depressive disorder (MDD; American Psychiatric Association 2013; Beck et al. 1993), and indeed, many adolescents with a history of STBs also have a history of MDD (Nock et al. 2013). Compared with adolescents without MDD, those with the disorder have significantly higher odds of experiencing SI (Connor and Rueter 2009) and attempting suicide (Goldston et al. 2009; Nrugham et al. 2008). Adolescents who have MDD in addition to certain other psychiatric disorders (e.g., social anxiety disorder, conduct disorder) show higher risk for a later SA than adolescents who have only social anxiety disorder or conduct disorder (Goldston et al. 2009; Stein et al. 2001). The effect of MDD on future STBs, however, may not be significant after accounting for past STBs or other relevant predictors such as hopelessness and NSSI (Goldston et al. 2009; Nrugham et al. 2008).

Other Psychiatric Disorders

Other psychiatric disorders have received less attention than MDD as risk factors for STBs in youth. For most other psychiatric disorders, only one or two studies exist that have tested the disorder as a risk factor for STBs in adolescent samples. In these studies, bipolar disorders (Lan et al. 2015), alcohol use disorder (Reinherz et al. 1995), and attention-deficit/hyperactivity disorder (ADHD; Swanson et al. 2014) have been shown to predict SI. ADHD (Swanson et al. 2014), borderline personality disorder (Yen et al. 2013), and conduct disorder (Wei et al. 2016) have been identified as risk factors for SAs or for hospitalization for severe SI. Although these are distinct disorders, one overlapping feature is impulsiveness

(American Psychiatric Association 2013). Impulsiveness has been shown to predict SI and SAs in adolescents (McKeown et al. 1998) and therefore may account for some of the association between these psychiatric disorders and future STBs.

Of note, adolescents who develop psychiatric disorders, including MDD, before age 14 appear to be at heightened risk for developing SI or attempting suicide later in adolescence (Reinherz et al. 1995). One potential explanation for this finding is that psychopathology may interfere with normative adolescent development (Cicchetti and Rogosch 2002). Given that the span from early to late adolescence is typified by rapid changes in cognitive, emotional, and social development (e.g., Crone and Dahl 2012; Somerville et al. 2010; Steinberg 2005), having a psychiatric disorder during this period may damage the development of normative processes such as social competence (Masten and Cicchetti 2010).

Depressive Symptoms

Symptoms of MDD have received greater attention than MDD diagnoses as risk factors for STBs. This may be because symptom severity and manifestation (i.e., number and type of symptoms) vary across individuals and across time within the same individual, making them more useful for clinical intervention than simply knowing the patient's MDD diagnosis. Several studies have indicated that depressive symptom severity predicts future SI (Giletta et al. 2015; Ran et al. 2015; Vander Stoep et al. 2011), recurrent SI (Adrian et al. 2016; Vander Stoep et al. 2011), and SAs (Goldston et al. 2006; Thompson et al. 2012; Vander Stoep et al. 2011). One recent study found that fluctuations in depressive symptom severity around an adolescent's own average level of depression (i.e., within-person variation rather than between-person variation) were especially predictive of SI and were predictive of SAs in girls with a history of physical or sexual abuse (Miller et al. 2017). Notably, the effect of depressive symptom severity on SI and SAs has been shown to remain significant after controlling for a history of STBs (Giletta et al. 2015; Miller et al. 2017; Nrugham et al. 2008). Nrugham et al. (2008) examined specific depressive symptoms as risk factors for SAs. They found that feelings of worthlessness, but not other depressive symptoms, predicted a future SA after controlling for previous STBs and NSSI. A study by Yen and colleagues (2013) showed that low positive affect (i.e., anhedonia), but not negative affect, predicted SA after controlling for past SI.

Taken together, these findings highlight the importance of examining specific depressive symptoms (notably, feelings of worthlessness and anhedonia) in addition to MDD diagnosis. Moreover, this research highlights that the odds of future STBs may differ not only based on how severely depressed an adolescent is compared with others (e.g., Giletta et al. 2015) but also on how severe the adolescent's depressive symptoms are compared with how they usually feel (Miller et al. 2017). This suggests that clinicians who are concerned about patients' potential suicide risk may benefit from monitoring *changes* in their patients' level of depression from their baseline, or typical, level of depression.

Hopelessness

Hopelessness (i.e., pessimistic beliefs about one's future) has strong empirical and theoretical connections to depression. In fact, it was after recording depressed patients' hopeless thoughts (and noting that patients with such thoughts reported suicidal thoughts more often than other patients) that Dr. Aaron Beck first proposed hopelessness as a mechanism linking depression to suicide (Beck 1963). Since then, hopelessness has played a central role in many contemporary suicide theories (e.g., Abramson et al. 2000; Baumeister 1990; Beck 1986; Van Orden et al. 2010). Longitudinal studies of adults have shown that hopelessness is a significant predictor of STBs (e.g., Beck et al. 1985; Klonsky et al. 2012; Kuo et al. 2004). Similar support has been found in samples of college students (Miranda et al. 2013; Smith et al. 2006). However, findings are mixed regarding the utility of hopelessness for predicting STBs among adolescents. One longitudinal study by Tsypes and Gibb (2016) found that hopelessness predicted first-onset SI, controlling for past depressive symptoms. However, several other prospective studies found that hopelessness, although a significant predictor when examined alone, did not predict future STBs after controlling for past STBs and depressive symptoms (Mazza and Reynolds 1998; Myers et al. 1991; Prinstein et al. 2008). Interestingly, a recent study by Horwitz et al. (2017) categorized hopelessness according to two components: *positive expectancy* (i.e., the belief that good things will happen in the future) and *negative expectancy* (i.e., the belief that bad things will happen in the future). They found that low positive expectancy, but not high negative expectancy, predicted future suicidal behavior (i.e., SAs, aborted attempts, preparations for attempts). This result held when controlling for past depressive symptoms and SI. Taken together, these findings suggest that by identifying the specific facets of hopelessness that are related to STBs, clinicians could tailor their interventions to target suicide-specific hopeless cognitions.

Cognitive-Affective Processes

In addition to hopelessness, other maladaptive cognitive processes, or thinking patterns, have shown predictive utility for SI and SAs in adolescents. As with hopelessness, early research on depression targeted negative thinking patterns as mechanisms underlying the elevated risk for suicide among depressed individuals (Joiner and Rudd 1995; Miranda and Nolen-Hoeksema 2007; Smith et al. 2006). Recent longitudinal research with adolescents has examined a range of negative thinking patterns as risk factors for STBs. Burke and colleagues (2016) found that *negative self-referential thinking* (i.e., a bias toward processing negative information about oneself more quickly than positive information) and *negative inferential style* (i.e., believing negative events have negative implications for future events and for the self) each predicted future SI when controlling for past MDD diagnosis and SI. They also found that *rumination* (i.e., repetitive thinking about one's feelings and problems) independently predicted future SI; however, the effect of rumination was no longer significant after controlling for negative inferential style and negative self-relevant thinking (Burke et al. 2016). Using a sample of older children and younger adolescents (ages 8–14 years at baseline), Tsypes et al. (2016) found that participants who misinterpret emotion shown in facial expressions (e.g., interpreting anger as sadness) had higher odds of experiencing SI 2 years later, controlling for participants' MDD diagnosis. Tsypes et al. (2016) suggested these results might indicate a bias toward avoiding (and therefore not inspecting carefully) social signals of rejection (e.g., an angry face). Taken together, these findings highlight the importance of attending to adolescents' cognitive-affective biases when assessing risk for SI.

Another promising line of research has examined the relation of adolescent STBs to implicit cognitive processes (i.e., processes occurring outside of one's conscious awareness; Greenwald et al. 1998). Specifically, two studies have measured how adolescents' implicit self-identification with self-injury or death/suicide (i.e., Self-Injury Implicit Association

Test [IAT] or Death IAT) may indicate risk for STBs. Instead of asking individuals to self-report their suicidal thinking, these IATs measure implicit identification with self-harm and death/suicide through the strength of associations (i.e., reaction times on a computer task) between images/words related to self-injury/suicide and words related to the self. For instance, faster reaction times on trials where self-injurious images and self-relevant words are paired indicate stronger implicit identification with self-injury. As such, implicit measures like the IAT do not rely on introspection and therefore may be less susceptible to reporting bias compared with explicit self-reports (Greenwald et al. 1998). Using the Self-Injury IAT, Nock and Banaji (2007) found that adolescents who exhibited stronger implicit identification with self-injury were more likely to report future SI. Similar results were found using the Death IAT. Adolescents who demonstrated stronger implicit associations with death/suicide (i.e., faster reaction times on trials where "death" and "me" were paired) at hospital admission were more likely to report SI at hospital discharge (C.R. Glenn et al. 2017). Notably, results from both studies held after controlling for past SI. Findings from these studies suggest that implicit measures, like the IAT, may be potentially powerful tools for examining risk for STBs. Because implicit associations are thought to occur outside of conscious awareness, they may provide an objective method for assessing risk for STBs when an adolescent is unable or unwilling to verbally communicate their current SI (J.J. Glenn et al. 2017).

Behavioral Risk Factors, Including Nonsuicidal Self-Injury

There is limited prospective research on behavioral risk factors for adolescent STBs. A few studies have examined underage cigarette use and found that the behavior predicts both SI (Bronisch et al. 2008; Zhang and Wu 2014) and SAs (Riala et al. 2007). There is evidence, however, that the effect of cigarette smoking on STBs diminishes after controlling for relevant covariates such as symptoms of depression and anxiety and low parental attachment (e.g., McGee et al. 2005).

In addition to cigarette smoking, aggressive behavior in adolescence has been shown to predict STBs. One longitudinal study found that children with elevated scores on a composite of aggression and attention problems were more likely to experience SI or attempt suicide by the time they were 19 years old (Holtmann et al. 2011). Two other studies found that aggression specifically predicted future SI (Myers et al. 1991) and SAs (Yen et al. 2013), controlling for past SI. These preliminary findings indicate the importance of focusing on externalizing behaviors in predicting STBs. Future research is needed to clarify the contexts in which these behaviors occur (e.g., the settings in which an adolescent is aggressive) and examine other variables, such as impulsiveness, that may potentiate or explain the relation of these behaviors to STBs (García-Forero et al. 2009).

To date, NSSI has received significant attention as a potential risk factor for STBs in adolescence. NSSI is distinct from suicidal behavior in several important ways. One central way the two differ is that when individuals engage in NSSI, they do not have an intention to die, but use NSSI primarily as a means of emotion regulation or self-punishment (e.g., Bentley et al. 2014; Grandclerc et al. 2016). Additionally, NSSI has a much higher prevalence rate, is engaged in more frequently, and typically has an earlier age of onset than suicidal behavior (Grandclerc et al. 2016).

In adults, NSSI is one of the strongest risk factors for STBs (Franklin et al. 2017). Although there are few prospective studies in adolescents, the existing research does suggest that NSSI may be an important risk factor for STBs in youth. Several studies have shown that NSSI predicts future SI (Guan et al. 2012) and SAs (Asarnow et al. 2011; Wilkinson et al. 2011; You and Lin 2015) after controlling for past SI and SAs. Horwitz et al. (2015) also found that among adolescents recently discharged from an inpatient psychiatric hospital, NSSI was a significant predictor of SAs when examined alone; however, the effects were not maintained after accounting for previous SI severity and SAs. Although this research indicates that NSSI is related to future STBs, we currently do not know *why* the two are related. According to the interpersonal theory, one explanation is that as individuals engage in NSSI more frequently, they build up a tolerance for pain and reduce their fear of death and potentially lethal self-injury, thereby acquiring a capability to engage in suicidal behavior (Van Orden et al. 2010). In support of this explanation, a study with college students found that the more frequently individuals engaged in NSSI, the higher their acquired capability for suicide was 1 year later (as indexed by a heightened tolerance of pain; Willoughby et al. 2015).

Although many people who engage in NSSI also have histories of STBs, especially in clinical samples (e.g., Grandclerc et al. 2016), it is important to note that the presence of NSSI does *not* mean an individual is suicidal (Kumar et al. 2004). Despite this, NSSI is sometimes interpreted as suicidal behavior, which may result in a treatment response that does not match the severity of the manifesting problem (e.g., inappropriate hospitalization) and may cause emotional or financial harm to a patient (Shaffer and Jacobson 2009). If a patient presents with NSSI, clinicians should not dismiss the probability of suicide risk, but they should take care not to misrepresent the behavior itself as an indicator of current suicidal intent.

Other Psychological Risk Factors

Several studies have examined other psychological risk factors for STBs that do not fit well under one of the previous categories. For example, Martin et al. (2015) found that elevated psychological distress (i.e., combination of current anxiety/depressive symptoms and social dysfunction) placed adolescents at elevated risk for a future SA. In two studies examining stress in girls who were recently discharged from an inpatient hospital, dependent stress experiences (i.e., stress caused or exacerbated by the girl's own behavior; Stone et al. 2014) and deviations from participants' typical level of stress (Miller et al. 2017) were shown to predict future SI or the occurrence of a suicide event (i.e., SI, SAs, inpatient hospitalization). These findings suggest that examining deviations from an adolescent's typical level of functioning and typical reaction to stressors may inform their risk for STBs.

Dispositional psychological characteristics such as *low self-esteem* (i.e., negative attitudes toward oneself; Lewinsohn et al. 1994; Martin et al. 2005; Thompson and Light 2011), *high neuroticism* (i.e., tendency to experience negative affect; Enns et al. 2003), and low extraversion in males (Vrshek-Schallhorn et al. 2011) have been associated with elevated risk for a future SA. However, these psychological characteristics predict a wide range of negative outcomes (e.g., internalizing disorders, ADHD; Isomaa et al. 2013; Miller et al. 2008) and may not predict STBs after controlling for other relevant predictors such as past STBs (e.g., Martin et al. 2005; Miller et al. 2017; Stone et al. 2014; Thompson and Light 2011; Vrshek-Schallhorn et al. 2011). As with MDD, these characteristics may broadly indicate elevated risk for STBs but may not be as useful for distinguishing those at highest risk.

Sleep Problems

Sleep problems (e.g., insomnia, poor sleep quality) are related to a range of negative outcomes in adolescents such as poor academic performance, obesity, and risk-taking behaviors (Shochat et al. 2014), and they have also emerged as a risk factor for adolescent STBs. Findings from two longitudinal studies indicated that general sleep problems (i.e., trouble sleeping) predicted SI over a 3- to 5-year follow-up period, even after controlling for relevant risk factors (e.g., depressive symptoms; Wong and Brower 2012; Wong et al. 2011). In addition, general sleep problems, and insomnia specifically, have also been found to predict future SAs (Roane and Taylor 2008; Wong and Brower 2012). The role of sleep problems as a specific risk factor for STBs in youth is promising, particularly because sleep difficulties are very amenable to intervention (e.g., cognitive-behavioral therapy for insomnia; Edinger et al. 2001).

History of Suicidal Thoughts and Behaviors

Of all the risk factors discussed in this chapter, a history of prior STBs is consistently found to be the strongest predictor of future STBs (Franklin et al. 2017). Several studies have demonstrated that youth with a history of SI have significantly higher odds of experiencing SI when assessed 6 months later (e.g., Giletta et al. 2015; Prinstein et al. 2008; Ran et al. 2015), and they are more likely to make a future SA than youth without a history of SI (e.g., Borges et al. 2008; Horwitz et al. 2015; You and Lin 2015). Adolescents who experience chronic SI may be at even greater risk of an SA in the future than individuals who experience SI less frequently (Czyz and King 2015). The odds of an SA are especially high for adolescents who have a history of a single SA (Borges et al. 2008; Horwitz et al. 2015; King et al. 2014) and may be greater still for adolescents who have a history of multiple SAs (Miranda et al. 2008).

One explanation for these findings is, like those who engage in NSSI, individuals who have attempted suicide have demonstrated a capability for acting on suicidal thoughts (Van Orden et al. 2010). In other words, individuals with a past SA may have less fear of death and a higher tolerance for pain, which may make it easier for them to overcome the powerful self-preservation instinct and engage in suicidal behavior (Van Orden et al. 2010).

Summary

The majority of research on risk factors for STBs in youth examines psychological characteristics such as psychiatric diagnoses and past STBs. Notably, depressive symptoms and sleep problems have received promising support as risk factors for STBs, and these risk factors may be especially amenable to clinical intervention. Although the existing evidence for psychological risk factors is a great starting point, additional research is needed to identify strong and reliable predictors of STBs, to clarify the mechanisms through which these risk factors exert their effects, and to clarify when and for whom these risk factors are especially predictive of STBs.

Early Environmental Risk Factors

This section will review the most common early environmental risk factors for STBs among adolescents: childhood maltreatment (i.e., sexual abuse, physical abuse, emotional abuse, neglect), accumulation of multiple types of maltreatment, and family history of STBs.

Childhood Sexual Abuse

Considerable research has demonstrated a connection between childhood sexual abuse (CSA) and future SAs in adolescence (e.g., Stewart et al. 2015). Several studies have demonstrated that more chronic CSA and perpetration by an immediate family member (i.e., parent, sibling, stepparent) carry the greatest risk for STBs, particularly for an SA (Brezo et al. 2008; Taussig et al. 2014; Ystgaard et al. 2004). Of note, CSA occurring prior to age 13 years has been shown to be related to both future and lifetime history of an SA, after controlling for the effects of physical abuse (Rabinovitch et al. 2015).

Childhood Physical Abuse

Like CSA, childhood physical abuse (CPA) confers substantial risk for STBs, specifically for future SAs in adolescence (e.g., Marshall et al. 2013; Salzinger et al. 2007). Generally, it appears that adolescents who experienced CPA have higher odds of SI (Dunn et al. 2013), a single SA (Hadland et al. 2015; Joiner et al. 2007), and, in one study, repeated SAs (Ystgaard et al. 2004). Experiencing physical abuse during early childhood or early adolescence has been shown to increase risk for SAs during late adolescence, even after controlling for relevant variables such as age, sex, psychopathology during childhood and adolescence, and parental psychopathology (Johnson et al. 2002).

Childhood Emotional Abuse

Compared with CSA and CPA, research on childhood emotional abuse (CEA) and STBs is more limited. Three studies have found that CEA prospectively predicts SI (Puzia et al. 2014) and SAs (Hadland et al. 2015). In contrast to CSA and CPA, this specific subtype of maltreatment is posited to confer risk for STBs through negative self-attributions that are internalized by the child (Rose and Abramson 1992). This limited research highlights the need for greater attention to CEA by a caregiver as a risk factor for STBs.

Polyvictimization

Studies often examine maltreatment types (i.e., CSA, CPA, CEA, neglect) separately or control for the overlap among maltreatment exposures. However, it is important to examine how these frequently co-occurring negative life events may combine to confer risk for future STBs. For instance, several studies have demonstrated a significant relationship between polyvictimization (i.e., experiencing multiple types of maltreatment) and future STBs (Friestad et al. 2014; Greger et al. 2015; Thompson et al. 2012). Polyvictimization has been related to both a past history of an SA (Guendelman et al. 2016) and a future SA (Friestad et al. 2014). One study found that all adolescents in residential psychiatric care with current SI and suicide plans reported exposure to multiple forms of maltreatment in childhood (Greger et al. 2015). Findings from these studies suggest that an important avenue for future research is to examine the combined rather than isolated effects of multiple forms of maltreatment and adverse childhood experiences.

Family History of Suicidal Thoughts and Behaviors

The familial transmission of suicide risk has been well documented over the past two decades (e.g., Brent et al. 2002; Lizardi et al. 2009). Although the transmission of suicide risk can be examined genetically, this section focuses on the occurrence and impact of familial STBs within the context of the adolescent's family environment. In terms of suicide death, Qin et al. (2002) demonstrated that a family history of suicide death predicted risk of suicide death across all offspring, including adolescents. Several studies have shown that offspring of parents who have attempted suicide before are more likely to attempt suicide themselves (Lizardi et al. 2009; Melhem et al. 2007) and report a greater number of SAs (Lizardi et al. 2009) than offspring with no family history of an SA. In a retrospective study, adolescent males who have attempted suicide and who also had a family history of SAs made a more medically serious SA compared with those without a family history of an SA (Rajalin et al. 2013). Similar results have been found when focusing specifically on maternal transmission of suicide risk, even after controlling for the presence of maternal depression and other types of psychopathology. A history of a maternal SA increased the risk for SI and SA in both male and female offspring (Lieb et al. 2005). In fact, an SA by a caregiver predicted an adolescent's SA over and above adolescent psychopathology (Roberts et al. 2010). With respect to SI in offspring, Abrutyn and Mueller (2014) found some notable gender differences, demonstrating that a family member's SA increased SI the following year among adolescent girls but not for adolescent boys. Taken together, these studies provide strong evidence for the familial transmission of suicide risk—an association not completely accounted for by the transmission of familial psychopathology.

Summary

A number of environmental risk factors have been linked to adolescent STBs, most notably childhood maltreatment and family history of STBs. Although these factors are not modifiable, they may indicate distal risk for STBs and identify individuals who may benefit from selective interventions. Within the interpersonal theory framework, childhood maltreatment may be negative experiences that increase adolescents' tolerance for pain and reduce their fear of death (i.e., acquired capability for suicide), placing them at higher risk for STBs (Van Orden et al. 2010).

Social Risk Factors

In this section, we review social risk factors for suicide, such as peer victimization, peer suicide exposure, and media exposure to suicide and other factors such as low social support.

Peer Victimization

Peer victimization (i.e., being the target of repeated, aggressive behavior by one's peers) is highly prevalent during adolescence, with rates in the United States as high as 30% between sixth and twelfth grade (Nansel et al. 2001). Although the association between peer victimization and STBs has received strong empirical support in retrospective and cross-sectional work (e.g., Holt et al. 2015; Selkie et al. 2016), few studies have examined the longitudinal effects on STBs of being bullied (Geoffroy et al. 2016; Klomek et al. 2008). The strongest evidence comes from Geoffroy et al. (2016), who found that greater peer victimization was associated with an elevated risk of both SI and SAs 2 years later, even after accounting for relevant covariates (e.g., socioeconomic status, maternal history of STBs, prior SI, prior mental health diagnoses). Additional longitudinal studies are needed to replicate these findings.

Future studies on peer victimization should consider two understudied aspects of the phenomenon. The first is how being a perpetrator of bullying relates to STBs. Several studies have found that being a bully predicts SI (Heikkilä et al. 2013; Holt et al. 2015; Winsper et al. 2012). Additionally, cross-sectional findings indicate that those who are both bully perpetrators *and* bully victims are more likely to attempt suicide compared with those who are only the victim or perpetrator of bullying (Holt et al. 2015; Selkie et al. 2016). Second, peer victimization comes in different forms, ranging from direct forms (e.g., physical aggression, teasing) to indirect forms (e.g., social exclusion, gossiping). Understanding the unique influence of peer victimization on STBs over and above other risk factors (e.g., depression) and identifying the differential impact of distinct forms of victimization can help clarify how peer victimization confers risk for adolescent STBs.

Cyber Victimization

One specific form of victimization that has received increased attention is victimization occurring online, or *cyber victimization*. Given adolescents' constant access to the internet and their high engagement with social media platforms, they have little reprieve from peer victimization even after the school day ends (Holt et al. 2015; Kowalski et al. 2014; van Geel et al.

2014). Among adolescents ages 13–17 years, 92% report going online daily and 56% report going online multiple times each day (Lenhart 2015). Cyberbullies have perceived anonymity online, which provides space for individuals to say and do things they would not necessarily do in person and limits the ability of the perpetrator to fully understand the impact of their behavior (Kowalski et al. 2014; Selkie et al. 2016). Cross-sectional research has begun to show that cyber victimization may be more strongly related to SI than traditional bullying (Gini and Espelage 2014; van Geel et al. 2014). Further longitudinal testing is needed to identify the mechanisms and clarify the temporal relation of cyber victimization and STBs.

Peer Suicide Exposure

Although strong social relationships may help protect against adolescent STBs (see section "Protective Factors"), these relationships may have adverse consequences when someone in an adolescent's social circle dies by suicide. Feigelman and Gorman (2008) found greater SI in the first year after a friend's suicide death, controlling for relevant variables such as family history of SAs. However, the effect of the friend's death was not significant after controlling for the adolescent's own SI prior to the friend's death. Conversely, Abrutyn and Mueller (2014) reported that having a friend attempt suicide predicted later SI and SA for adolescent females and SI for adolescent males, an effect which held after controlling for age, adolescent education, family structure, race/ethnicity, parents' education, and prior STBs.

Exposure to a peer's suicide is also a risk factor for "copycat" behaviors or a clustering of suicidal behaviors, particularly during adolescence, irrespective of whether or not the adolescent had a strong relationship with the peer who died (Gould 2001). A *point cluster* is defined as a significant increase in suicidal behavior localized in both time (e.g., 7–90 days; Gould et al. 1990b; Gould et al. 1994) and space (e.g., peer suicides in schools; Gould et al. 1990a; Niedzwiedz et al. 2014). Point clusters occur primarily during adolescence and young adulthood (ages 15–24 years; Gould et al. 1990b) and are often explained according to social learning theory as an example of behavior modeling (Gould 2001). More research is needed to clarify when, where, and among which social groups point clusters are likely to occur.

Media Exposure to Suicide

Unlimited multimedia access coupled with the increase in both nonfictional (e.g., adolescents live streaming their own suicide attempts and deaths) and fictional (e.g., the graphic suicide death portrayed in the Netflix series *13 Reasons Why*) depictions of suicide, which are available to youth, make it imperative to understand the potential impact of exposure to these portrayals on adolescents' suicide risk. A significant increase in suicidal behavior following media coverage of a suicide death is defined as a *mass cluster* (Gould et al. 2003). In contrast to a point cluster, a mass cluster is not confined to a specific space (e.g., school) or community but is more broadly defined (e.g., national or global increases in suicidal behavior following celebrity suicide, film portrayals of suicide; Niedzwiedz et al. 2014). Research indicates that the type of media portraying suicidal behavior may impact the effect of the exposure on STBs among adolescents (Gould et al. 2003). Studies specifically examining fictional portrayals of suicides (i.e., characters attempting or dying by suicide) have shown mixed effects on subsequent SAs (Gould 2001; Gould et al. 2003). It is essential to determine the specific content and circumstances surrounding media exposure that confer risk for suicide in youth (Gould 2001), especially given adolescents' constant access to media and the internet (Lenhart 2015; Robertson et al. 2012).

Other Social Factors

Other research has examined the impact of specific relationship characteristics on adolescent STBs. A few studies have found poor parental support predicts SI (Miller et al. 2014) and a greater number of SAs in adolescents (MacGregor et al. 2014). Low perceived peer support also has been found to predict SAs (Tuisku et al. 2014). Finally, in patients at high risk for serious mental illness, stress surrounding mental illness stigma has been significantly associated with SI, even after controlling for age, sex, depressive symptoms, and prior SI (Xu et al. 2016).

Summary

There is emerging evidence suggesting social phenomena, such as peer victimization and exposure to suicide in the media, may confer risk for STBs. Although research to date has been promising, prospective studies in this area are limited. Moving forward, it will be important to examine adolescent-specific social risk factors (e.g., relational aggression including social exclusion; Remillard and Lamb 2005), the mechanisms linking social risk factors to STBs in youth (e.g., thwarted belongingness in the interpersonal theory), and how these risk factors may disrupt normative social development during adolescence.

Protective Factors

A *protective factor* can be defined as a characteristic that lessens the likelihood of STBs in general or a factor that decreases risk among a high-risk group (Kazdin et al. 1997; Rutter 1987). This section is organized into internal and external protective factors. *Internal protective factors* are endogenous characteristics (e.g., self-compassion), whereas *external protective factors* are exogenous characteristics (e.g., social support).

Internal Factors

Few longitudinal studies have examined how internal factors in adolescents protect against STBs. In a 21-year longitudinal study among New Zealand youth with depression, Fergusson et al. (2003) found specific personality constructs contributed to resilience among those at risk for STBs. Specifically, low levels of neuroticism and low levels of *novelty seeking* (i.e., tendency toward intense excitement in response to novel stimuli) protected against the occurrence of future SI and SAs (Fergusson et al. 2003). High self-esteem also protected against a future SA (Fergusson et al. 2003). In another study, *self-compassion* (i.e., feelings of kindness toward one's perceived inadequacies while understanding that one is connected to the human experience) protected against thoughts of death and SI over and above mindfulness (Zeller et al. 2015). In terms of cognitive protective factors, problem solving and distraction in response to negative affect protected against SI in young adolescents ages 12–13 years (Burke et al. 2016). Other prospective research has found that higher levels of *grit* (i.e., perseverance through adversity, while maintaining effort and interest, to reach a long-term goal) buffered against the effect of negative life events on SI in an undergraduate population (Blalock et al. 2015). Grit may be a promising trait to investigate prospectively in adolescents.

External Factors

There is considerable evidence suggesting that social connectedness protects against STBs in adolescents. Several studies have demonstrated the buffering effects of peer and family connectedness in relation to STBs. Czyz et al. (2012) assessed inpatient suicidal adolescents over the 12 months following hospital discharge. Adolescents who reported improvements in peer connectedness over this time period were half as likely to attempt suicide, and adolescents who reported improved family connectedness were less likely to experience SI (Czyz et al. 2012). In another study, social connectedness with peers, parents, and school predicted reduced risk for an SA (Kidd et al. 2006; Nkansah-Amankra et al. 2012). Additionally, social connectedness appears to protect against suicide risk in minority populations. For example, family connectedness reduced the odds of SI and SAs in urban African American and Latinx youth (O'Donnell et al. 2004) and SAs in sexual minority youth (Mustanski and Liu 2013). Family connectedness, teacher caring, and school safety were protective against SI and SA in a sample of middle and high school students (Eisenberg et al. 2007). Peer support has also been found to protect against SA in adolescents living in impoverished communities (Farrell et al. 2015). Given that social connectedness, particularly peer relationships, becomes increasingly salient during adolescence (Crone and Dahl 2012), understanding *how* social relationships buffer against suicide risk may be a promising area for future prospective research.

In addition to connectedness, there is some research to suggest that religiosity may protect against STBs in adolescents. One study found that participation in religious or church activities protected against SAs in adolescents, and private religiosity, consisting of frequency of prayer and self-reported importance of religion, protected against SI (Nkansah-Amankra et al. 2012). Generally, religiosity has been found to protect against a range of adolescent risk behaviors, and this may be due to mediating factors such as moral opposition to suicide and increased social connectedness (Malone et al. 2000).

Summary

Relative to risk factors, prospective research on protective factors for adolescent STBs is limited (see sections "Limitations" and "Future Directions"). Currently, social connectedness and positive emotional and cognitive processes (e.g., high self-esteem, distraction from negative affect) have the largest amount of support as protective factors. It is important to note that the existing body of protective factor research, like the risk factor research, fails to provide insight into *why* and *how* these factors decrease risk for suicidal behavior. Research on protective mechanisms is essential in order to leverage this information to enhance interventions and preventions for suicidal youth.

Limitations

Although the studies reviewed in this chapter provide valuable evidence for risk and protective factors for adolescent STBs, there are several noteworthy limitations. Below, we discuss major limitations pertaining to measurement and research design in suicide research.

Measurement

Inaccurate Assessment of Suicidal Thoughts and Behaviors

Single-item self-report questionnaires of STBs are widely used yet can potentially produce misclassification due to lack of clarity (Millner et al. 2015). For example, in a large study of adults, 40% of those who endorsed "yes" to a single question assessing SAs later reported *not* having any intent to die during the self-injurious act (Nock and Kessler 2006). Another study found similar misclassification issues when using single-item SI measures (Millner et al. 2015). These examples demonstrate a common issue with single-item assessments: individuals responding to these items often vary in what they think "counts" as a suicidal thought or behavior. This variability can result in individuals endorsing "yes" to STBs that they may not have experienced or endorsing "no" to STBs they have experienced.

Clinical interviews (e.g., Columbia-Suicide Severity Rating Scale [Posner et al. 2011], Self-Injurious Thoughts and Behaviors Interview [Nock et al. 2007]) may help resolve issues of clarity and accuracy in STB assessment. Although this method places greater burden on the assessor (e.g., time required to train interviewers), clinical interviews allow researchers and clinicians to clearly describe definitions of STBs, answer respondents' clarifying questions, and follow up on adolescents' vague or unclear responses.

Reliance on Self-report

In addition to single-item measures, assessment of STBs and their associated risk and protective factors rely heavily on self-report. Although self-reports provide valuable information about an individual's experience, these tools may be problematic for the assessment of STBs. For example, reporting biases due to perceived stigma or motivations to conceal SI to avoid hospitalization could prevent at-risk adolescents from being identified and receiving care. Most of the studies reviewed in this chapter used self-report or interview measures to obtain information about STB risk. Given the noted limitations, our field may benefit from exploring additional methods of risk assessment such as behavioral measures (e.g., Death IAT; C.R. Glenn et al. 2017; J.J. Glenn et al. 2017). By augmenting self-report measures with more objective tools, adolescents' risk for SI and SAs may be more accurately determined.

Research Design

Difficulties With Recruitment in Suicide Research

Although STBs are impairing among youth, rates of suicidal behavior in any given sample of youth is relatively low, given their low base rates (Centers for Disease Control and Prevention 2018). As a result, studies on STBs that recruit from a community sample require sample sizes that are larger than typically needed for studies of other psychological phenomena (e.g., depression). Because this approach is time-consuming and costly, an alternative is to recruit samples of adolescents at high risk for STBs (e.g., by using the risk factors reviewed in this chapter). Recruiting high-risk samples with higher rates of STBs would increase the statistical power for risk estimation (i.e., increase probability of detecting effects where they exist). In addition, recruiting high-risk samples enables examination of how risk changes over the short term and over other meaningful periods of time (e.g., throughout treatment, postdischarge from inpatient hospitalization). A better understanding of what signals short-term suicide risk and how risk changes over critical time periods is crucial for developing more sensitive suicide risk assessment protocols and effective interventions.

Distal Risk Factors

Most research on risk factors for adolescent STBs has focused on distal (i.e., more than 6 months from the occurrence of the risk factor) rather than proximal factors (i.e., closer than 6 months from the occurrence of the risk factor). Although distal risk factors are valuable for estimating risk for STBs over the long term, they are less useful for identifying *which* adolescents are at risk for STBs (as distal risk factors relate to a number of poor clinical outcomes) and *when* they are at risk (e.g., in the next hours, days, weeks). To date, the shortest periods of time between measurements of risk factors and STBs have been 3 months (acquired capability in males, depressive symptoms; Czyz and King 2015; Giletta et al. 2015) and 6 months (e.g., past SI, aggression, anhedonia; Ran et al. 2015; Yen et al. 2013). Such research is valuable, but shorter assessment periods (e.g., days, weeks) are needed to improve understanding of short-term risk.

No Identified Causal Risk Factors

No study to date has identified *causal* risk or protective factors for STBs in adolescence. The lack of causal factors for STBs suggests that, as clinicians, we know little about the mechanisms underlying increases and decreases in suicide risk. Indeed, this may explain why many existing treatments for STBs in adolescence have demonstrated limited effectiveness (Brent et al. 2013; Glenn et al. 2015). To establish causality, a risk or protective factor must be manipulated and result in a change in risk for an STB (Kraemer et al. 1997). Therefore, research using experimental designs is needed to identify: 1) which factors may be causally related to future STBs and 2) which of these factors may have the *greatest* impact on increasing or decreasing risk for STBs among adolescents. Identifying causal risk factors is necessary to develop more effective, STB-specific interventions for at-risk adolescents.

Future Directions

The limitations of prior research on adolescent STBs suggest some important areas for future research directions. Below, we suggest five areas for future research.

Suicide-Specific Mechanisms of Risk

Most research has focused on risk factors that predict a range of negative outcomes in addition to STBs. Although these risk factors are an important starting place, they have limited utility for predicting adolescent STBs specifically. Identifying suicide-specific risk factors and understanding *how* widely harmful factors (e.g., peer victimization) confer specific risk for STBs are crucial for developing more effective risk assessment tools and targeted interventions for STBs.

Proximal Risk Factors

Research has mainly focused on distal risk factors (i.e., distant in time from suicidal behavior). However, the most challenging task for clinicians is to identify short-term risk for suicidal behavior (i.e., risk within the next minutes, hours, or days; Rudd et al. 2006). Therefore, the field is in great need of research that provides information on behavioral, affective, and cognitive signs that may signal short-term risk for STBs (e.g., Bagge et al. 2017). Given that most adolescents who act on their suicidal thoughts do so within the first year after the onset of SI (Nock et al. 2013), it will be important for short-term risk factor research to elucidate *why* and *when* adolescents transition from thinking about suicide to attempting suicide. Currently, we know that SI is one of the strongest predictors of SAs, but prior studies have not had the temporal resolution needed to identify the mechanisms underlying the transition from SI to an SA (e.g., intensely following adolescents currently thinking about suicide over short periods of time).

Protective Factors

Existing prospective research on protective factors for adolescent STBs is extremely limited. The identification of protective factors for STBs is a crucial step in identifying effective prevention and intervention targets. Future research may benefit from examining internal factors, such as self-compassion, or external factors, such as peer and familial connectedness, both of which may be targeted in clinical interventions such as interpersonal therapy, dialectical behavior therapy, or attachment-based family therapy.

Differential Effects of Risk Factors

Future research is needed to explore how risk factors function differently among individuals, because they may not have a uniform effect for everyone. For example, existing studies have found differences in psychological risk factors by sex (e.g., low extraversion predicts SA in boys only; Vrshek-Schallhorn et al. 2011). Risk factors may also not have the same effects over time within the same person. Instead, as an individual's risk factor changes in severity or form, its ability to predict that individual's future STBs may also change. For example, Miller and colleagues (2017) found that fluctuations around an adolescent's *own* average level of depression, rather than an adolescent's level of depression relative to others, were particularly predictive of future STBs.

Developmentally Sensitive Framework for Suicide

The onset and rise in STBs occur during a developmental period marked by rapid psychological, social, and biological changes (Steinberg 2005). Such changes are not readily accounted for by existing suicide theories, which were developed to explain suicidal behavior among adults. The field would benefit from a developmentally sensitive framework to understand the onset and maintenance of STBs during adolescence.

Conclusion

In this chapter, we provide an overview of existing prospective research on risk and protective factors for STBs in adolescents. See Table 2–1 for a listing of risk and protective factors. Of the evidence reviewed, psychological characteristics such as depressive symptoms, aggression, sleep problems, and NSSI demonstrate promising evidence as strong risk factors for STBs and may be useful targets for intervention. Other findings indicate that adolescents with a history of child abuse and maltreatment, those who have had a friend or family member die by suicide, and those who have been both perpetrators and victims of bullying may be at distal risk for STBs and in greatest need of selective preventions. Finally, although there is less research dedicated to protective factors, the findings noted in this chapter indicate that it may be useful to bolster characteristics such as connectedness, self-compassion, and religiosity in patients at risk for STBs. Taken together, the existing evidence for risk and protective factors provides a useful foundation for informing clinical risk assessment and safety management (reviewed in Chapter 3, "Safety Planning and Risk Management") and new and more effective interventions and preventions for adolescent STBs.

TABLE 2-1.   Risk and protective factors for suicidal thoughts and behaviors in adolescents

Risk factors	Protective factors
Psychological	Internal
Aggression	Distraction/problem-solving skills
Alcohol use disorder	Grit
Anhedonia	Neuroticism (low)
Misinterpretation of emotion in facial expression	Novelty seeking (low)
Bipolar disorder	Self-esteem/self-compassion (high)
Borderline personality disorder	External
Cigarette smoking	Family connectedness
Conduct disorder	Peer connectedness
Extraversion (low)	Religiosity
History of suicidal thoughts and behaviors	Teacher caring
Hopelessness	School connectedness/safety
Implicit associations with death/suicide or self-injury	
Impulsiveness	
Major depression/depressive symptoms	
Negative self-referential thinking	
Neuroticism	
Nonsuicidal self-injury	
Psychological distress	
Rumination	
Self-esteem (low)	
Sleep problems	
Social anxiety	
Stress	
Worthlessness (feelings of)	

TABLE 2-1.	Risk and protective factors for suicidal thoughts and behaviors in adolescents *(continued)*	
Risk factors	Protective factors
Early Environmental	
Childhood maltreatment (physical, sexual, emotional, neglect)	
Family history of suicidal thoughts and behaviors	
Social	
Exposure to peer suicide	
Media exposure to suicide	
Parental/peer support (low)	
Peer victimization (including cyber)	
Stigma of mental illness	

References

Abramson LY, Alloy LB, Hogan ME, et al: The hopelessness theory of suicidality, in Suicide Science: Expanding the Boundaries. Edited by Joiner TE, Rudd MD. New York, Kluwer Academic/Plenum Publishers, 2000, pp 17–32

Abrutyn S, Mueller AS: Are suicidal behaviors contagious in adolescence? Using longitudinal data to examine suicide suggestion. Am Sociol Rev 79(2):211–227, 2014 26069341

Adrian M, Miller AB, McCauley E, et al: Suicidal ideation in early to middle adolescence: sex-specific trajectories and predictors. J Child Psychol Psychiatry 57(5):645–653, 2016 26610726

American Psychiatric Association: Diagnostic and Statistical Manual of Mental Disorders, 5th Edition. Arlington, VA, American Psychiatric Association, 2013

Asarnow JR, Porta G, Spirito A, et al: Suicide attempts and nonsuicidal self-injury in the treatment of resistant depression in adolescents: findings from the TORDIA study. J Am Acad Child Adolesc Psychiatry 50(8):772–781, 2011 21784297

Bagge CL, Littlefield AK, Glenn CR: Trajectories of affective response as warning signs for suicide attempts. Clin Psychol Sci 5:259–271, 2017

Baumeister RF: Suicide as escape from self. Psychol Rev 97(1):90–113, 1990 2408091

Beck AT: Thinking and depression I. Idiosyncratic content and cognitive distortions. Arch Gen Psychiatry 9:324–333, 1963 14045261

Beck AT: Hopelessness as a predictor of eventual suicide. Ann N Y Acad Sci 487:90–96, 1986 3471167

Beck AT, Steer RA, Kovacs M, et al: Hopelessness and eventual suicide: a 10-year prospective study of patients hospitalized with suicidal ideation. Am J Psychiatry 142(5):559–563, 1985 3985195

Beck AT, Steer RA, Beck JS, et al: Hopelessness, depression, suicidal ideation, and clinical diagnosis of depression. Suicide Life Threat Behav 23(2):139–145, 1993 8342213

Bentley KH, Nock MK, Barlow DH: The four-function model of nonsuicidal self-injury: key directions for future research. Clin Psychol Sci 2:638–656, 2014

Blalock DV, Young KC, Kleiman EM: Stability amidst turmoil: grit buffers the effects of negative life events on suicidal ideation. Psychiatry Res 228(3):781–784, 2015 26070767

Borges G, Angst J, Nock MK, et al: Risk factors for the incidence and persistence of suicide-related outcomes: a 10-year follow-up study using the National Comorbidity Surveys. J Affect Disord 105(1–3):25–33, 2008 17507099

Brent DA, Moritz G, Liotus L, et al: Familial risk factors for adolescent suicide, in Suicide Prevention. Edited by Kosky RJ, Eshkevari HS, Goldney RD, et al. Boston, MA, Springer, 2002, pp 41–50

Brent DA, McMakin DL, Kennard BD, et al: Protecting adolescents from self-harm: a critical review of intervention studies. J Am Acad Child Adolesc Psychiatry 52(12):1260–1271, 2013 24290459

Brezo J, Paris J, Vitaro F, et al: Predicting suicide attempts in young adults with histories of childhood abuse. Br J Psychiatry 193(2):134–139, 2008 18669998

Bronisch T, Höfler M, Lieb R: Smoking predicts suicidality: findings from a prospective community study. J Affect Disord 108(1–2):135–145, 2008 18023879

Burke TA, Connolly SL, Hamilton JL, et al: Cognitive risk and protective factors for suicidal ideation: a two year longitudinal study in adolescence. J Abnorm Child Psychol 44(6):1145–1160, 2016 26597963

Centers for Disease Control and Prevention (CDC): Web-Based Injury Statistics Query and Reporting System (WISQARS). National Center for Injury Prevention and Control. May 3, 2018. Available at: www.cdc.gov/injury/wisqars/index.html. Accessed June 20, 2018.

Cicchetti D, Rogosch FA: A developmental psychopathology perspective on adolescence. J Consult Clin Psychol 70(1):6–20, 2002 11860057

Connor J, Rueter M: Predicting adolescent suicidality: comparing multiple informants and assessment techniques. J Adolesc 32(3):619–631, 2009 18708245

Crone EA, Dahl RE: Understanding adolescence as a period of social-affective engagement and goal flexibility. Nat Rev Neurosci 13(9):636–650, 2012 22903221

Czyz EK, King CA: Longitudinal trajectories of suicidal ideation and subsequent suicide attempts among adolescent inpatients. J Clin Child Adolesc Psychol 44(1):181–193, 2015 24079705

Czyz EK, Liu Z, King CA: Social connectedness and one-year trajectories among suicidal adolescents following psychiatric hospitalization. J Clin Child Adolesc Psychol 41(2):214–226, 2012 22417194

Czyz EK, Berona J, King CA: A prospective examination of the interpersonal-psychological theory of suicidal behavior among psychiatric adolescent inpatients. Suicide Life Threat Behav 45(2):243–259, 2015 25263410

Dunn EC, McLaughlin KA, Slopen N, et al: Developmental timing of child maltreatment and symptoms of depression and suicidal ideation in young adulthood: results from the National Longitudinal Study of Adolescent Health. Depress Anxiety 30(10):955–964, 2013 23592532

Durkheim E: Le Suicide: Étude de Sociologie. Paris, F Alcan, 1897

Edinger JD, Wohlgemuth WK, Radtke RA, et al: Does cognitive-behavioral insomnia therapy alter dysfunctional beliefs about sleep? Sleep 24(5):591–599, 2001 11480656

Eisenberg ME, Ackard DM, Resnick MD: Protective factors and suicide risk in adolescents with a history of sexual abuse. J Pediatr 151(5):482–487, 2007 17961690

Enns MW, Cox BJ, Inayatulla M: Personality predictors of outcome for adolescents hospitalized for suicidal ideation. J Am Acad Child Adolesc Psychiatry 42(6):720–727, 2003 12921480

Farrell CT, Bolland JM, Cockerham WC: The role of social support and social context on the incidence of attempted suicide among adolescents living in extremely impoverished communities. J Adolesc Health 56(1):59–65, 2015 25438969

Feigelman W, Gorman BS: Assessing the effects of peer suicide on youth suicide. Suicide Life Threat Behav 38(2):181–194, 2008 18444776

Fergusson DM, Beautrais AL, Horwood LJ: Vulnerability and resiliency to suicidal behaviours in young people. Psychol Med 33(1):61–73, 2003 12537037

Franklin JC, Ribeiro JD, Fox KR, et al: Risk factors for suicidal thoughts and behaviors: a meta-analysis of 50 years of research. Psychol Bull 143(2):187–232, 2017 27841450

Friestad C, Åse-Bente R, Kjelsberg E: Adverse childhood experiences among women prisoners: relationships to suicide attempts and drug abuse. Int J Soc Psychiatry 60(1):40–46, 2014 23045353

García-Forero C, Gallardo-Pujol D, Maydeu-Olivares A, et al: Disentangling impulsiveness, aggressiveness and impulsive aggression: an empirical approach using self-report measures. Psychiatry Res 168(1):40–49, 2009 19464063

Geoffroy MC, Boivin M, Arseneault L, et al: Associations between peer victimization and suicidal ideation and suicide attempt during adolescence: results from a prospective population-based birth cohort. J Am Acad Child Adolesc Psychiatry 55(2):99–105, 2016 26802776

Giletta M, Calhoun CD, Hastings PD, et al: Multi-level risk factors for suicidal ideation among at-risk adolescent females: the role of hypothalamic-pituitary-adrenal axis responses to stress. J Abnorm Child Psychol 43(5):807–820, 2015 24958308

Gini G, Espelage DL: Peer victimization, cyberbullying, and suicide risk in children and adolescents. JAMA 312(5):545–546, 2014 25096695

Glenn CR, Franklin JC, Nock MK: Evidence-based psychosocial treatments for self-injurious thoughts and behaviors in youth. J Clin Child Adolesc Psychol 44(1):1–29, 2015 25256034

Glenn CR, Kleiman EM, Coppersmith DDL, et al: Implicit identification with death predicts change in suicide ideation during psychiatric treatment in adolescents. J Child Psychol Psychiatry 8(12):1219–1229 2017 28675456

Glenn JJ, Werntz AJ, Slama SJ, et al: Suicide and self-injury-related implicit cognition: a large-scale examination and replication. J Abnorm Psychol 126(2):199–211, 2017 27991808

Goldston DB, Reboussin BA, Daniel SS: Predictors of suicide attempts: state and trait components. J Abnorm Psychol 115(4):842–849, 2006 17100542

Goldston DB, Daniel SS, Erkanli A, et al: Psychiatric diagnoses as contemporaneous risk factors for suicide attempts among adolescents and young adults: developmental changes. J Consult Clin Psychol 77(2):281–290, 2009 19309187

Gould MS: Suicide and the media. Ann N Y Acad Sci 932:200–221, discussion 221–224, 2001 11411187

Gould MS, Wallenstein S, Kleinman M: Time-space clustering of teenage suicide. Am J Epidemiol 131(1):71–78, 1990a 2293755

Gould MS, Wallenstein S, Kleinman MH, et al: Suicide clusters: an examination of age-specific effects. Am J Public Health 80(2):211–212, 1990b 2297071

Gould MS, Petrie K, Kleinman MH, et al: Clustering of attempted suicide: New Zealand national data. Int J Epidemiol 23(6):1185–1189, 1994 7721521

Gould MS, Jamieson P, Romer D: Media contagion and suicide among the young. Am Behav Sci 46:1269–1284, 2003

Grandclerc S, De Labrouhe D, Spodenkiewicz M, et al: Relations between nonsuicidal self-injury and suicidal behavior in adolescence: a systematic review. PLoS One 11(4):e0153760, 2016 27089157

Greenwald AG, McGhee DE, Schwartz JLK: Measuring individual differences in implicit cognition: the implicit association test. J Pers Soc Psychol 74(6):1464–1480, 1998 9654756

Greger HK, Myhre AK, Lydersen S, et al: Previous maltreatment and present mental health in a high-risk adolescent population. Child Abuse Negl 45:122–134, 2015 26003821

Guan K, Fox KR, Prinstein MJ: Nonsuicidal self-injury as a time-invariant predictor of adolescent suicide ideation and attempts in a diverse community sample. J Consult Clin Psychol 80(5):842–849, 2012 22845782

Guendelman MD, Owens EB, Galán C, et al: Early adult correlates of maltreatment in girls with attention-deficit/hyperactivity disorder: increased risk for internalizing symptoms and suicidality. Dev Psychopathol 28(1):1–14, 2016 25723055

Hadland SE, Wood E, Dong H, et al: Suicide attempts and childhood maltreatment among street youth: a prospective cohort study. Pediatrics 136(3):440–449, 2015 26240210

Heikkilä HK, Väänänen J, Helminen M, et al: Involvement in bullying and suicidal ideation in middle adolescence: a 2-year follow-up study. Eur Child Adolesc Psychiatry 22(2):95–102, 2013 23053774

Holt MK, Vivolo-Kantor AM, Polanin JR, et al: Bullying and suicidal ideation and behaviors: a meta-analysis. Pediatrics 135(2):e496–e509, 2015 25560447

Holtmann M, Buchmann AF, Esser G, et al: The Child Behavior Checklist-Dysregulation Profile predicts substance use, suicidality, and functional impairment: a longitudinal analysis. J Child Psychol Psychiatry 52(2):139–147, 2011 20854363

Horwitz AG, Czyz EK, King CA: Predicting future suicide attempts among adolescent and emerging adult psychiatric emergency patients. J Clin Child Adolesc Psychol 44(5):751–761, 2015 24871489

Horwitz AG, Berona J, Czyz EK, et al: Positive and negative expectations of hopelessness as longitudinal predictors of depression, suicidal ideation, and suicidal behavior in high-risk adolescents. Suicide Life Threat Behav 47(2):168–176, 2017 27371943

Isomaa R, Väänänen JM, Fröjd S, et al: How low is low? Low self-esteem as an indicator of internalizing psychopathology in adolescence. Health Educ Behav 40(4):392–399, 2013 22872582

Johnson JG, Cohen P, Gould MS, et al: Childhood adversities, interpersonal difficulties, and risk for suicide attempts during late adolescence and early adulthood. Arch Gen Psychiatry 59(8):741–749, 2002 12150651

Joiner TE: Why People Die by Suicide. Cambridge, MA, Harvard University Press, 2005

Joiner TE Jr, Rudd MD: Negative attributional style for interpersonal events and the occurrence of severe interpersonal disruptions as predictors of self-reported suicidal ideation. Suicide Life Threat Behav 25(2):297–304, 1995 7570789

Joiner TE Jr, Sachs-Ericsson NJ, Wingate LR, et al: Childhood physical and sexual abuse and lifetime number of suicide attempts: a persistent and theoretically important relationship. Behav Res Ther 45(3):539–547, 2007 16765909

Kazdin AE, Kraemer HC, Kessler RC, et al: Contributions of risk-factor research to developmental psychopathology. Clin Psychol Rev 17(4):375–406, 1997 9199858

Kidd S, Henrich CC, Brookmeyer KA, et al: The social context of adolescent suicide attempts: interactive effects of parent, peer, and school social relations. Suicide Life Threat Behav 36(4):386–395, 2006 16978093

King CA, Jiang Q, Czyz EK, et al: Suicidal ideation of psychiatrically hospitalized adolescents has one-year predictive validity for suicide attempts in girls only. J Abnorm Child Psychol 42(3):467–477, 2014 23996157

Klomek AB, Sourander A, Kumpulainen K, et al: Childhood bullying as a risk for later depression and suicidal ideation among Finnish males. J Affect Disord 109(1–2):47–55, 2008 18221788

Klonsky ED, May AM: The three-step theory (3ST): a new theory of suicide rooted in the "ideation-to-action" framework. Int J Cogn Ther 8:114–129, 2015

Klonsky ED, Kotov R, Bakst S, et al: Hopelessness as a predictor of attempted suicide among first admission patients with psychosis: a 10-year cohort study. Suicide Life Threat Behav 42(1):1–10, 2012 22320192

Kowalski RM, Giumetti GW, Schroeder AN, et al: Bullying in the digital age: a critical review and meta-analysis of cyberbullying research among youth. Psychol Bull 140(4):1073–1137, 2014 24512111

Kraemer HC, Kazdin AE, Offord DR, et al: Coming to terms with the terms of risk. Arch Gen Psychiatry 54(4):337–343, 1997 9107150

Kumar G, Pepe D, Steer RA: Adolescent psychiatric inpatients' self-reported reasons for cutting themselves. J Nerv Ment Dis 192(12):830–836, 2004 15583504

Kuo WH, Gallo JJ, Eaton WW: Hopelessness, depression, substance disorder, and suicidality—a 13-year community-based study. Soc Psychiatry Psychiatr Epidemiol 39(6):497–501, 2004 15205735

Lan WH, Bai YM, Hsu JW, et al: Comorbidity of ADHD and suicide attempts among adolescents and young adults with bipolar disorder: a nationwide longitudinal study. J Affect Disord 176:171–175, 2015 25723560

Lenhart A: Teen, social media, and technology overview 2015. Pew Research Center, April 9, 2015. Available at: http://www.pewinternet.org/2015/04/09/teens-social-media-technology-2015/. Accessed June 22, 2018.

Lewinsohn PM, Rohde P, Seeley JR: Psychosocial risk factors for future adolescent suicide attempts. J Consult Clin Psychol 62(2):297–305, 1994 8201067

Lieb R, Bronisch T, Höfler M, et al: Maternal suicidality and risk of suicidality in offspring: findings from a community study. Am J Psychiatry 162(9):1665–1671, 2005 16135626

Lizardi D, Sher L, Sullivan GM, et al: Association between familial suicidal behavior and frequency of attempts among depressed suicide attempters. Acta Psychiatr Scand 119(5):406–410, 2009 19367777

Ma J, Batterham PJ, Calear AL, et al: A systematic review of the predictions of the Interpersonal-Psychological Theory of Suicidal Behavior. Clin Psychol Rev 46:34–45, 2016 27155061

MacGregor EK, Grunebaum MF, Galfalvy HC, et al: Depressed parents' attachment: effects on offspring suicidal behavior in a longitudinal family study. J Clin Psychiatry 75(8):879–885, 2014 25098943

Malone KM, Oquendo MA, Haas GL, et al: Protective factors against suicidal acts in major depression: reasons for living. Am J Psychiatry 157(7):1084–1088, 2000 10873915

Marshall BDL, Galea S, Wood E, et al: Longitudinal associations between types of childhood trauma and suicidal behavior among substance users: a cohort study. Am J Public Health 103(9):e69–e75, 2013 23865651

Martin G, Richardson AS, Bergen HA, et al: Perceived academic performance, self-esteem and locus of control as indicators of need for assessment of adolescent suicide risk: implications for teachers. J Adolesc 28(1):75–87, 2005 15683636

Martin G, Thomas H, Andrews T, et al: Psychotic experiences and psychological distress predict contemporaneous and future non-suicidal self-injury and suicide attempts in a sample of Australian school-based adolescents. Psychol Med 45(2):429–437, 2015 25065410

Masten AS, Cicchetti D: Developmental cascades. Dev Psychopathol 22(3):491–495, 2010 20576173

Mazza JJ, Reynolds WM: A longitudinal investigation of depression, hopelessness, social support, and major and minor life events and their relation to suicidal ideation in adolescents. Suicide Life Threat Behav 28(4):358–374, 1998 9894304

McGee R, Williams S, Nada-Raja S: Is cigarette smoking associated with suicidal ideation among young people? Am J Psychiatry 162(3):619–620, 2005 15741485

McKeown RE, Garrison CZ, Cuffe SP, et al: Incidence and predictors of suicidal behaviors in a longitudinal sample of young adolescents. J Am Acad Child Adolesc Psychiatry 37(6):612–619, 1998 9628081

Menninger KA: Man Against Himself. New York, Harcourt, Brace, 1938

Melhem NM, Brent DA, Ziegler M, et al: Familial pathways to early onset suicidal behavior: familial and individual antecedents of suicidal behavior. Am J Psychiatry 164(9):1364–1370, 2007 17728421

Miller AB, Adams LM, Esposito-Smythers C, et al: Parents and friendships: a longitudinal examination of interpersonal mediators of the relationship between child maltreatment and suicidal ideation. Psychiatry Res 220(3):998–1006, 2014 25454119

Miller AB, Eisenlohr-Moul T, Giletta M, et al: A within-person approach to risk for suicidal ideation and suicidal behavior: examining the roles of depression, stress, and abuse exposure. J Consult Clin Psychol 85(7):712–722, 2017 28425734

Miller CJ, Miller SR, Newcorn JH, et al: Personality characteristics associated with persistent ADHD in late adolescence. J Abnorm Child Psychol 36(2):165–173, 2008 17701339

Millner AJ, Lee MD, Nock MK: Single-item measurement of suicidal behaviors: validity and consequences of misclassification. PLoS One 10(10):e0141606, 2015 26496707

Miranda R, Nolen-Hoeksema S: Brooding and reflection: rumination predicts suicidal ideation at 1-year follow-up in a community sample. Behav Res Ther 45(12):3088–3095, 2007 17825248

Miranda R, Scott M, Hicks R, et al: Suicide attempt characteristics, diagnoses, and future attempts: comparing multiple attempters to single attempters and ideators. J Am Acad Child Adolesc Psychiatry 47(1):32–40, 2008 18174823

Miranda R, Tsypes A, Gallagher M, et al: Rumination and hopelessness as mediators of the relation between perceived emotion dysregulation and suicidal ideation. Cognit Ther Res 37:786–795, 2013

Mustanski B, Liu RT: A longitudinal study of predictors of suicide attempts among lesbian, gay, bisexual, and transgender youth. Arch Sex Behav 42(3):437–448, 2013 23054258

Myers K, McCauley E, Calderon R, et al: The 3-year longitudinal course of suicidality and predictive factors for subsequent suicidality in youths with major depressive disorder. J Am Acad Child Adolesc Psychiatry 30(5):804–810, 1991 1938798

Nansel TR, Overpeck M, Pilla RS, et al: Bullying behaviors among US youth: prevalence and association with psychosocial adjustment. JAMA 285(16):2094–2100, 2001 11311098

Niedzwiedz C, Haw C, Hawton K, et al: The definition and epidemiology of clusters of suicidal behavior: a systematic review. Suicide Life Threat Behav 44(5):569–581, 2014 24702173

Nkansah-Amankra S, Diedhiou A, Agbanu SK, et al: A longitudinal evaluation of religiosity and psychosocial determinants of suicidal behaviors among a population-based sample in the United States. J Affect Disord 139(1):40–51, 2012 22483954

Nock MK: Why do people hurt themselves? Curr Dir Psychol Sci 18(2):78–83, 2009 20161092

Nock MK, Banaji MR: Prediction of suicide ideation and attempts among adolescents using a brief performance-based test. J Consult Clin Psychol 75(5):707–715, 2007 17907852

Nock MK, Kessler RC: Prevalence of and risk factors for suicide attempts versus suicide gestures: analysis of the National Comorbidity Survey. J Abnorm Psychol 115(3):616–623, 2006 16866602

Nock MK, Holmberg EB, Photos VI, et al: Self-Injurious Thoughts and Behaviors Interview: development, reliability, and validity in an adolescent sample. Psychol Assess 19(3):309–317, 2007 17845122

Nock MK, Borges G, Bromet EJ, et al: Suicide and suicidal behavior. Epidemiol Rev 30:133–154, 2008 18653727

Nock MK, Green JG, Hwang I, et al: Prevalence, correlates, and treatment of lifetime suicidal behavior among adolescents: results from the National Comorbidity Survey Replication Adolescent Supplement. JAMA Psychiatry 70(3):300–310, 2013 23303463

Nrugham L, Larsson B, Sund AM: Specific depressive symptoms and disorders as associates and predictors of suicidal acts across adolescence. J Affect Disord 111(1):83–93, 2008 18395267

O'Connor RC: Towards an integrated motivational–volitional model of suicidal behavior, in International Handbook of Suicide Prevention: Research, Policy, and Practice. Edited by O'Connor RC, Platt S, Gordon J. Hoboken, NJ, Wiley, 2011, pp 181–198

O'Donnell L, O'Donnell C, Wardlaw DM, et al: Risk and resiliency factors influencing suicidality among urban African American and Latino youth. Am J Community Psychol 33(1–2):37–49, 2004 15055753

Posner K, Brown GK, Stanley B, et al: The Columbia-Suicide Severity Rating Scale: initial validity and internal consistency findings from three multisite studies with adolescents and adults. Am J Psychiatry 168(12):1266–1277, 2011 22193671

Prinstein MJ, Nock MK, Simon V, et al: Longitudinal trajectories and predictors of adolescent suicidal ideation and attempts following inpatient hospitalization. J Consult Clin Psychol 76(1):92–103, 2008 18229987

Puzia ME, Kraines MA, Liu RT, et al: Early life stressors and suicidal ideation: mediation by interpersonal risk factors. Pers Individ Dif 56:68–72, 2014

Qin P, Agerbo E, Mortensen PB: Suicide risk in relation to family history of completed suicide and psychiatric disorders: a nested case-control study based on longitudinal registers. Lancet 360(9340):1126–1130, 2002 12387960

Rabinovitch SM, Kerr DC, Leve LD, et al: Suicidal behavior outcomes of childhood sexual abuse: longitudinal study of adjudicated girls. Suicide Life Threat Behav 45(4):431–447, 2015 25370436

Rajalin M, Hirvikoski T, Jokinen J: Family history of suicide and exposure to interpersonal violence in childhood predict suicide in male suicide attempters. J Affect Disord 148(1):92–97, 2013 23273935

Ran MS, Zhang Z, Fan M, et al: Risk factors of suicidal ideation among adolescents after Wenchuan earthquake in China. Asian J Psychiatr 13:66–71, 2015 25845324

Reinherz HZ, Giaconia RM, Silverman AB, et al: Early psychosocial risks for adolescent suicidal ideation and attempts. J Am Acad Child Adolesc Psychiatry 34(5):599–611, 1995 7775355

Remillard AM, Lamb S: Adolescent girls' coping with relational aggression. Sex Roles 53:221–229, 2005

Riala K, Alaräisänen A, Taanila A, et al: Regular daily smoking among 14-year-old adolescents increases the subsequent risk for suicide: the Northern Finland 1966 Birth Cohort Study. J Clin Psychiatry 68(5):775–780, 2007 17503989

Roane BM, Taylor DJ: Adolescent insomnia as a risk factor for early adult depression and substance abuse. Sleep 31(10):1351–1356, 2008 18853932

Roberts RE, Roberts CR, Xing Y: One-year incidence of suicide attempts and associated risk and protective factors among adolescents. Arch Suicide Res 14(1):66–78, 2010 20112145

Robertson L, Skegg K, Poore M, et al: An adolescent suicide cluster and the possible role of electronic communication technology. Crisis 33(4):239–245, 2012 22562859

Rose DT, Abramson LY: Developmental predictors of depressive cognitive style: research and theory, Rochester Symposium of Developmental Psychopathology, IV. Edited by Cicchetti D, Toth S. Rochester, NY, University of Rochester Press, 1992, pp 323–349

Rudd MD, Berman AL, Joiner TE Jr, et al: Warning signs for suicide: theory, research, and clinical applications. Suicide Life Threat Behav 36(3):255–262, 2006 16805653

Rutter M: Psychosocial resilience and protective mechanisms. Am J Orthopsychiatry 57(3):316–331, 1987 3303954

Salzinger S, Rosario M, Feldman RS, et al: Adolescent suicidal behavior: associations with preadolescent physical abuse and selected risk and protective factors. J Am Acad Child Adolesc Psychiatry 46(7):859–866, 2007 17581450

Selkie EM, Fales JL, Moreno MA: Cyberbullying prevalence among US middle and high school-aged adolescents: a systematic review and quality assessment. J Adolesc Health 58(2):125–133, 2016 26576821

Shaffer D, Jacobson C: Proposal to the DSM-V Childhood Disorder and Mood Disorder Work Groups to Include Non-Suicidal Self-Injury (NSSI) as a DSM-V Disorder. Washington, DC, American Psychiatric Association, 2009

Shneidman ES: Suicide as psychache. J Nerv Ment Dis 181(3):145–147, 1993 8445372

Shochat T, Cohen-Zion M, Tzischinsky O: Functional consequences of inadequate sleep in adolescents: a systematic review. Sleep Med Rev 18(1):75–87, 2014 23806891

Smith JM, Alloy LB, Abramson LY: Cognitive vulnerability to depression, rumination, hopelessness, and suicidal ideation: multiple pathways to self-injurious thinking. Suicide Life Threat Behav 36(4):443–454, 2006 16978098

Somerville LH, Jones RM, Casey BJ: A time of change: behavioral and neural correlates of adolescent sensitivity to appetitive and aversive environmental cues. Brain Cogn 72(1):124–133, 2010 19695759

Stein MB, Fuetsch M, Müller N, et al: Social anxiety disorder and the risk of depression: a prospective community study of adolescents and young adults. Arch Gen Psychiatry 58(3):251–256, 2001 11231832

Steinberg L: Cognitive and affective development in adolescence. Trends Cogn Sci 9(2):69–74, 2005 15668099

Stewart JG, Kim JC, Esposito EC, et al: Predicting suicide attempts in depressed adolescents: clarifying the role of disinhibition and childhood sexual abuse. J Affect Disord 187:27–34, 2015 26318268

Stewart SM, Eaddy M, Horton SE, et al: The validity of the interpersonal theory of suicide in adolescence: a review. J Clin Child Adolesc Psychol 46(3):437–449, 2017 25864500

Stone LB, Liu RT, Yen S: Adolescent inpatient girls' report of dependent life events predicts prospective suicide risk. Psychiatry Res 219(1):137–142, 2014 24893759

Swanson EN, Owens EB, Hinshaw SP: Pathways to self-harmful behaviors in young women with and without ADHD: a longitudinal examination of mediating factors. J Child Psychol Psychiatry 55(5):505–515, 2014 25436256

Taussig HN, Harpin SB, Maguire SA: Suicidality among preadolescent maltreated children in foster care. Child Maltreat 19(1):17–26, 2014 24567247

Thompson MP, Light LS: Examining gender differences in risk factors for suicide attempts made 1 and 7 years later in a nationally representative sample. J Adolesc Health 48(4):391–397, 2011 21402269

Thompson R, Litrownik AJ, Isbell P, et al: Adverse experiences and suicidal ideation in adolescence: exploring the link using the LONGSCAN samples. Psychol Violence 2(2):211–225, 2012 24349862

Tsypes A, Gibb BE: Cognitive vulnerabilities and development of suicidal thinking in children of depressed mothers: a longitudinal investigation. Psychiatry Res 239:99–104, 2016 27137968

Tsypes A, Burkhouse KL, Gibb BE: Classification of facial expressions of emotion and risk for suicidal ideation in children of depressed mothers: evidence from cross-sectional and prospective analyses. J Affect Disord 197:147–150, 2016 26991369

Tuisku V, Kiviruusu O, Pelkonen M, et al: Depressed adolescents as young adults—-predictors of suicide attempt and non-suicidal self-injury during an 8-year follow-up. J Affect Disord 152–154:313–319, 2014 24144580

van Geel M, Vedder P, Tanilon J: Relationship between peer victimization, cyberbullying, and suicide in children and adolescents: a meta-analysis. JAMA Pediatr 168(5):435–442, 2014 24615300

Van Orden KA, Witte TK, Cukrowicz KC, et al: The interpersonal theory of suicide. Psychol Rev 117(2):575–600, 2010 20438238

Vander Stoep A, Adrian M, McCauley E, et al: Risk for suicidal ideation and suicide attempts associated with co-occurring depression and conduct problems in early adolescence. Suicide Life Threat Behav 41(3):316–329, 2011 21463356

Vrshek-Schallhorn S, Czarlinski J, Mineka S, et al: Prospective predictors of suicidal ideation during depressive episodes among older adolescents and young adults. Pers Individ Dif 50(8):1202–1207, 2011 21814297

Wei HT, Lan WH, Hsu JW, et al: Risk of suicide attempt among adolescents with conduct disorder: a longitudinal follow-up study. J Pediatr 177:292–296, 2016 27453371

Wenzel A, Beck AT: A cognitive model of suicidal behavior: theory and treatment. Appl Prev Psychol 12:189–201, 2008

Wilkinson P, Kelvin R, Roberts C, et al: Clinical and psychosocial predictors of suicide attempts and nonsuicidal self-injury in the Adolescent Depression Antidepressants and Psychotherapy Trial (ADAPT). Am J Psychiatry 168(5):495–501, 2011 21285141

Willoughby T, Heffer T, Hamza CA: The link between nonsuicidal self-injury and acquired capability for suicide: a longitudinal study. J Abnorm Psychol 124(4):1110–1115, 2015 26372006

Winsper C, Lereya T, Zanarini M, et al: Involvement in bullying and suicide-related behavior at 11 years: a prospective birth cohort study. J Am Acad Child Adolesc Psychiatry 51(3):271–282.e3, 2012 22365463

Wong MM, Brower KJ: The prospective relationship between sleep problems and suicidal behavior in the National Longitudinal Study of Adolescent Health. J Psychiatr Res 46(7):953–959, 2012 22551658

Wong MM, Brower KJ, Zucker RA: Sleep problems, suicidal ideation, and self-harm behaviors in adolescence. J Psychiatr Res 45(4):505–511, 2011 20889165

World Health Organization (WHO): Age—not the whole story. 2014. Available at: http://apps.who.int/adolescent/second-decade/section2/page2/age-not-the-whole-story.html. Accessed June 22, 2018.

Xu Z, Müller M, Heekeren K, et al: Pathways between stigma and suicidal ideation among people at risk of psychosis. Schizophr Res 172(1–3):184–188, 2016 26843510

Yen S, Weinstock LM, Andover MS, et al: Prospective predictors of adolescent suicidality: 6-month post-hospitalization follow-up. Psychol Med 43(5):983–993, 2013 22932393

You J, Lin MP: Predicting suicide attempts by time-varying frequency of nonsuicidal self-injury among Chinese community adolescents. J Consult Clin Psychol 83(3):524–533, 2015 25774785

Ystgaard M, Hestetun I, Loeb M, et al: Is there a specific relationship between childhood sexual and physical abuse and repeated suicidal behavior? Child Abuse Negl 28(8):863–875, 2004 15350770

Zalsman G, Hawton K, Wasserman D, et al: Suicide prevention strategies revisited: 10-year systematic review. Lancet Psychiatry 3(7):646–659, 2016 27289303

Zeller M, Yuval K, Nitzan-Assayag Y, et al: Self-compassion in recovery following potentially traumatic stress: longitudinal study of at-risk youth. J Abnorm Child Psychol 43(4):645–653, 2015 25234347

Zhang X, Wu LT: Suicidal ideation and substance use among adolescents and young adults: a bidirectional relation? Drug Alcohol Depend 142:63–73, 2014 24969957

Safety Planning and Risk Management

Michele Berk, Ph.D.
Stephanie Clarke, Ph.D.

Introduction

Regardless of the particular treatment setting or approach, there are several strategies that can be used to enhance safety that should be routinely applied when working with suicidal adolescents and their families. These strategies are relatively brief, are easy to implement, and have the enormous potential to save lives. Given the absence of research data enabling clinicians to accurately predict which adolescents at risk will attempt suicide at any given time, as well as the limits of existing treatment approaches, the use of basic safety interventions to reduce risk is of critical importance. In Table 3–1, we provide a user-friendly checklist of these interventions, as a reference guide for the clinician to use during treatment sessions.

Suicide Risk Assessment With Adolescents

A thorough risk assessment should be conducted during every contact with an adolescent at risk for suicide, particularly those with a history of prior

TABLE 3-1.   Checklist of safety-based interventions

	Specific steps to be taken	Check if completed
Restriction of lethal means	Discussed importance of removal of firearms from the home	
	Reviewed removal of lethal means with parent	
	Reviewed access to lethal means with teen	
	Asked teen if he or she has any lethal means hidden "just in case" he or she wants to use them in the future	
Parental monitoring	Reviewed need for close monitoring and discussed amount of close monitoring currently needed	
	If 24/7 monitoring needed, a plan set up to reassess safety within the next 1–2 days	
Creation of a written safety plan	Written safety plan completed with teen	
	Written safety plan reviewed with parent	
Creation of a hope box	Hope box completed	
Providing emergency contact information	Parent and teen provided with emergency cards with 24/7 emergency hotline numbers/911	
Reduction of family conflict	Parents informed of the importance of reducing family conflict until the teen is no longer suicidal	
Educating parents	Parents informed to take all communications about suicidal thoughts or urges seriously and to implement appropriate safety interventions as needed	
Reducing contagion	Plan discussed with parent and teen for limiting access to internet content related to suicide and communication about suicidality/self-harm with peers	

suicide attempts (SAs) and/or nonsuicidal self-injuries (NSSI), which are robust risk factors for future suicide attempts (Asarnow et al. 2011; Bridge et al. 2006; Wilkinson et al. 2011). Suicidal and self-harm urges and behaviors may wax and wane over time; hence, measurement of current risk is recommended during every patient contact. Core components of risk assessment include, but are not limited to, 1) current and recent suicidal ideation, intent, and plan; 2) the ability to commit to using a safety plan if suicidal urges occur between clinical contacts; 3) access to lethal means; 4) safety of the home environment (i.e., parents' ability to closely monitor youth and restrict access to lethal means); 5) current status of risk and protective factors; and 6) current stressors/potential triggering events. There are several structured clinical interviews available to assist clinicians in conducting and documenting a comprehensive risk assessment, such as the Columbia-Suicide Severity Rating Scale (C-SSRS; Posner et al. 2011), the Linehan Risk Assessment and Management Protocol (LRAMP; Linehan et al. 2012), and the Collaborative Assessment and Management of Suicidality Framework (CAMS) Suicide Status Form (Jobes 2006). Self-report forms, such as the dialectical behavior therapy (DBT) "diary card" (see Chapter 4, "Dialectical Behavior Therapy for Suicidal Multiproblem Adolescents," for a description of a diary card), the Suicide Ideation Questionnaire (SIQ; Reynolds 1987), and the Beck Depression Inventory (BDI), may also be used to gather information.

As described in detail in Chapter 2, "Risk and Protective Factors for Suicidal Thoughts and Behaviors in Adolescents," numerous risk factors for death by suicide and suicide attempts in adolescents have been identified in the research literature. These risk factors include, but are not limited to, 1) prior suicidality and self-harm behavior (e.g., suicidal ideation, NSSI, prior suicide attempt[s]); 2) psychiatric disorders (e.g., mood disorders, substance abuse and dependence, conduct disorder, borderline personality disorder, anxiety disorders, psychotic disorders); 3) cognitive/emotional/behavioral states and traits (e.g., hopelessness, poor problem-solving skills, perception of being a burden to others, emotion dysregulation, impulsivity, risk-taking behavior, anger, aggression, acute insomnia with agitation, acute psychosis); 4) environmental circumstances (loneliness, social isolation, negative life events, access to lethal means, family conflict, contagion, bullying); 5) identification as lesbian, gay, bisexual, transgender (LGBT); 6) genetic factors (family history of suicide); and 7) gender (males are more likely to die by suicide) and age (suicide is the second leading cause of death for ages 10–34 years in the United States [Centers for Disease Control and Prevention 2016]). Despite the identification of multiple risk factors, it remains impossible for clinicians to accurately predict which individuals with these risk factors will go on to attempt suicide at any given time or ultimately die by suicide (Fowler 2012). Risk increases with the number of risk factors present; however, no algorithms exist to predict which combinations of risk factors are most likely to lead to suicidal behavior at any given time (Franklin et al. 2017). Hence, the clinician must ultimately rely on clinical judgment to determine risk.

At times, obtaining the information needed to assess risk can be challenging. Adolescents may have difficulty sharing information related to risk with the clinician for multiple reasons, including 1) fear of hospitalization, 2) genuine uncertainty about their current degree of suicidality, and 3) a desire to conceal a planned suicide attempt. We caution against interpreting difficulty communicating risk as "gamey" or "manipulative" (Linehan 1993). This may lead to invalidating and hostile interactions with patients (which may further exacerbate the problem), overlooking valid concerns on the part of the teen that need to be addressed in order for safety planning to be effective, and underestimating the actual risk. It is important for the clinician to work with the teen to identify and resolve roadblocks to sharing information by, for example, providing clear information about when hospitalization would be considered and teaching skills for identifying and labeling thoughts and feelings. The parent/caregiver can also be very helpful in this type of situation by providing the therapist with information about the teen's level of risk from his or her perspective and determining if the teen can be kept safe via environmental interventions in the home (e.g., parental close monitoring, restriction of lethal means; see subsections "Restriction of Lethal Means" and "Parental Monitoring") or if the teen requires an inpatient or residential level of care. To avoid lengthy, confusing, and potentially frustrating conversations about risk with a teen who is having difficulty providing information, an advance agreement may also be useful (such as, "If you are unable to report your level of risk to me, I will need to speak with your parent and determine with him or her if you can be kept safe at home or will need hospitalization"). Other options that may be helpful are determining if other observable suicide risk factors are elevated and administering self-report measures, because patients may be more willing to endorse an item on a written form than to state it verbally.

Hospitalization

As described in the American Academy of Child and Adolescent Psychiatry's (AACAP) *Practice Parameter for the Assessment and Treatment of Children and Adolescents With Suicidal Behavior* (Shaffer et al. 2001), if the teen is determined to be at high risk of imminent suicidal behavior, psychiatric hospitalization should be considered. Potential benefits of hospitalization include increased safety due to decreased access to potentially lethal means, close supervision by mental health professionals, immediate access to mental health treatment, and short-term removal from problematic environments that are acutely maintaining symptoms (e.g., a conflictual home environment). However, decisions about hospitalization should be made conservatively and should prioritize the best interest of the teen over concerns about liability, as hospitalization is not a benign intervention. There are no research data supporting the effectiveness of hospitalization at reducing suicidal behavior, and it has been suggested that hospitalization may even be iatrogenic under certain circumstances (Linehan 1993). Results of a recent meta-analysis of 100 studies of patients hospitalized for suicidality found that rates of completed suicide were highest in the first 3 months following hospital discharge, at 100 times the global suicide rate (Chung et al. 2017). Additionally, data have failed to show the benefit of hospitalization with regard to reduced suicidal ideation and attempts when compared with intensive outpatient treatments (Huey et al. 2004; Knesper et al. 2010) and rehospitalization rates are high (e.g., 13% at 90-day follow-up, Vigod et al. 2013; 38% at 6-month follow-up, Owen et al. 1997; and 30%–43% at 1-year follow-up, Loch 2014). Taken together, these findings suggest that hospitalization is ineffective at lowering the risk of subsequent suicidal behavior.

One primary concern about hospitalization is the increased risk of future SA or NSSI if the hospitalization is reinforcing for the patient (e.g., provides desired outcomes; Linehan 1993). For example, hospitalization may be reinforcing by removing the teen from an aversive situation (e.g., home, school, peer interactions) or leading to an increase in positive interpersonal responses (e.g., nurturing, caretaking, increased attention/concern). Moreover, hospitalization removes the patient from the natural environment and deprives him or her of the opportunity to learn how to cope effectively with suicidal and self-harm urges and behaviors, leaving him or her vulnerable to rehospitalization in the future. Repeated hospitalizations also disrupt peer relationships and academic functioning, which are central aspects of an adolescent's "life worth living" (Linehan 1993) and thus serve a critical protective function. Another downside of hospitalization is the potential for contagion among teens on the inpatient unit, particularly regarding sharing of methods of SA and NSSI and the portrayal of suicidal behavior as a desirable option. Teens are particularly vulnerable to contagion (Insel and Gould 2008). Moreover, psychiatric hospitalization may be stigmatizing to teens and lead to decreased self-esteem and self-efficacy with regard to their ability to cope (Comtois and Linehan 2006).

In summary, although hospitalization may sometimes be unavoidable and is recommended when the youth is in imminent danger of attempting suicide, decisions about hospitalization should be made conservatively and carefully, after weighing the pros and cons for each individual teen. The interventions discussed in the remainder of this chapter address how to create a safe environment for the youth outside of the hospital setting and may reduce the need for hospitalization. These safety interventions largely overlap with those recommended in the recently released expert guidelines by the Suicide Prevention Resource Center (2015) for discharging suicidal adults home from the emergency department (ED) (versus hospitalization), as well as the AACAP Practice Parameter noted above. Several of the treatments discussed in later chapters of this book also provide examples of enhanced outpatient care that may serve as safe alternatives to hospitalization.

Safety Interventions

As shown in Table 3–1, the following safety interventions will be discussed: 1) restriction of lethal means; 2) parental monitoring; 3) creation of a written safety plan; 4) creation of a hope box; 5) providing emergency contact numbers; 6) reducing family conflict; 7) educating parents to take suicidal thoughts and behaviors seriously; and 8) reducing contagion.

Restriction of Lethal Means

Means restriction refers to removing or limiting access to dangerous or potentially life-threatening objects or settings, such as firearms, sharps (e.g., knives, razors, scissors), bridges, tall buildings, and any medications and toxic substances that could be used to overdose (Miller 2013). It has been documented that removing the suicidal individual's access to lethal means is a highly effective suicide prevention strategy (Barber and Miller 2014). In fact, means restriction is one of the only approaches to suicide prevention that has a robust empirical basis (Mann et al. 2005), and therefore, the 2012 National Strategy for Suicide Prevention (U.S. Department of Health and Human Services Office of the Surgeon General and National Action Alliance for Suicide Prevention 2012) includes means restriction assessment and education as a central strategy for suicide prevention.

Access to lethal means should be assessed repeatedly, in every contact with a suicidal teen, as new means may be acquired between sessions or it may be revealed that the teen has been hiding means that he or she was not yet willing to give up. We have found that using the following metaphor works well to illustrate the risk of impulsive suicidal behavior when means are readily available, "If you were on a diet, would you be more likely to break your diet if you did or did not have a chocolate cake in your kitchen?" Although the teen can always acquire additional means for self-harm, removing easily available means for an impulsive suicide attempt may give the patient time to reconsider, seek help, and/or be interrupted by others (e.g., "you can always go to the store to buy a chocolate cake, but that would take much more time and effort and you would have more opportunities to change your mind or for somebody else to stop you"). Unwillingness to remove lethal means can often reveal important therapeutic issues. For example, it may suggest that the teen is not fully committed to giving up suicide or self-harm as an option, and this would become a critical treatment goal.

Although some general discussion of restriction of access to lethal means can be conducted with the parent and adolescent together, it is recommended that the clinician speak with each individually, because the clinician must balance the importance of conducting a thorough assessment of access to lethal means with the risk of unintentionally introducing the teen to methods of suicide that he or she may not have previously considered. In our clinic, when we discuss restriction of lethal means with teens, we ask open-ended questions about whether or not they have access to ways of killing themselves and ask specific questions only about methods they have already identified or used in the past (e.g., for a teen with a history of NSSI by cutting with razors, "Do you have currently have any razors?"). It is imperative that the clinician gather detailed information about methods used in past SAs or NSSI and methods the teen may have considered for future attempts and to ensure that he or she does not have access to those items. We have also found that it is important to ask the adolescent about any means he or she may have hidden away "just in case" for use in the future. In many cases, this question will lead the teen to reveal possession of additional items not previously disclosed. The clinician should work with the teen and parent to identify the location of those items and dispose of them.

Typically, our discussion about lethal means with parents is much more detailed and includes review of all potentially lethal means and discussion about how to identify these items and remove them from the home. Parents should be told that, ideally, all potentially lethal means should be confiscated and removed from the home. If this is not possible, then needed items (e.g., prescription medications) should be kept in a locked box or safe. However, these options are less desirable than removal, as adolescents are often able to find and access these items. In our clinic, we also instruct parents to look through the adolescent's room and belongings (e.g., backpack, purse) to determine if there are any hidden lethal means. This may need to be done repeatedly, as the adolescent may acquire new lethal means while out of the home. Although this can raise privacy issues between adolescents and parents, we choose to err on the side of caution and prioritize safety over privacy for teens at risk of suicide and/ or serious self-harm. Obtaining increased privacy from parents can also serve as a powerful contingency, motivating teens to reduce suicidal and self-harm behavior.

Although restriction of lethal means may appear simple, in our experience, parents often struggle with this task because it can trigger anxiety, shame, and the perception that the clinician is blaming the parent for the teen's prior self-harm behaviors. Parents may also become overwhelmed at the idea of having to be responsible for removing all possible items and/ or feel hopeless that they can do so properly. We have found it helpful to reassure parents that it is impossible to remove access to everything (e.g., the adolescent can always find a way to obtain something if they are really determined) and that the primary goal is to reduce the likelihood of impulsive suicide attempts and increase the window of time for the teen to seek help and for others to intervene. Repeating the dieting metaphor described above can also be helpful.

In cases where the parent's reluctance to remove lethal means is more entrenched, it may be useful to assess possible misperceptions about suicide (e.g., "Nobody can stop another person from killing themselves," "If you take away one method, he or she will just find another one," "My son or daughter just needs to learn more self-control") and provide appropriate psychoeducation. At times, a parent's resistance to removal of lethal means may indicate parental neglect and/or severe family pathology, and the clinician should consider whether or not a different living situation is needed. The ability of the parent to restrict access to lethal means in the home (along with performing other safety interventions) can be a determining factor in whether or not the adolescent can receive outpatient versus inpatient or residential treatment.

Specific Means/Methods to Assess

Owing to the high lethality of firearms, it is essential that suicidal individuals do not have access to guns. It has been shown that adolescents who died by suicide were twice as likely to have lived in a home with a gun, compared with a control group of adolescents recruited from an inpatient psychiatric unit, both with and without histories of suicide attempts (Brent et al. 1991). We refer readers to the excellent Means Matter website for detailed information about speaking to families about removal and/or safe storage of firearms (www.hsph.harvard.edu/means-matter/). Parents should be informed unequivocally that the safest option is to completely remove firearms from the home. In the study by Brent et al. (1991), it was found that safe storage of guns (e.g., locked, ammunition stored separately) did not reduce rates of suicides using firearms. If parents are unable or unwilling to remove firearms from the home, then the clinician should focus on ensuring that the gun is stored safely and providing information about safe storage practices. For information on how to safely remove and/or store a firearm, see www.hsph.harvard.edu/means-matter/recommendations/families/#QUESTIONS.

In addition to guns, parents should be directed to remove all other potentially lethal means, including medications, sharps, methods of suffocation/hanging, household poisons, and alcohol and other substances. Parents should be asked to remove all medications as is possible (both prescription and over-the-counter medications) and to lock up (e.g., purchase a safe or lockbox to which the adolescent does not have access) any needed medications, as well as to keep only small amounts on hand to reduce the likelihood of a lethal overdose if the teen obtains access. We routinely caution parents about medications containing acetaminophen (e.g., Tylenol), because many parents are not aware that even small dosages are potentially life-threatening and require immediate medical attention. We also recommend that parents safely store and dispense any medications the teen has been prescribed (e.g., psychiatric medications) one pill at a time and observe the adolescent taking the medication to prevent him or her from saving pills for a future suicide attempt via overdose.

Parents should also be instructed to remove access to sharp objects the adolescent can use to cut himself or herself. These items include (but are not limited to) knives, razors, scissors, and blades from pencil and eye makeup sharpeners. If needed, the parent can purchase an electric razor for the teen. Other items to address include household cleaners/poisons and items that can be used for hanging/suffocation (e.g., belts, ties, scarves, plastic bags). In addition, the parent may consider placing locks on doors and windows leading out of the home, particularly on higher stories of a house or apartment, removal of car keys and/or driving privileges, and removal of locks from bathroom or bedroom doors or even removal of the bedroom door altogether. Finally, it may also be necessary to block access to "suicide hotspots," such as bridges, tall buildings, cliffs, and trains, if these exist in the teen's local community (see report of Public Health England [2015]).

Parental Monitoring

An adolescent who is residing in the home (versus in hospital or residential treatment setting) and who is at risk of attempting suicide should be monitored closely by parents. Depending on the level of risk, parental monitoring may include frequent check-ins with the adolescent, not allowing the adolescent to be alone in his or her room or in an isolated part of the home, not allowing the youth to lock the door to his or her bedroom or the bathroom, not allowing the adolescent to leave the home, or not allowing the adolescent to be alone at all (constant monitoring, including sleeping in the same room or bed with the adolescent). Given that 24/7 monitoring by parents is not sustainable for extended periods of time, an adolescent who requires 24/7 monitoring should be reevaluated frequently by the clinician to determine if the crisis has resolved to the extent that parents can reduce monitoring or if the youth needs to be transferred to an inpatient level of care. The clinician's recommendation for the amount of parental monitoring should be commensurate with the clinician's assessment of current risk and, hence, may vary over time. *Parental monitoring* is defined as both awareness of the teen's activities and close physical monitoring; low levels of parental monitoring are associated with increased risk for suicide among adolescents (King et al. 2001; Kostenuik and Ratnapalan 2010). The AACAP Practice Parameter for suicidal youth also recommends that youth be monitored by a supportive and trustworthy person (Shaffer et al. 2001). With teens, the ability of the parent to provide close monitoring in the home may be a deciding factor in whether or not the youth requires hospitalization or can be safely managed through a crisis in a less restrictive setting.

Creation of a Written Safety Plan

It is often difficult for patients to plan and implement adaptive coping strategies in the place of self-harm when they are in the midst of a suicidal crisis and overwhelmed by strong negative emotions (Wenzel et al. 2009). For this reason, it is important to develop a detailed, written crisis plan that the teen can immediately access and follow in future crisis situations (Berk et al. 2004; Stanley et al. 2009; Wenzel et al. 2009). Stanley and Brown (2012) have developed a safety plan template and intervention that has been identified as a "best practice" by the Suicide Prevention Resource Center/American Foundation for Suicide Prevention that can be adapted across settings and populations. A generic template is available online at www.sprc.org/sites/default/files/Brown_StanleySafetyPlanTemplate.pdf. The safety plan template provides the basis for a collaborative, in-depth discussion with adolescents and parents about ways to keep the adolescent safe during a suicidal crisis. The safety plan template is organized in a stepwise manner and starts with strategies that the youth can implement himself or herself at home and ends with 24/7 emergency contact numbers that can be used when there is imminent danger and emergency services are needed.

Step 1 of the safety plan consists of warning signs that a suicidal crisis may be developing. The therapist should work with the teen to identify and list situations, thoughts, feelings, body sensations, and behaviors that typically precede suicidality. For example, the teen may recall that he or she often develops suicidal ideation after getting a poor grade on a test at school and having the thought "Nothing will ever get better for me." The parent should be informed of the warning signs the teen has listed so he or she can help the teen stay safe when these warning signs are present. The parent can also be asked to contribute warning signs he or she has observed in the teen before prior suicidal crises.

Step 2 consists of internal coping strategies that the youth can perform on his or her own to take his or her mind off problems and/or suicidal thoughts. These strategies may include engaging in distracting activities, self-soothing, relaxation techniques, and physical activities. We have found the DBT distress tolerance skills handouts to be useful in providing youth with suggestions for internal coping skills (i.e., TIP: changing your body chemistry, distracting, self-soothing and improving the moment; Linehan 2015; Rathus and Miller 2015). In order to help teens identify distracting activities that are engaging enough to divert their attention away from suicidal thoughts and urges, we have often used the following prompt, "What activities do you do that you become so involved or engrossed in that you wouldn't even hear somebody calling your name to dinner?" We have also found it helpful to introduce basic internal coping skills with adolescents, such as distraction and self-soothing, with the rationale that the goal of using these strategies is to reduce distress enough to make safe choices not to solve longer-term problems (Linehan 2015). We have encountered teens who reported feeling invalidated by the suggestion that a relatively simple skill, such as watching a funny video or doing a crossword puzzle, is sufficient to solve their problems. Hence, we clarify from the outset that this is not what we are saying to offset premature rejection of these skills and potential rupture in the therapeutic relationship.

Step 3 consists of listing people and social settings that can be used for distraction. Step 4 is a list of people whom the teen can reach out to for help in an emergency. In both cases, the teen should be asked to put the phone numbers for these individuals on the list for easy access in a crisis (or to make sure these contacts are added to his or her mobile phone), to avoid having to access this information from memory when emotionally dysregulated. Step 5 is a list of mental health providers and 24/7 emergency contact numbers that the adolescent can use in a suicidal crisis. In our clinics, we already have this information printed on copies of our safety plan template. The teen should be instructed to keep copies of his or her safety plan easily accessible at all times. Step 6 provides space to list steps that need to be taken to keep the environment safe (e.g., restriction of lethal means), and finally, there is space to list reminders of reasons to live.

Both the youth and parent should be given a copy of the completed safety plan at the end of the session. Both should be instructed to keep copies of the plan accessible at all times, and we have suggested having each take pictures of the plan to store on their mobile phones as a way to ensure this. It is important to review the completed safety plan with the parent, so that he or she is aware of the components of the plan and can support the teen in using it. Parents should also be asked to verify that the coping skills are feasible and the contact people the youth listed are appropriate. If the teen has listed a coping skill that the parent determines is not feasible (e.g., involves spending money on an item or activity that the family cannot afford), then the therapist should work with the adolescent and parent to come up with alternative ideas that the youth is willing to do. The therapist, according to his or her clinical judgment, may choose to complete the safety plan with the adolescent separately from the parent and review afterward or may choose to involve the parent in the creation of the safety plan.

Creation of a Hope Box

We have also found that the creation of a "hope box" is a useful companion to the safety plan (see Asarnow et al. 2009; Berk et al. 2004, 2008, 2009; Brown et al. 2005; Wenzel et al. 2009). Similar to the written safety plan, the hope box is a way to prepare in advance for a suicidal crisis by placing tangible reminders of the coping skills listed in the safety plan, as well as materials needed to use them and reminders of the teen's reasons to live, in a box that can be easily accessed in a suicidal crisis. Items that may be placed in the hope box include photographs of favorite people and places, postcards, letters, self-soothing items such as scented candles and music, and distracting tasks such as paints and paper for painting or a funny DVD the youth can watch. Copies of the written safety plan and emergency contact numbers can also be placed in the hope box. The teen should be told to put the hope box in a place where they can easily access it when feeling suicidal. There is also a "Virtual Hope Box" app that can be downloaded for free from the National Center for Telehealth and Technology (T2), under the auspices of Defense Health Agency (DHA) Connected Health (http://t2health.dcoe.mil/apps/virtual-hope-box).

The hope box should be created as part of the safety plan established in the initial sessions, and the adolescent should continue to add items to the hope box as new coping strategies are identified during the course of treatment. Distraction methods (e.g., listening to a favorite song, word search puzzles) and self-soothing techniques (e.g., techniques that improve mood via hearing, smell, sound, taste, and touch) typically used in the "Distress Tolerance" module of DBT (Linehan 2015) are particularly amenable to the hope box. The hope box can be assigned for homework, with the youth instructed to bring it to the next session to review with the clinician. We have found that reviewing the hope box often serves as a useful bonding experience between the therapist and the teen; the teen is able to show the therapist who and what is really important to them. The clinician should check that all items selected by the youth will trigger positive affect and coping. Youth should not be allowed to put negative/destructive items or reminders of negative events/behaviors in their hope box. If the clinician is unclear whether the item is positive or negative (e.g., a favorite song that mentions suicide), this should be explored in detail with the youth (e.g., "Does this song make you feel inspired or remind you that you don't want to hurt yourself or will it end up putting the idea of suicide at the front of your mind when you are already upset and vulnerable?").

The parent should be informed of the hope box and asked to remind his or her teen to use it during a crisis. When clinically indicated, the parent may also participate in the creation of the hope box by taking the youth to obtain items to include, such as going to the bookstore to buy a favorite book or magazine to put in the hope box. It can also be helpful to have parents write down positive statements on index cards that the youth can put in the hope box (e.g., "I will always love you, no matter what happens").

Providing Emergency Contact Numbers

As shown in Figure 3–1, we provide all suicidal adolescents and parents with wallet-sized cards with the phone numbers of mobile crisis teams, 24/7 crisis hotlines, and 911, which they can keep with them at all times. It is important to provide the family with emergency contact information and explicit instructions for when to use various resources discussed. Parents should be informed that if they are concerned that their adolescent may be in imminent danger of harming himself or herself and/or if they

In case of emergency:

Call 911 or go to the nearest emergency room

Or call one of the 24/7 hotline numbers below:

- Santa Clara County Child and Adolescent Mobile Crisis Program (EMQ): **1-877-41-CRISIS**
- San Mateo County Crisis Intervention and Suicide Prevention Center: **(650) 579-0350**
- National Suicide Prevention Lifeline: **1 (800) 273-TALK**
- Crisis Text Line: **Text START to 741-741**

Stanford Children's Health — Division of Child and Adolescent Psychiatry

FIGURE 3-1. **Emergency card.**

feel they can no longer keep the teen safe in the home, then they should call 911 or take the adolescent to the nearest ED. If they are unsure if they are able to transport the adolescent safely themselves (e.g., the adolescent is combative or might run away or jump out of the car), then they should call 911 to have an ambulance or police transport the adolescent to the ED. Adolescents should be told to inform their parents or a trusted adult immediately, call 911 or go to the nearest ED, and/or use other 24/7 crisis hotline numbers provided if they feel they can no longer keep themselves safe. Parents and teens should also be given clear information about the therapist's after-hours availability and be instructed to call emergency contact numbers if the adolescent is in imminent danger and the therapist is not immediately reachable. Parents should be told to check in with the adolescent regularly about whether or not he or she is having thoughts about suicide as well as to be observant regarding the specific warning signs identified in the safety plan and elevation of general suicide risk factors (see Chapter 2 for detailed discussion of risk factors). It is important to provide psychoeducation to parents to clarify that simply asking about suicidal thoughts does not increase the likelihood of the adolescent having suicidal thoughts and/or behaviors, which is a relatively common misconception (Gould et al. 2005).

Reduction of Family Conflict

Improving family functioning is a critical treatment target for suicidal youth (Brent et al. 2013). Family conflict has been identified as a key risk factor for adolescent suicide and suicidal behavior, and family cohesion has been identified as a protective factor (Bridge et al. 2006). Importantly, parents/caregivers play a significant role in maintaining the safety of suicidal youth. Removing lethal means from the home, closely monitoring the youth, and seeking emergency services when needed are critical functions conducted by parents that may prevent suicidal behavior. Strengthening relationships between parents and teens is essential in enabling parents to perform these safety functions effectively and in increasing the likelihood that the adolescent will reach out to the parent for help when in a suicidal crisis. In fact, research consistently demonstrates the essential role that parents and family play in the success of interventions for suicidal adolescents, and all of the evidence-based treatments discussed in the remainder of this book include significant parent and family-based components.

Parents should be informed that family conflict is a well-known risk factor for adolescent suicidal behavior and that reducing parent-teen conflict should be an urgent priority. We typically tell parents that the number one goal at the beginning of treatment is to establish a positive relationship with their teen, so that the teen will go to them for help if they feel suicidal instead of concealing this information from them. Accordingly, parents should be educated about the importance of maintaining an open, positive, and nonjudgmental relationship with their child. It can be helpful to validate parents' concerns about other difficulties the teen may be having (e.g., not completing chores, doing poorly in school), which often impact the family and cause parents a great deal of distress and lead to conflict. However, it is important to emphasize that the first priority is to decrease family conflict, so any issues that do not directly impact safety should be of lower priority until suicide risk has decreased. We typically recommend that parents "pick their battles" and limit arguments and disagreements to issues directly related to safety. We also reassure parents that the other problems they have identified will definitely be addressed in treatment in the future, after safety has been established.

Educating Parents to Take Suicide Attempts/ Suicidal Ideation Seriously

Parents should be told to take *all* communications by the adolescent about suicidality seriously. In our work, we have found that parents often experience the teen's suicidality as "attention seeking" or "manipulative." Parents may minimize risk for many reasons, such as lack of knowledge/ education about suicidal behavior, fear, helplessness, and desire to believe that their child is okay. We recommend informing parents that it is very rare for a teen to "pretend" to be suicidal to get attention or get his or her way and that any child who is repeatedly talking about suicide/self-harm for any reason is at risk. Even in the unlikely event that the adolescent is lying or exaggerating for personal gain, we would consider this approach to getting his or her needs met to be highly problematic and requiring mental health treatment. It should be emphasized to parents that it is safer to take suicidality seriously and be wrong than not to take it seriously and have something terrible happen (i.e., "better safe than sorry").

Suicide Contagion and Use of Social Media/ Electronic Devices

Suicide contagion is defined as "the exposure to suicide or suicidal behaviors within one's family, one's peer group, or through media reports of suicide and can result in an increase in suicide and suicidal behaviors" (U.S. Department of Health and Human Services, www.hhs.gov/answers/mental-health-and-substance-abuse/what-does-suicide-contagion-mean/index.html). The notion of contagion is derived from social learning theory, which posits that human behavior is learned observationally through modeling the behavior of others (Bandura 1971). Research has shown that people are more likely to imitate the behavior of a model when they have things in common with that person (e.g., they are the same age and gender), when the model is perceived to have positive qualities, and when the behavior of the model results in desired outcomes (Insel and Gould 2008). Adolescents, who are forming their identities and often rely on the behaviors of others to guide their choices, are particularly vulnerable to contagion (Insel and Gould 2008). In severe cases, contagion may lead to "suicide clusters," in which multiple deaths by suicide occur among group of individuals within a specific location and time frame (Gould et al. 1990). Increased use of social media and communication via electronic devices by adolescents has also increased the potential for contagion (Singaravelu et al. 2015; Whitlock et al. 2006), and few guidelines for parents exist on how to most effectively limit usage of social media to reduce contagion.

To reduce risk of contagion, adolescents who are at risk for suicidal and/or self-harm behavior should be cautioned against sharing information with peers about these behaviors, as well as from receiving this information from peers, including via social networking platforms and websites. Many adolescents we have treated have reported to us that they believe it is very helpful to speak with peers who also struggle with suicidality, both because that peer uniquely understands their experience and because they feel they can be helpful to their peer. Accordingly, in getting teens to agree to reduce communication of suicidality to peers, we have found it helpful to first validate their desire to help their friend and/or reach out to their friend for help for themselves. We then inform them that even though it may feel helpful, talking with friends about the topic of suicidality or self-harm is actually destructive to both of them, as the mere words themselves are very triggering and may lead to contagion. In other words, if one person is trying to eat healthy and the other person wants to have a conversation about chocolate cake, then the person who is trying to eat healthy is really going to want to eat chocolate cake! We brainstorm other ways the teen can support their friends and get support for themselves without discussing these topics, as well as how to get adults involved and the importance of adults, rather than teens, in handling suicidal crises. We have found that many teens have even been willing to make an agreement with their friends that they will not discuss suicidality and/or self-harm with each other so they can continue to be helpful and not harmful to each other.

Conclusion

Safety-based interventions are essential when working with adolescents at risk for suicide, and they play a central role in suicide prevention. The safety measures described in this chapter should be used with every suicidal individual, regardless of treatment orientation or approach; they are designed to reduce the risk of suicidal behavior and block the ability to carry out suicidal actions. This chapter outlines several evidence-based safety interventions for suicidal youth and their parents/caregivers along with suggestions about how to implement them in clinical practice. For readers who would like additional information on safety practices with suicidal youth, we provide a list of recommended readings below.

Recommended Readings

Freedenthal S: Helping the Suicidal Person: Tips and Techniques for Professionals. New York, Routledge, 2017

Means Matter website: https://www.hsph.harvard.edu/means-matter/

Shaffer D, Pfeffer CR; The Work Group on Issues, American Academy of Child and Adolescent Psychiatry: Practice parameter for the assessment and treatment of children and adolescents with suicidal behavior. J Am Acad Child Adolesc Psychiatry 40 (7 Suppl):24S–51S, 200111434483

Suicide Prevention Resource Center: Caring for adult patients with suicide risk: a consensus guide for emergency departments. 2015. Available at: http://www.sprc.org/sites/default/files/EDGuide_full.pdf. Accessed June 22, 2018.

References

Asarnow JR, Berk MS, Baraff LJ: Family intervention for suicide prevention: a specialized emergency department intervention for suicidal youth. Prof Psychol Res Pr 40:118–125, 2009

Asarnow JR, Porta G, Spirito A, et al: Suicide attempts and nonsuicidal self-injury in the treatment of resistant depression in adolescents: findings from the TORDIA study. J Am Acad Child Adolesc Psychiatry 50(8):772–781, 2011 21784297

Bandura A: Social Learning Theory. New York, General Learning Press, 1971

Barber CW, Miller MJ: Reducing a suicidal person's access to lethal means of suicide: a research agenda. Am J Prev Med 47(3)(Suppl 2):S264–S272, 2014 25145749

Berk MS, Henriques GR, Warman DM, et al: Cognitive therapy for suicide attempters: overview of the treatment and case examples. Cognit Behav Pract 11:265–277, 2004

Berk MS, Brown GK, Wenzel A, et al: A cognitive therapy intervention for adolescent suicide attempters: an empirically informed treatment, in Handbook of Evidence-Based Treatment Manuals for Children and Adolescents. Edited by Lecroy C. New York, Oxford University Press, 2008, pp 431–455

Berk MS, Grosjean M, Warnick HD: Beyond threats: risk factors for suicide in borderline personality disorder. Curr Psychiatr 8:32–41, 2009

Brent DA, Perper JA, Allman CJ, et al: The presence and accessibility of firearms in the homes of adolescent suicides. A case-control study. JAMA 266(21):2989–2995, 1991 1820470

Brent DA, McMakin DL, Kennard BD, et al: Protecting adolescents from self-harm: a critical review of intervention studies. J Am Acad Child Adolesc Psychiatry 52(12):1260–1271, 2013 24290459

Bridge JA, Goldstein TR, Brent DA: Adolescent suicide and suicidal behavior. J Child Psychol Psychiatry 47(3–4):372–394, 2006 16492264

Brown GK, Ten Have T, Henriques GR, et al: Cognitive therapy for the prevention of suicide attempts: a randomized controlled trial. JAMA 294(5):563–570, 2005 16077050

Centers for Disease Control and Prevention: 10 leading causes of death by age group, United States—2016, 2016. Available at: https://www.cdc.gov/injury/wisqars/pdf/leading_causes_of_death_by_age_group_2016-508.pdf. Accessed November 26, 2018.

Chung DT, Ryan CJ, Hadzi-Pavlovic D, et al: Suicide rates after discharge from psychiatric facilities: a systematic review and meta-analysis. JAMA Psychiatry 74(7):694–702, 2017 28564699

Comtois KA, Linehan MM: Psychosocial treatments of suicidal behaviors: a practice-friendly review. J Clin Psychol 62(2):161–170, 2006 16342292

Fowler JC: Suicide risk assessment in clinical practice: pragmatic guidelines for imperfect assessments. Psychotherapy (Chic) 49(1):81–90, 2012 22369082

Franklin JC, Ribeiro JD, Fox KR, et al: Risk factors for suicidal thoughts and behaviors: a meta-analysis of 50 years of research. Psychol Bull 143(2):187–232, 2017 27841450

Gould MS, Wallenstein S, Kleinman M: Time-space clustering of teenage suicide. Am J Epidemiol 131(1):71–78, 1990 2293755

Gould MS, Marrocco FA, Kleinman M, et al: Evaluating iatrogenic risk of youth suicide screening programs: a randomized controlled trial. JAMA 293(13):1635–1643, 2005 15811983

Huey SJ Jr, Henggeler SW, Rowland MD, et al: Multisystemic therapy effects on attempted suicide by youths presenting psychiatric emergencies. J Am Acad Child Adolesc Psychiatry 43(2):183–190, 2004 14726725

Insel BJ, Gould MS: Impact of modeling on adolescent suicidal behavior. Psychiatr Clin North Am 31(2):293–316, 2008 18439450

Jobes DA: Managing Suicidal Risk: A Collaborative Approach. New York, Guilford, 2006

King RA, Schwab-Stone M, Flisher AJ, et al: Psychosocial and risk behavior correlates of youth suicide attempts and suicidal ideation. J Am Acad Child Adolesc Psychiatry 40(7):837–846, 2001 11437023

Knesper DJ, American Association of Suicidology, Suicide Prevention Resource Center: Continuity of care for suicide prevention and research: suicide attempts and suicide deaths subsequent to discharge from the emergency department or psychiatry inpatient unit. Education Development Center, 2010. Available at: http://www.sprc.org/sites/default/files/migrate/library/continuityofcare.pdf. Accessed June 22, 2018.

Kostenuik M, Ratnapalan M: Approach to adolescent suicide prevention. Can Fam Physician 56(8):755–760, 2010 20705879

Linehan MM: Cognitive-Behavioral Treatment of Borderline Personality Disorder. New York, Guilford, 1993

Linehan MM: DBT Skills Training Handouts and Worksheets. New York, Guilford, 2015

Linehan MM, Comtois KA, Ward-Ciesielski EF: Assessing and managing risk with suicidal individuals. Cognit Behav Pract 19(2):218–232, 2012

Loch AA: Discharged from a mental health admission ward: is it safe to go home? A review on the negative outcomes of psychiatric hospitalization. Psychol Res Behav Manag 7:137–145, 2014 24812527

Mann JJ, Apter A, Bertolote J, et al: Suicide prevention strategies: a systematic review. JAMA 294(16):2064–2074, 2005 16249421

Miller DN: Lessons in suicide prevention from the Golden Gate Bridge: means restriction, public health, and the school psychologist. Contemp Sch Psychol 17:71–79, 2013

Owen C, Rutherford V, Jones M, et al: Psychiatric rehospitalization following hospital discharge. Community Ment Health J 33(1):13–24, 1997 9061259

Posner K, Brown GK, Stanley B, et al: The Columbia-Suicide Severity Rating Scale: initial validity and internal consistency findings from three multisite studies with adolescents and adults. Am J Psychiatry 168(12):1266–1277, 2011 22193671

Public Health England: Preventing suicides in public places: a practice resource. London, Public Health England, November 2015. Available at https://assets.publishing.service.gov.uk/government/uploads/system/uploads/attachment_data/file/481224/Preventing_suicides_in_public_places.pdf. Accessed November 26, 2018.

Rathus JH, Miller AL: DBT Skills Manual for Adolescents. New York, Guilford, 2015

Reynolds WM: Suicidal Ideation Questionnaire. Lutz, FL, Psychological Assessment Resources, 1987

Shaffer D, Pfeffer CR; The Work Group on Quality Issues, American Academy of Child and Adolescent Psychiatry: Practice parameter for the assessment and treatment of children and adolescents with suicidal behavior. J Am Acad Child Adolesc Psychiatry 40 (7 Suppl):24S–51S, 2001 11434483

Singaravelu V, Stewart A, Adams J, et al: Information-Seeking on the Internet. Crisis 36(3):211–219, 2015 26088826

Stanley B, Brown K: Safety planning intervention: a brief intervention to mitigate suicide risk. Cognit Behav Pract 19:256–264, 2012

Stanley B, Brown G, Brent DA, et al: Cognitive-behavioral therapy for suicide prevention (CBT-SP): treatment model, feasibility, and acceptability. J Am Acad Child Adolesc Psychiatry 48(10):1005–1013, 2009 19730273

Suicide Prevention Resource Center: Caring for Adult Patients with Suicide Risk: A Consensus Guide for Emergency Departments. 2015. Available at: http://wwwsprcorg/sites/default/files/EDGuide_fullpdf. Accessed June 22, 2018.

U.S. Department of Health and Human Services Office of the Surgeon General and National Action Alliance for Suicide Prevention: 2012 National Strategy for Suicide Prevention: Goals and Objectives for Action. Washington, DC, U.S. Department of Health and Human Services, 2012

Vigod SN, Kurdyak PA, Dennis CL, et al: Transitional interventions to reduce early psychiatric readmissions in adults: systematic review. Br J Psychiatry 202(3):187–194, 2013 23457182

Wenzel A, Brown GK, Beck AT: Cognitive Therapy for Suicidal Patients: Scientific and Clinical Applications. Washington, DC, American Psychological Association, 2009

Whitlock JL, Powers JL, Eckenrode J: The virtual cutting edge: the internet and adolescent self-injury. Dev Psychol 42(3):407–417, 2006 16756433

Wilkinson P, Kelvin R, Roberts C, et al: Clinical and psychosocial predictors of suicide attempts and nonsuicidal self-injury in the Adolescent Depression Antidepressants and Psychotherapy Trial (ADAPT). Am J Psychiatry 168(5):495–501, 2011 21285141

PART II

Treatment Approaches

Dialectical Behavior Therapy for Suicidal Multiproblem Adolescents

Alec L. Miller, Psy.D.

Jill H. Rathus, Ph.D.

Michele Berk, Ph.D.

Amy S. Walker, Ph.D.

Overview of Treatment Approach

Marsha Linehan (1993) originally developed dialectical behavior therapy (DBT) to treat suicidal adult women diagnosed with borderline personality disorder. Prior to the development of DBT, these individuals were often viewed by clinicians as being too challenging to help. Linehan's compassionate therapeutic approach, which balanced the core dialectic of acceptance and change, revolutionized the field of cognitive-behavioral therapy for this population. The DBT comprehensive treatment package provided individual therapy, skills training, and phone coaching to effectively treat multiproblem clients who felt invalidated by treatment strategies focused solely on change. Since that time, DBT has been expanded into a more transdiagnostic treatment, including a treatment model used to treat multiproblem adolescents across settings (Miller et al. 2007; Rathus and Miller 2015; Ritschel et al. 2013).

Prior to the 1990s, the assessment and treatment of suicidal and nonsuicidal self-injury (NSSI) was not a common professional specialty. Recent studies have indicated that adolescent suicide is the second leading cause of death among 10 to 24 year-olds in the United States (Centers for Disease Control and Prevention 2016), with rates continuing to rise in this age group. Further research indicates that in 2015, 18% of ninth to twelfth graders seriously contemplated attempting suicide, 15% made a plan for how they would attempt suicide, and 8.6% attempted suicide (Kann et al. 2016). Furthermore, 15%–30% of adolescents in community samples reported engaging in NSSI (Miller and Smith 2008). DBT has been found to be an effective treatment with suicidal multiproblem adolescents to reduce suicidal ideation, NSSI, emotion dysregulation, depression, and borderline personality disorder symptoms (McCauley et al. 2016; Mehlum et al. 2014, 2016; Miller et al. 2007; Rathus and Miller 2002).

In this chapter, we begin by discussing the rationale for using DBT with adolescents. We then review the theoretical model underlying DBT, empirical evidence for the approach, and the treatment structure and primary interventions/strategies used. We conclude this chapter with a brief case description illustrating the implementation of DBT with adolescents in an outpatient setting and discuss future adaptations of DBT with adolescents in different treatment settings.

In adapting DBT for adolescents, the differential developmental needs of adolescents and families compared with adults were recognized; hence, there were many factors to consider when adapting DBT for this population (Miller et al. 2007; Rathus and Miller 2002). As adolescents reside at home with their families and attend school throughout the day, it is important to consider how these different environments contribute to the development and maintenance of emotion dysregulation over time. Through a review of the literature on adolescent development, client feedback, and clinical observation (Miller et al. 1997, 2007; Rathus and Miller 2002), the original DBT comprehensive model was modified to address the unique needs of multiproblem youth. Specific attention was given to the biosocial theory, which informed the development of the modes and functions of DBT (e.g., multifamily skills group, phone coaching for both adolescents and parents, and parent/family sessions) to address teen and parent needs and concerns. Furthermore, adolescent-family secondary treatment targets were identified, and common dialectical dilemmas for teens and parents were established (Rathus and Miller 2000). Owing to the unique needs of the adolescent population, a family-based skills module, called "walking the middle path," was created to address skills deficits relevant to adolescents and their families with regard to teaching dialectical thinking and acting, validation of self and other, and learning principles such as positive reinforcement and shaping (Rathus and Miller 2015).

Theoretical Model and Proposed Mechanism of Change

Linehan's (1993) biosocial theory suggests that chronic problems of emotion dysregulation stem from a biological vulnerability to emotion dysregulation transacting with an invalidating environment.

Biological Vulnerability

Emotional vulnerability is defined as a high sensitivity to emotional stimuli, high reactivity (i.e., intense emotional responses), and a slow return to emotional baseline. In addition to this vulnerability, these adolescents also have difficulty regulating emotional reactions and do not exhibit the skill set for effectively managing their emotions in the moment.

The Invalidating Environment

The *invalidating environment* is defined as the tendency of people in the emotionally vulnerable person's environment to pervasively dismiss, negate, trivialize, punish, or respond erratically to the person's private experiences (e.g., emotions, thoughts, behaviors). For teens, the invalidating environment may be composed of a variety of individuals including family members, teachers, peers, or other health professionals. In an invalidating environment, one's emotional experiences and interpretations are not perceived as valid responses and are, instead, often trivialized, dismissed, or punished. These emotional experiences may also be attributed to socially unacceptable characteristics such as manipulation, overreactivity, or attention seeking. At times, individuals in the environment may also inadvertently reinforce emotional escalations by providing soothing responses, accommodations, or expanded limits after suicidal communication or other communications of distress. This response can be problematic, because individuals then learn that to have their distress "heard," they may have to heighten their emotional display of distress.

Invalidating environments emphasize controlling emotional expressiveness (e.g., "Stop worrying! It's not a big deal"), oversimplify the ease of problem solving (e.g., "Just study more next time, then you will pass the test"), and are generally intolerant of negative affect displays (e.g., "Put a smile on your face. Don't ruin this for your sister"). Individuals in invalidating environments do not receive effective coaching in emotion regulation, and, instead, maladaptive learning takes place. These individuals may learn that "emotions are bad," "I shouldn't feel the way I feel," or "In order to be taken seriously, I have to show them how distressed I really am; they need to know!"

The transaction between biological emotional vulnerability and the invalidating environment occurs over time and adversely shapes each side of the relationship. The "match" between the individual and their environment becomes an important factor as to how this transaction influences development of chronic emotion dysregulation. An individual with extreme emotional vulnerability, who might be described as "sensitive," may develop emotion dysregulation in a family with "normal" levels of invalidation (e.g., the well-meaning parent who doesn't understand why their child with attention-deficit/hyperactivity [ADHD] can't sit still while doing homework and ultimately yells at them, "Stop fidgeting and sit still for once!"). Another scenario would be an individual with a lower level of emotional vulnerability living in a highly invalidating environment who develops persistent emotional dysregulation as a result of the transaction (e.g., the sports coach throughout high school who screams, says taking breaks is a sign of weakness, dismisses emotional displays, and tells injured plays to "suck it up and get back in there") (Rathus et al. 2017). Finally, the most extreme form of invalidation arguably among youth is physical and sexual abuse (Miller et al. 2007).

Over time, the transaction between one's biological vulnerability and the invalidating environment leads to an inability to regulate arousal, tolerate distress, or trust internal emotional responses (Linehan 1993). As a result of this transaction and the invalidating environment's response to emotional expression, the individual vacillates between emotional suppression and extreme emotional displays. Maladaptive behaviors such as self-harm, substance use, or school avoidance may function to regulate emotions and may be inadvertently reinforced by the environment.

In DBT, the primary mechanism of change is teaching DBT skills to improve one's ability to effectively regulate emotions. A unique component of DBT for adolescents is including families as a whole in treatment and having teens and their parents learn the skills together in the multifamily skills group. This treatment modality allows for the whole family to learn not only the skills but also the DBT language and to create a more validating environment. The resulting validating environment allows teens to more effectively regulate their emotions.

In DBT for adolescents, we discuss the biosocial theory with both teens and their parents in the multifamily skills group (Rathus and Miller 2015). It is important to present the theory in a nonjudgmental way and to elicit a discussion of how each family thinks the model applies to them. Normalizing the transaction aids this discussion and helps create a link between how families have reached this point and how DBT skills can be effective in addressing this dilemma.

Review of Empirical Evidence

DBT for adults has been well established as an effective treatment for problems associated with borderline personality disorder through dozens of randomized control trials (RCTs; Koons et al. 2001; Linehan et al. 1991, 2006; Verheul et al. 2003). To date, three published RCTs have been conducted to help establish the efficacy and effectiveness of DBT for adolescents (Goldstein et al. 2015; McCauley et al. 2018; Mehlum et al. 2014).

Mehlum et al. (2014) completed a large RCT in Oslo, Norway, comparing 19 weeks of outpatient DBT with enhanced usual care (EUC) for suicidal and self-harming adolescents. EUC consisted of any non-DBT therapy in addition to suicide risk assessment protocol training. The DBT condition consisted of weekly individual therapy, weekly multifamily skills training groups, telephone coaching for adolescents, clinically indicated family sessions, and weekly therapist consultation meetings. Participants included 77 adolescents (ages 12–18 years) with reported recent and repetitive self-harm behavior who also endorsed at least three out of nine borderline personality features. Participants engaged in DBT or EUC at several different child and adolescent psychiatric outpatient clinics.

DBT was superior to EUC in reducing the frequency of self-harm behavior, severity of suicidal ideation, and depressive symptoms. The DBT condition yielded large effect sizes for treatment outcomes, whereas the EUC condition yielded weak to moderate outcomes. Results from a 1-year follow-up study (Mehlum et al. 2016) indicated that DBT remained superior to EUC in reducing the frequency of self-harm episodes. However, intergroup differences were not observed on outcomes such as suicidal ideation, hopelessness, and depressive or borderline symptoms. Additional long-term follow-up research is underway, and the authors hope to complete additional studies at 2-year and 10-year time points.

McCauley and colleagues (2018) conducted a multisite, randomized controlled trial with adolescents at high risk of suicide, looking specifically at whether or not DBT is effective at decreasing suicide attempts. One hundred and seventy-three adolescents, ages 12–18 years, with 1) at least one lifetime history of a suicide attempt; 2) three or more lifetime episodes of self-harm (either suicide attempts or NSSI), with at least one occurring within the past 12 weeks; 3) elevated suicidal ideation; and 4) at least three criteria for borderline personality disorder (including the self-injury criterion), participated in the study. Youth were randomly assigned to 6 months of either DBT (consisting of weekly individual therapy, weekly multifamily skills training, telephone coaching for adolescents and parents, family sessions as needed, and a weekly therapist consultation team meeting) or individual and group supportive therapy (IGST), which was a manualized, client-centered approach that also included individual and group components. To enhance internal validity, IGST was matched with DBT for hours of treatment, treatment modalities (e.g., both individual and group therapy), therapy drop-out policies, therapist expertise, and availability of supervision (Berk et al. 2014). Results showed that youth in the DBT condition experienced significantly lower rates of suicide attempts, NSSI, and suicidal ideation at the end of the 6-month treatment period than youth who received IGST; however, both groups showed improvement at 12-month follow-up, with no differences between groups (McCauley et al. 2018).

Goldstein et al. (2015) conducted a small RCT of DBT ($n=14$) versus psychosocial treatment as usual ($n=6$) for adolescents diagnosed with bipolar disorder. The DBT condition included 36 sessions (18 individual and 18 family skills training sessions), alternating weekly over the course of 1 year. The treatment as usual condition was an eclectic psychotherapy approach including psychoeducational, supportive, and cognitive-behavioral therapy techniques. Results indicated that individuals in the DBT condition had greater treatment adherence and reductions in depressive symptoms over time. Additional results indicated trends toward greater reductions in suicidal ideation and emotion dysregulation in the DBT condition.

In addition to the previously discussed RCTs, two reviews and one meta-analysis have been conducted studying the outcomes of DBT for adolescent treatment programs in various settings (Cook and Gorraiz 2016; Groves et al. 2011; MacPherson et al. 2013). MacPherson et al.'s (2013) review indicated that 18 open and quasi-experimental trials with DBT for adolescents have been conducted.

Quasi-experimental studies on DBT with adolescents indicate that DBT was effective in reducing various target behaviors (e.g., nonsuicidal self-injurious behavior, suicidal ideation, suicidal behavior, emotion dysregulation) in suicidal, multiproblem youth across treatment settings (Fleischhaker et al. 2011; Katz et al. 2004; McDonell et al. 2010; Rathus and Miller 2002). Open trials of DBT with adolescents indicate successful applications to 1) multiple diagnoses with suicidal and nonsuicidal self-injurious behavior (Courtney and Flament 2015; Fleischhaker et al. 2006; James et al. 2008; Sunseri 2004; Woodberry and Popenoe 2008), 2) bipolar disorder (Goldstein et al. 2007), 3) externalizing disorders in forensic (Trupin et al. 2002) and outpatient settings (Marco et al. 2013; Nelson-Gray et al. 2006), 4) eating disorders (Fischer and Peterson 2015; Safer et al. 2007; Salbach-Andrae et al. 2008, 2009), 5) school refusal (Chu et al. 2015), and 6) trichotillomania (Welch and Kim 2012).

Taken together, outcome data from studies investigating the efficacy and effectiveness of applying DBT to various adolescent populations indicate that DBT reduces suicidal behavior, NSSI, depression, and borderline personality features. In addition, these studies provide evidence for treatment feasibility across cultures and treatment settings.

Treatment Components and Primary Intervention Strategies

DBT Treatment Stages

DBT conceptualizes treatment as occurring over the course of four treatment stages that relate to the client's manifesting problem severity and complexity. Each of these treatment stages has its own *treatment targets*: behaviors or patterns that are identified and highlighted for treatment focus through a collaborative process with client and therapist. In addition to the four stages, there is a pretreatment stage in which the therapist and client collaboratively develop treatment goals and build commitment to the treatment model. Each stage is described below.

Pretreatment Orientation and Commitment to Treatment, Agreement on Goals

The main goals of the pretreatment stage are to orient the client to the DBT treatment model and build commitment to treatment. The pretreatment stage typically lasts for four to six sessions. During these sessions, the therapist and client discuss the possibility of working together, come to a mutual decision to do so, and begin to establish treatment goals that will help build a life worth living. In addition, consent for treatment is obtained from both the adolescent and family during this stage.

Stage 1: Attaining Basic Capacities, Increasing Safety, Reducing Behavioral Dyscontrol

The main goal of stage 1 is stabilization and reduction of suicidal and self-harm behaviors by building basic capacities, establishing a sense of safety, and increasing behavioral control. These goals are obtained through four hierarchically arranged treatment targets: (1) reducing life-threatening behavior, (2) reducing therapy-interfering behavior, (3) reducing quality-of-life–interfering behavior, and (4) increasing behavioral skills. In adolescent DBT, the client and family are asked for a 6-month commitment during stage 1. For some clients, this is enough time to address these four target areas. For others, an additional 6 months of stage 1 treatment or a graduate group is recommended to further address these concerns (Miller et al. 2007).

Stage 1 treatment includes both individual therapy and skills training (multifamily skills group or individual family skills training). In individual therapy, clients self-monitor their specific behavioral targets through the use of a DBT diary card that is modified based on individual needs. The completed diary card is reviewed at the beginning of each session, and then the information is used to create the individual session agenda. Target behaviors are addressed hierarchically with life-threatening behaviors being discussed first, followed by therapy-interfering behaviors, quality-of-life–interfering behaviors, and behavioral skills. Therapists use behavioral chain and solution analyses to address the problem behaviors identified. Chain analyses assess antecedents and consequences of problem behaviors in painstaking detail; solution analyses highlight which DBT problem-solving strategies may be employed (e.g., skills training, exposure, cognitive modification, contingency management). Table 4–1 provides an overview of the DBT treatment stages and their respective treatment targets specific to adolescents.

Stage 2: Increasing Nonanguished Emotional Experiencing: Reducing Traumatic Stress

Once the client's behaviors have improved and he or she is exhibiting behavioral control, the client can be transitioned to the next stage of treatment. Stage 2 treatment may differ according to the client's needs and the treatment setting. Standard DBT stage 2 addresses emotionally processing past trauma, grief, and loss through evidence-based exposure therapy. For others who do not have a trauma history, stage 2 might include a graduate group or evidence-based treatments for other psychiatric disorders (Miller et al. 2007).

Stages 3 and 4

Stages 3 and 4 aim to address normal problems in living, increase self-respect, and increase finding freedom and joy (see Table 4–1 for specific treatment targets during these stages).

Modes and Functions of DBT

Stage 1 DBT treatment serves five functions: 1) improving motivation to change, 2) enhancing capabilities, 3) ensuring skill generalization, 4) structuring the environment, and 5) improving therapists' motivation and capabilities. These functions are critical to an effective, comprehensive DBT program. The various modes of treatment that employ these functions can look different across various settings (e.g., outpatient, inpatient, therapeutic school programs). In the following section, we discuss outpatient modes of adolescent DBT.

TABLE 4-1.   Standard dialectical behavior therapy (DBT) stages and their hierarchies of primary treatment targets

---

Pretreatment stage: orientation and commitment to treatment, agreement on goals

Targets

  Inform adolescent about and orient adolescent to DBT.

  Inform adolescent's family about and orient family to DBT.

  Secure adolescent's commitment to treatment.

  Secure adolescent's family's commitment to treatment.

  Secure therapist's commitment to treatment.

Stage 1: Attaining basic capacities, increasing safety, reducing behavioral dyscontrol

Hierarchy of primary targets in individual DBT therapy

  1. Decreasing life-threatening behaviors

     a. Suicidal/homicidal crisis behaviors

     b. Suicide attempts

     c. Nonsuicidal self-injury

     d. Suicidal ideation or communication

  2. Decreasing therapy-interfering behaviors

     a. By the adolescent

     b. By the therapist

     c. By participating family members

  3. Decreasing quality-of-life–interfering behaviors

     a. High-risk, impulsive behaviors

     b. Dysfunctional interpersonal interactions

     c. Substance-abuse-related behaviors

     d. School problems

  4. Increasing behavioral skills

Hierarchy of primary targets in DBT skills training:

  1. Decreasing behaviors likely to destroy therapy

  2. Increasing skill acquisition, strengthening, and generalization

     a. Core mindfulness skills

     b. Interpersonal effectiveness

     c. Emotion regulation

TABLE 4-1. Standard dialectical behavior therapy (DBT) stages and their hierarchies of primary treatment targets *(continued)*

---

     d. Distress tolerance

     e. Walking the middle path

   3. Decreasing therapy-interfering behaviors

Stage 2: Increasing nonanguished emotional experiencing: reducing traumatic stress

Primary target in individual DBT

     1. Decreasing avoidance of emotional experience and posttraumatic stress

Stage 3: Increasing self-respect and achieving individual goals, addressing normal problems in living

Primary targets in individual DBT

     1. Increasing respect for self

     2. Achieving individual goals

Stage 4:

Primary targets in individual DBT

     1. Resolving a sense of incompleteness

     2. Finding freedom and joy

Source. Adapted from Miller AL, Rathus JH, Linehan MM: *Dialectical Behavior Therapy With Suicidal Adolescents*, New York, Guilford, 2007, p. 45, Table 3–1, p. 47 and Table 3–2. Copyright © 2007 Guilford Press. Used with permission.

Components of Comprehensive DBT for Adolescents

Components of comprehensive DBT for adolescents are the following:

- Individual therapy
- Multifamily skills group
- Phone coaching
- Family and parent sessions as clinically indicated
- Consultation team

Individual Therapy

The primary function of the individual therapy sessions is to improve the client's motivation to change. (These sessions also help to enhance the client's capabilities and ensure skill generalization, although these functions are primarily met in skills group and phone coaching, respectively.) Individual therapy sessions are the primary mode of treatment in which clients start to learn how to apply the skills they learn in skills group to their own lives to address their specific behavioral treatment targets. It is the responsibility of the individual therapist to 1) assess problem behaviors and skills deficits, 2) problem solve, and 3) organize other modes of treatment to address the client's problem behaviors and targets (Miller et al. 2007).

As stated previously, the agenda for the individual session is guided by the diary card, a self-monitoring tool completed by the client. The therapeutic focus within and across sessions is determined by the highest-priority treatment target at the moment. Issues concerning life-threatening behavior (e.g., suicidal ideation/behavior, NSSI) are addressed first, followed by therapy-interfering behavior (on the part of either the client or the therapist), quality-of-life–interfering behavior (e.g., substance use, interpersonal conflict, academic concerns, peer conflict), and skill development. Typically, multiple targets can be addressed in one session, although any life-threatening issue takes precedence. In adolescent DBT, therapy-interfering behaviors that are often identified are the following: not completing the diary card, arriving late to session, missing a session, and being on a cell phone during session. Common quality-of-life–interfering behaviors are concerns related to academic adjustment, conflict with peers, conflict with family members, and substance use.

Multifamily Skills Group

The main function of the multifamily skills group (MFSG) is to enhance capabilities, and it is the primary mode for teaching behavioral skills. Although other skills training options are available (e.g., teen-only groups, concurrent teen and parent groups, individual/family skills training), we recommend a multifamily group format when conducting skills training for teens and their families. The multifamily group format allows for a more didactic experience, enhances motivation in families, and offers a support network (Rathus et al. 2017). The MFSG curriculum takes place over 24 weeks and includes five skills modules. The five skills modules are emotion regulation, interpersonal effectiveness, distress tolerance, walking the middle path, and core mindfulness. These skills modules directly map onto the five problem areas adolescents typically present with when DBT is recommended. Table 4–2 lists areas of behavioral dysregulation and the corresponding skills modules. For additional information regarding adolescent DBT skills, please refer to the *DBT Skills Manual for Adolescents* (Rathus and Miller 2015).

Phone Coaching

The main function of phone coaching is to facilitate skill generalization, although it has other important functions as well. Once clients are fully committed to DBT and begin to learn skills, they are oriented to phone coaching. Between-session phone calls provide opportunities for skill generalization through in vivo skills coaching when the client is experiencing distress, with the purpose being that the client can ask for help prior to engaging in a maladaptive behavior. Such calls might also include crisis intervention. To ensure safety during crisis intervention, other family members might participate in the phone calls. Another function of phone coaching is to allow clients to reach out with good news, helping to break the relationship between suicidal or maladaptive behavior and therapist attention and support. Last, phone coaching might be used to repair the relationship between the client and therapist so that neither individual has to wait until the next session to resolve a problem. In settings where between-session contact is not possible, in vivo skills coaching can be provided through a brief structured intervention. For example, with an adolescent anxiously anticipating results of an audition for the school show or another teen worried about being rejected when asking a peer to prom, the skills group leader or individual DBT therapist might propose using the "cope ahead" skill (in which the teen plans in advance how he or she will cope with his or her most feared outcome) to most effectively manage emotions in each context.

Parent/Family Sessions

Parent and family sessions primarily address the function of structuring the environment and are scheduled in adolescent DBT when clinically indicated. Family sessions may also address improving motivation to change, enhancing capabilities, and ensuring skill generalization. Family sessions work to ensure skill generalization by providing a forum for in vivo practice

TABLE 4-2.   Characteristics of dysregulation and corresponding dialectical behavior therapy (DBT) skills modules

Some characteristics of dysregulation	DBT skills modules
Emotion dysregulation	
Emotional vulnerability; emotional reactivity; emotional lability; angry outbursts; steady negative emotional states such as depression, anger, shame, anxiety, and guilt; deficits in positive emotions; difficulty in modulating emotions; mood-dependent behaviors	Emotion regulation
Interpersonal dysregulation	
Unstable relationships, interpersonal conflicts, chronic family disturbance, social isolation, difficulties getting needs met and keeping self-respect in relationships, loneliness	Interpersonal effectiveness
Behavioral dysregulation	
Impulsive behaviors such as cutting classes, blurting out in class, spending money; risky sexual behavior; risky online behaviors; bingeing and/or purging; drug and alcohol abuse; aggressive behaviors; suicidal and nonsuicidal self-injurious behavior; escaping or avoiding emotional experiences	Distress tolerance
Cognitive dysregulation and family conflict	
Nondialectical thinking and acting (i.e., extremes, polarized, or black-or-white), poor perspective taking and conflict resolution, invalidation of self and others, absence of flexibility, difficulty effectively influencing own and other's behaviors (i.e., obtaining desired changes)	Walking the middle path
Self-dysregulation	
Lack of awareness of emotions, thoughts, action urges; poor attentional control; inability to reduce one's suffering while also having difficulty accessing pleasure; identity confusion, sense of emptiness, and dissociation	Core mindfulness

Source.   Reprinted from Miller AL, Rathus JH, Linehan MM: *Dialectical Behavior Therapy With Suicidal Adolescents*, New York, Guilford, 2007, p. 36, Table 2–1. Copyright © 2007 Guilford Press. Used with permission.

of skills in a therapeutic setting (Miller et al. 2007). In addition, when parents take part in skills training, they are able to adopt the same DBT language and provide a model of effective skill use at home.

As adolescents are typically still living in the invalidating environments that contributed to the development of behavioral dysregulation, structuring the environment and conducting family sessions becomes necessary for effective treatment (Miller et al. 2007). Family sessions may be scheduled for a variety of reasons, including invalidating behavior between family members and interpersonal conflict that directly relates to the client's target behavior. Walking the middle path and interpersonal effectiveness skills (Rathus and Miller 2015) are often reviewed in family sessions to address these concerns.

Specialized parent sessions may be needed to teach parents behavior management strategies to more effectively structure the environment to reinforce adaptive behavior and ignore maladaptive or ineffective behavior. Some adolescent DBT programs also provide parent phone coaching as an adjunctive service to the multifamily skills group in order to promote skill generalization for the parents outside of the therapeutic setting. In vivo skills coaching helps parents to more effectively implement behavior management strategies and employ DBT skills in the moment.

Consultation Team

All clinicians serving as treatment providers within a standard DBT program are required to participate in a weekly consultation team meeting, which provides support to DBT clinicians and also their DBT therapeutic skills. The main functions of the consultation team are to enhance therapist capabilities and to improve therapist motivation. Treating clients presenting with suicidal ideation/behavior, NSSI, and emotion dysregulation can be extremely challenging and stressful, making it difficult to adhere to the full DBT framework. As a result, an essential component of comprehensive DBT with adolescents and adults is a weekly therapist consultation meeting. The consultation team is meant to provide "therapy to the therapists" to help reduce therapist burnout and increase adherence to DBT principles. The structure of the consultation team is the same across client populations, and consultation items are addressed in a hierarchy similar to that used in individual therapy (i.e., addressing life-threatening concerns first).

DBT Treatment Strategies in Individual Therapy

DBT uses specific treatment and stylistic strategies to address treatment targets in individual sessions. The strategies described below are used in both adult and adolescent DBT.

Dialectical Strategies

In DBT, therapists use dialectical strategies to structure the therapeutic interactions and balance dialectical tensions. The main dialectic addressed in DBT is the balance between acceptance and change. The goal in highlighting dialectical tensions in treatment is to highlight all sides of the situation and provide a space for synthesis, or "middle path." There are eight dialectical treatment strategies utilized in DBT: (1) entering the paradox, (2) metaphors, (3) devil's advocate, (4) extending, (5) activating the client's wise mind, (6) making lemonade out of lemons, (7) allowing natural change, and (8) assessing dialectically by asking "What is being left out?" (Linehan 1993). In adolescent DBT, metaphors are a particularly useful strategy because they help to highlight and teach the skills in a more interesting and relatable manner. Skills group leaders often use metaphors or stories to help clients understand and connect to the material.

Validation

Validation is the core acceptance strategy and communicates that another person's feelings, thoughts, or actions make sense. Validation is a helpful tool for lowering the emotional intensity of the interaction and ensuring that the other person will stay in the conversation. When using validation as a treatment strategy, it is important to validate the valid, not the invalid. For example, a teen becomes very upset that she is not invited to a party all of her friends are attending and throws her shoe at the wall, creating a hole. The therapist can validate the feeling of anger but should not validate the physical aggression.

Problem Solving

Problem-solving strategies fall within the change side of the core dialectic. Behavioral chain analyses highlight the chain of events leading to and following problematic target behaviors and inform which problem-solving strategies might be warranted. DBT has four problem-solving strategies: (1) skills training, (2) contingency management, (3) exposure, and (4) cognitive modification.

Stylistic Strategies

Stylistic strategies pertain more to the style of therapist communication than to the technique used. There are two types of communication styles used in DBT: reciprocal and irreverent. Reciprocal communication is responsive in nature and reflects warmth and genuineness. Reciprocal communication can also include self-involving self-disclosure, in which a therapist shares how the client and/or his or her behavior is impacting the therapist in the moment. Irreverence is a strategy used to catch the client off guard, to capture their attention. For example, a client might say "DBT sucks, nothing is working." An irreverent response would be, "You seem surprised that the skills don't work when you don't use them." Irreverence is a key technique when working with teens as it tends to be a different response style from what they are used to from other adults in their lives. As a result, it helps to strengthen the therapist-client relationship.

Case Management

Case management strategies come into play when there are problems in the client's environment (e.g., home, school) that are impeding the client's daily functioning. There are two types of case management strategies: consultation to the client and consultation to the environment. When engaging in consultation to the client, the therapist acts as a consultant to the patient rather than intervening directly with individuals in the client's environment. The purpose of the strategy is to help coach the client to effectively advocate for their needs. Although the consultation-to-the-client strategy is preferred, there are times when consultation to the environment is warranted. If the stakes are too high, the risk to the client is too great, or if the client has repeatedly attempted to advocate with no success, the therapist may consult directly to the environment. Even when the therapist consults directly to the environment, it is recommended that the teen be part of the consultation in order to model effective skill use. In general, consultation to the client is the preferred case management strategy for increasing the client's skill set and helping him or her build mastery.

Case Example

Jan was a 17-year-old white female who presented to outpatient treatment with preexisting diagnoses of major depressive disorder, ADHD, and a specific learning disorder for mathematical reasoning. At intake, Jan was also diagnosed with borderline personality disorder. She was referred for comprehensive adolescent DBT after an increase in NSSI, temper outbursts, and significant interpersonal conflict with her parents. Jan's parents divorced when she was 11 years old, and Jan's relationship with her father has continued to be strained as a result of the divorce. Jan reported that she was seeking DBT because her previous therapy experiences were not effective.

Jan and her mother reported a significant history of emotional dysregulation. Jan's mother, Susan, reported that Jan was always "sensitive" and first started exhibiting temper outbursts when she was a young child. Although the temper outbursts decreased in frequency over the years (from 10 times per week to 1–2 times per week), they continued to cause significant distress within the family. Jan reported that she often felt "triggered" by others not understanding what she was going through and felt frustrated by others' actions (e.g., worry thoughts related to parents lying, brother's substance use, being asked to do something she does not want to do or something that feels "unfair"). She stated that during an outburst, she would often yell, curse, name call, and throw objects. In addition to the temper outbursts, Jan reported difficulty with persistent sad mood, irritability, poor sleep hygiene, disordered eating behavior, poor academic adjustment, and significant interpersonal conflict with family members. She first started to engage in NSSI as a way to "release emotional pain." Per Jan's report, over time the NSSI became more of a "habit" and a strategy she used on a regular basis to regulate her emotions and "feel something different." In addition, she endorsed significant distress related to her academic achievement. Jan reported that she always found school to be challenging and had to work significantly harder than her peers to achieve good grades. Throughout her years attending school, she often felt invalidated by school personnel with respect to her learning difficulties and mental health concerns. Jan additionally reported that she smoked marijuana on a daily basis as a way to "calm down" and decrease her experience of anxiety.

Jan and Susan reported that despite their very close relationship, they experienced significant interpersonal conflict on a daily basis. Susan reported difficulty understanding Jan's experience of intense emotions and felt scared and threatened during the outbursts. Susan reported that because of this fear, she did not set limits with Jan and typically let her "do what she wanted" to avoid the conflict. Susan additionally reported that she would often become more attentive and present after Jan's outbursts because she wanted Jan to feel better in the moment.

Jan identified reasons for living and long-term goals, including living for her mother, brother, and dog; graduating from high school; completing college; and beginning a career in the mental health field. Her immediate treatment goals were to feel better (i.e., decrease experience of depression/anxiety), improve interpersonal relationships with peers and family members, and decrease NSSI and suicidal ideation.

When building commitment in the first session, Jan's difficulties were categorized according to the five adolescent DBT problem areas. She endorsed problems in all five problem areas:

1. Reduced focus, reduced awareness, and confusion about self: not knowing why she engages in problem behavior (i.e., lack of awareness), rumination (i.e., difficulty maintaining attention)
2. Impulsivity: NSSI, substance use, physical/verbal aggression
3. Emotion dysregulation: inability to regulate emotions effectively, persistent negative mood (e.g., hopelessness, shame, isolation), problematic eating behavior, poor sleep hygiene
4. Interpersonal problems: difficulty maintaining relationships with peers, feeling rejected by peers, difficulty advocating for needs with others
5. Teen and family challenges: family conflict, nondialectical thinking and acting, invalidation of lower levels of emotional expression, reinforcement of higher levels of emotional expression, inconsistent parental responses to problem behaviors

These behavioral difficulties were further sorted into the DBT target hierarchy:

- Decrease life-threatening behavior
    Decrease suicidal ideation/threats
    Decrease NSSI

- Decrease therapy-interfering behaviors

    Increase completion of diary card (i.e., honest reporting of target behaviors)

    Decrease active passivity (helplessness, wanting and/or asking others to solve one's problems)

- Decrease quality-of-life–interfering behaviors

    Decrease negative moods

    Decrease experience of anxiety

    Decrease family conflict and increase positive communication

    Maintain relationships with peers and make new ones

    Increase healthy eating behavior

    Improve sleep hygiene

    Decrease daily substance use

    Improve academic performance

    Decrease temper outbursts

- Increase behavioral skills

    Increase skills in mindfulness, emotion regulation, distress tolerance, interpersonal effectiveness, walking the middle path

Course of Treatment

The therapist oriented Jan to the comprehensive DBT program including weekly individual therapy, weekly 2-hour MFSG, 24-hour skills coaching for Jan, 24-hour skills coaching for the parents, and parenting/family sessions as needed. Jan's parents agreed to participate in the full comprehensive program during the initial intake session. Once Jan learned that both of her parents would be attending the MFSG, she said she would only commit to the individual sessions because she did not want to attend a group with her father. The therapist used commitment strategies including pros and cons, "freedom to choose" and "absence of alternatives," devil's advocate, and "foot in the door" to get Jan to actively participate in treatment. For example, Jan completed a pros and cons list of having both of her parents as part of the MFSG and realized that her father might be able to change some of his behaviors that Jan would find difficult if he attended the skills group. During the pretreatment stage, Jan did commit to weekly individual therapy with phone coaching and 24 weeks of the MFSG with both of her parents. Jan's parents received parent coaching by a skills group leader separate from Jan's individual therapist. Family sessions were conducted by Jan's individual therapist, as clinically indicated, to focus on walking the middle path and interpersonal effectiveness skills.

When Jan first entered treatment, she reported that the NSSI had become a "habit," and all of the strategies she had been given by previous therapists to address this target behavior were not effective. As a result, Jan expressed reluctance to track this target behavior on the diary card. She had difficulty recognizing urges to self-harm and further expressed that it was hard to even remember when she did engage in the target behavior (which was identified as a therapy-interfering behavior that was addressed in order to effectively target reduction of NSSI). To help increase her awareness, the therapist reviewed the core mindfulness skills. After some time, Jan did effectively track both self-harm urges and behaviors on a daily basis. In conducting behavioral chain analysis, one theme that consistently emerged was that Jan engaged in self-harm (target behavior) following interpersonal interactions with her family. On one occasion when Jan reported engaging in self-harm, she identified that she had been having trouble sleeping (vulnerability), was ruminating about poor grades at school (vulnerability), and was having concerns about her weight (vulnerability). Jan returned home from school one day with a failing grade in English class, and her mother asked if Jan would be willing to revisit the discussion regarding transferring to a different school with more academic support (prompting event). This led to intense shame (critical link), anger toward mother, urges to engage in verbal/physical aggression (critical link), and worry thoughts related to her academic future. After engaging in self-harm behavior, Jan reported that she felt angry at herself (consequence) for engaging in self-harm and went to her mother for comfort. Jan's mom saw the cuts on her forearm and apologized for upsetting her (consequence). After completing the chain, the therapist and Jan collaborated on a solution analysis by identifying skills to address each critical link in the chain. For example, to address the emotion of shame, the therapist and Jan identified the following skills: "ride the wave," "opposite action," and "check the facts." Jan reported that in feeling shame, her action urge was to continue to avoid the topic and pretend there was nothing wrong. In order to "act opposite" to shame, Jan engaged in a conversation first with the therapist and then a peer identifying her academic difficulties and related worry thoughts about changing schools. With regard to the urges to engage in verbal/physical aggression, TIPP (a set of skills designed to reduce distress and arousal by changing body chemistry), "wise mind ACCEPTS" (consisting of a variety of methods of temporary distraction from distressing situations), and opposite action were identified as skills to be used in the moment. Jan identified that when she is at her skills breaking point and is having urges to engage in verbal/physical aggression, she could TIPP her body chemistry with temperature or engage in intense exercise. In addition, Susan was referred to her parent coach to schedule a parent session to learn positive behavior management strategies and to respond in a neutral manner following Jan's self-harm to avoid reinforcing it.

Outcomes

At the 6-month mark, when Jan and her parents were graduating from the MFSG, Jan had been free from NSSI and suicidal ideation for 1 month and her temper outbursts had been significantly reduced to approximately two per month (from one to two per week). Jan reported that she was engaging in healthy eating and exercise behavior. Jan had fewer conflicts with her parents, and her family was able to regulate their conflict more effectively by using validation skills, dialectical thinking, interpersonal effectiveness skills, and effective behavior management strategies to shape and increase positive behaviors. To continue to address other quality-of-life–interfering behaviors (e.g., marijuana use, sleep hygiene, academic adjustment, isolation from peers), Jan continued in individual therapy and joined a DBT graduate group to collaboratively generalize skills with other teens who had successfully completed an MFSG.

Recommendations for Clinicians Interested in Using This Treatment Approach

Adopting and Adapting the Treatment Across Various Practice Settings

When DBT for adolescents is adapted for different settings, a set of questions must be answered, such as the following: Who will be treated? Who will compose the treatment team? What modes of DBT will be implemented? Should any adaptations to standard DBT be made? Whether a DBT program is being developed in an outpatient, inpatient, or school setting, these questions will need to be addressed to establish an effective DBT program.

Studies have shown that DBT can be effectively implemented in inpatient settings while providing skills training in various formats (Katz et al. 2004; McDonell et al. 2010). In an acute inpatient setting, Katz et al. (2004) implemented a 2-week DBT program with 10 manualized DBT skills training sessions. Group leaders chose to focus on core mindfulness and selected distress tolerance and emotion regulation skills in 45-minute group sessions every other day. On the alternate days, patients attended a homework-review group in which skills taught the previous day were reviewed. McDonell et al. (2010) implemented a comprehensive model of adolescent DBT in a long-term inpatient care setting. All elements of comprehensive DBT were offered; however, patients received various modes based on clinical need. Providers working in inpatient settings may want to consider how to incorporate patients' families in treatment to increase the generalization of skills once they are discharged from the hospital.

In addition to various classic treatment settings, adaptations of DBT to different school settings have become popular in recent years to help address growing rates of mental health concerns in school-age populations. Two general options are available when considering DBT in schools: comprehensive school-based DBT (including individual therapy, skills group, coaching, and consultation team) as a secondary and tertiary prevention model (A.L. Miller, K. Graling, J.J. Mazza et al., "Delivering Comprehensive DBT in Schools," unpublished manuscript, 2018) and a primary prevention model using Skills Training for Emotional Problem Solving for Adolescents (DBT STEPS-A; Mazza et al. 2016). Common barriers to implementation of comprehensive DBT in schools are student's unwillingness to engage in treatment, skills groups lasting under 45 minutes based on class period length, availability of skills coaches, and not enough protected time for DBT-related tasks during the school day (e.g., individual sessions on a weekly basis, skills group, consultation team). Preliminary studies indicate that comprehensive DBT in schools has reduced the number of disciplinary referrals at school (Catucci 2011) as well as influenced an improvement in various psychosocial measures (e.g., anxiety, depression, social stress, anger), school attendance, and grade point averages (J.B. Hanson, "Dialectical Behavior Therapy in Public Schools," PowerPoint presentation, Portland Public Schools, 2012). The STEPS-A primary prevention program (Mazza et al. 2016) was developed to enhance social-emotional learning in school settings across the student population. The newly published STEPS-A skills manual outlines a skills curriculum that guides teachers on how to teach the DBT-A skills to middle and high school students in a general education classroom setting. Because this model is newly available, research is warranted to assess the implementation and feasibility of the primary prevention model across school-based settings.

It is recommended that those who want to use DBT in a new setting or with a novel population try to "adopt" before you "adapt." Adopting means using the original treatment manual precisely how it is written before making a single change and adapting it. Miller and Rathus adhered to this principle of adopting first, then obtaining feedback from teens and parents, and then gradually adapting only where needed (Miller et al. 2007; Rathus and Miller 2015). Over time, Miller et al. (2007 made adaptations by adding a multifamily skills group and providing coaching for parents, adding new skills module relevant to teens and families, and simplifying the language and the handouts, to name a few.

Some providers in private practice and organizations without the staffing and resources to operate a comprehensive adolescent DBT program may start by initiating a small consultation team and/or co-leading a small skills group or—if that is too much—teaching DBT skills individually or with a single family at a time. In teaching DBT skills individually or with a single family, it is important to bear in mind that there are no data to support this format, although it may still work. Ideally, over time, the therapist would possibly add individual DBT therapy and intersession coaching and then family sessions. Some non-DBT therapists may choose to select specific DBT skills (Rathus and Miller 2015) to weave into their individual therapy sessions or medication management sessions as they see fit.

Clinical Implementation

Table 4–3 lists the treatment elements that can be easily implemented in everyday clinical practice.

Conclusion

In conclusion, DBT with suicidal adolescents is a multimodal psychosocial intervention that is an established evidence-based treatment. Most of the research has been conducted in outpatient settings; however, there is an in-

---

TABLE 4-3. Elements of the treatment that can be easily implemented in everyday practice

---

- DBT-A should only be implemented as a complete treatment package, as described in Miller et al. (2007) and supported by research (Mehlum et al. 2014).
- Basic DBT principles, such as reducing emotion dysregulation, balancing acceptance and change, and helping suicidal individuals "build a life worth living" (Linehan 1993), may be considered for use in everyday practice, but are not presently supported by research apart from the comprehensive treatment model.

---

creasing body of research demonstrating the effectiveness of DBT in other clinical and nonclinical settings and for youth with a variety of emotional and behavioral problems beyond suicidal and nonsuicidal self-injurious behavior. For those who are interested in applying DBT to teens, we suggest obtaining intensive training and ongoing consultation/supervision to ensure fidelity to the model.

Resources for Additional Training and Suggested Readings

For those interested in training in DBT with adolescents, there are several training companies that are supported by the treatment developer that provide adolescent-focused DBT trainings. Although learning the original adult model developed by Linehan (1993) is important for obtaining a comprehensive understanding of the theoretical background and rationale for the various components of the treatment, it is also critical to focus on adolescent-specific DBT trainings and materials. For these reasons, we recommend that readers interested in learning how to do individual DBT therapy with adolescents read the adolescent-focused text by Miller et al. (2007 and that those interested in learning how to teach DBT skills to teens read the adolescent skills manual by Rathus and Miller (2015). For educators who work in school settings, we recommend reading *DBT Skills in Schools: The Skills Training for Emotional Problem Solving for Adolescents (DBT STEPS-A)* (Mazza et al. 2016). Suggested empirical and theoretical articles are listed in the reference section below.

Links to Training Resources

DBT Training

- Behavioral Tech, A Linehan Institute Training Company, available at behavioraltech.org

Comprehensive School-Based DBT

- Cognitive Behavioral Consultants, available at cbc-psychology.com
- DBT STEPS-A: Mazza Consulting, available at www.mazzaconsulting.com/

Suggested Readings

Linehan MM: Cognitive-Behavioral Treatment of Borderline Personality Disorder. New York, Guilford, 1993

Mazza JJ, Dexter-Mazza ET, Miller AL, et al: DBT Skills Training in Schools: The Skills Training for Emotional Problem Solving for Adolescents (DBT STEPS-A). New York, Guilford, 2016

Miller AL, Rathus JH, Linehan MM: Dialectical Behavior Therapy With Suicidal Adolescents. New York, Guilford, 2007

Rathus JH, Miller AL: DBT Skills Manual for Adolescents. New York, Guilford, 2015

References

Berk M, Adrian M, McCauley E, et al: Conducting research on adolescent suicide attempters: dilemmas and decisions. Behav Ther (N Y N Y) 37(3):65–69, 2014 24954969

Catucci D: Dialectical behavior therapy with multi-problem adolescents in school setting. New York School Psychologist Newsletter, pp. 12-14, 2011 Retrieved from http://nyasp.org/newsletters/news2011fall.pdf

Centers for Disease Control and Prevention: 10 leading causes of death by age group, United States—2016. 2016. Available at: https://www.cdc.gov/injury/images/lc-charts/leading_causes_of_death_age_group_2016_1056w814h.gif. Accessed November 18, 2018.

Chu BC, Rizvi SL, Zendegui EA, Bonavitacola L: Dialectical behavior therapy for school refusal: treatment development and incorporation of web-based coaching. Cogn Behav Pract 22(3):317–330, 2015

Cook NE, Gorraiz M: Dialectical behavior therapy for nonsuicidal self-injury and depression among adolescents: preliminary meta-analytic evidence. Child Adolesc Ment Health 21(2):81–89, 2016

Courtney DB, Flament MF: Adapted dialectical behavior therapy for adolescents with self-injurious thoughts and behaviors. J Nerv Ment Dis 203(7):537–544, 2015 26075841

Fischer S, Peterson C: Dialectical behavior therapy for adolescent binge eating, purging, suicidal behavior, and non-suicidal self-injury: a pilot study. Psychotherapy (Chic) 52(1):78–92, 2015 24773094

Fleischhaker C, Munz M, Böhme R, et al: Dialectical behaviour therapy for adolescents (DBT-A)—a pilot study on the therapy of suicidal, parasuicidal, and self-injurious behaviour in female patients with a borderline disorder [in German]. Z Kinder Jugendpsychiatr Psychother 34(1):15–25, quiz 26–27, 2006 16485610

Fleischhaker C, Böhme R, Sixt B, et al: Dialectical behavioral therapy for adolescents (DBT-A): a clinical trial for patients with suicidal and self-injurious behavior and borderline symptoms with a one-year follow-up. Child Adolesc Psychiatry Ment Health 5(1):3, 2011 21276211

Goldstein TR, Axelson DA, Birmaher B, Brent DA: Dialectical behavior therapy for adolescents with bipolar disorder: a 1-year open trial. J Am Acad Child Adolesc Psychiatry 46(7):820–830, 2007 17581446

Goldstein TR, Fersch-Podrat RK, Rivera M, et al: Dialectical behavior therapy for adolescents with bipolar disorder: results from a pilot randomized trial. J Child Adolesc Psychopharmacol 25(2):140–149, 2015 25010702

Groves SS, Backer HS, van den Bosch LMC, Miller AL: Dialectical behavior therapy with adolescents: a review. Child Adolesc Ment Health https://doi.org/10.1111/j.1475-3588.2011.00611.x 2011

James AC, Taylor A, Winmill L, Alfoadari K: A preliminary community study of dialectical behaviour therapy (DBT) with adolescent females demonstrating persistent, deliberate self-harm (DSH). Child Adolesc Ment Health 13(3):148–152, 2008

Kann L, McManus T, Harris WA, et al; Center for Disease Control (CDC): Youth risk behavior surveillance - United States, 2015. MMWR Surveill Summ 65(6):1–174, 2016 27280474

Katz LY, Cox BJ, Gunasekara S, Miller AL: Feasibility of dialectical behavior therapy for suicidal adolescent inpatients. J Am Acad Child Adolesc Psychiatry 43(3):276–282, 2004 15076260

Koons C, Robins CJ, Tweed JL, et al: Efficacy of dialectical behavior therapy in women veterans with borderline personality disorder. Behav Ther 32(2):371–390, 2001

Linehan MM: Cognitive-Behavioral Treatment of Borderline Personality Disorder. New York, Guilford, 1993

Linehan MM, Armstrong HE, Suarez A, et al: Cognitive-behavioral treatment of chronically parasuicidal borderline patients. Arch Gen Psychiatry 48:1060–1064, 1991 1845222

Linehan MM, Comtois KA, Murray AM, et al: Two-year randomized controlled trial and follow-up of dialectical behavior therapy vs therapy by experts for suicidal behaviors and borderline personality disorder. Arch Gen Psychiatry 63(7):757–766, 2006 16818865

MacPherson HA, Cheavens JS, Fristad MA: Dialectical behavior therapy for adolescents: theory, treatment adaptations, and empirical outcomes. Clin Child Fam Psychol Rev 16(1):59–80, 2013 23224757

Marco JH, García-Palacios A, Botella C: Dialectical behavioural therapy for oppositional defiant disorder in adolescents: a case series. Psicothema 25(2):158–163, 2013 23628528

Mazza JJ, Dexter-Mazza ET, Miller AL, et al: DBT Skills Training in Schools: The Skills Training for Emotional Problem Solving for Adolescents (DBT STEPS-A). New York, Guilford, 2016

McCauley E, Berk MS, Asarnow JR, et al: Collaborative adolescent research on emotions and suicide (CARES): a randomized controlled trial of DBT with highly suicidal adolescent, in New Outcome Data on Treatments for Suicidal Adolescents. Symposium conducted at the meeting of the 50th Annual Convention of the Association for Behavioral and Cognitive Therapies (ABCT), New York, 2016

McCauley E, Berk MS, Asarnow JR, et al: Efficacy of dialectical behavior therapy for adolescents at high risk for suicide: a randomized clinical trial. JAMA Psychiatry 75(8):777–785, 2018 29926087

McDonell MG, Tarantino J, Dubose AP, et al: A pilot evaluation of dialectical behavioral therapy in adolescent long-term inpatient care. Child Adolesc Ment Health 15(4):193–196, 2010

Mehlum L, Tørmoen A, Ramberg M, et al: Dialectical behavior therapy for adolescents with repeated suicidal and self-harming behavior: a randomized trial. J Am Acad Child Adolesc Psychiatry 53:1082–1091, 2014 25245352

Mehlum L, Ramberg M, Tørmoen AJ, et al: Dialectical behavior therapy compared with enhanced usual care for adolescents with repeated suicidal and self-harming behavior: outcomes over a one-year follow-up. J Am Acad Child Adolesc Psychiatry 55(4):295–300, 2016 27015720

Miller AL, Smith HL: Adolescent non-suicidal self-injurious behavior: the latest epidemic to assess and treat. Appl Prev Psychol 12(4):178–188, 2008

Miller AL, Rathus JH, Linehan MM, et al: Dialectical behavior therapy adapted for suicidal adolescents. J Psychiatr Pract 3:78–86, 1997

Miller AL, Rathus JH, Linehan MM: Dialectical Behavior Therapy With Suicidal Adolescents. New York, Guilford, 2007

Nelson-Gray RO, Keane SP, Hurst RM, et al: A modified DBT skills training program for oppositional defiant adolescents: promising preliminary findings. Behav Res Ther 44(12):1811–1820, 2006 16579964

Rathus JH, Miller AL: DBT for adolescents: dialectical dilemmas and secondary treatment targets. Cogn Behav Pract 7(4):425–434, 2000

Rathus JH, Miller AL: Dialectical behavior therapy adapted for suicidal adolescents. Suicide Life Threat Behav 32(2):146–157, 2002

Rathus JH, Miller AL: DBT Skills Manual for Adolescents. New York, Guilford, 2015

Rathus JH, Miller AL, Bonavitacola L: DBT with Adolescents. Handbook of DBT. Oxford, UK, Oxford University Press, 2017

Ritschel L, Miller AL, Taylor V: DBT with multi-diagnostic youth, in Transdiagnostic Mechanisms and Treatment for Youth Psychopathology. Edited by Ehrenreich-May J, Chu B. New York, Guilford, 2013

Safer DL, Couturier JL, Lock J: Dialectical behavior therapy modified for adolescent binge eating disorder: a case report. Cogn Behav Pract 14(2):157–167, 2007

Salbach-Andrae H, Bohnekamp I, Pfeiffer E, et al: Dialectical behavior therapy of anorexia and bulimia nervosa among adolescents: a case series. Cogn Behav Pract 15:415–425, 2008

Salbach-Andrae H, Schneider N, Seifert K, et al: Short-term outcome of anorexia nervosa in adolescents after inpatient treatment: a prospective study. Eur Child Adolesc Psychiatry 18(11):701–704, 2009 19399545

Sunseri PA: Preliminary outcomes on the use of dialectical behavior therapy to reduce hospitalization among adolescents in residential care. Resid Treat Child Youth 21(4):59–76, 2004

Trupin EW, Stewart DG, Beach B, Boesky L: Effectiveness of a dialectical behaviour therapy program for incarcerated female juvenile offenders. Child Adolesc Ment Health 7(3):121–127, 2002

Verheul R, van den Bosch LMC, Koeter MWJ, et al: Dialectical behaviour therapy for women with borderline personality disorder: 12-month, randomised clinical trial in The Netherlands. Br J Psychiatry 182:135–140, 2003 12562741

Welch SS, Kim J: DBT-enhanced cognitive behavioral therapy for adolescent trichotillomania: an adolescent case study. Cogn Behav Pract 19(3):483–493, 2012

Woodberry KA, Popenoe EJ: Implementing dialectical behavior therapy with adolescents and their families in a community outpatient clinic. Cogn Behav Pract 15(3):277–286, 2008

5

Mentalization-Based Therapy for Adolescents

Peter Fonagy, Ph.D., FBA, FMedSci, FAcSS
Chloe Campbell, Ph.D.
Trudie Rossouw, M.B.Ch.B, FFPsych, MRCPsych, M.D. (Res)
Anthony Bateman, M.A., FRCPsych

Overview of Treatment Approach

Mentalizing is defined as the capacity to perceive and interpret human behavior—both other people's and one's own—in terms of intentional mental states such as feelings, beliefs, needs, reasons, or purposes. Mentalizing is what makes it possible to navigate the social world and to make sense of others' behaviors in a functional and proportionate way. It also helps us make sense of what is going on in our own minds by allowing us to regulate our affect, to recognize the reasons for our behavior, and to understand that there is a difference between what might be going on in our own minds and in someone else's. Mentalizing, therefore, underpins adaptive social behavior, whether it is a matter of appropriately modifying one's own behavior according to the social context (or being able to hold confidence in one's stance) or being able to understand, tolerate, and accommodate the complexity of other people's thoughts and actions. Mentalizing is an imaginative process, and effective mentalizing involves an awareness that states of mind are not fixed and unchangeable and that it is not possible to know what is going on in someone else's mind with absolute certainty. Effective mentalizing, therefore, also involves an appreciation of the fallibility of one's own inferences.

Mentalization-based therapy (MBT) originated as a day-hospital treatment program for borderline personality disorder (BPD) in adults (Bateman and Fonagy 1999, 2001). The approach has subsequently been developed as an outpatient treatment for a range of different disorders, including antisocial personality disorder (Bateman and Fonagy 2016), depression, anxiety, and eating disorders. MBT has also been adapted as a treatment approach for adolescents (MBT-A; Fonagy et al. 2014; Hutsebaut et al. 2012; Laurenssen et al. 2014; Rossouw and Fonagy 2012), and for families (MBT-F; Asen and Fonagy 2012a, 2012b, 2017a, 2017b). MBT-A is a yearlong program involving weekly individual MBT-A sessions and monthly family MBT (MBT-F) sessions. It is a manualized psychodynamic psychotherapeutic approach that focuses on impulsivity and affect regulation. Individual MBT-A sessions are 50 minutes long and are held on a weekly basis at the same time and place. MBT-F sessions tend to be at the same time and day, and the dates are known to the family well in advance to try to ensure attendance. A more intensive version of the program—such as an inpatient or day patient program—may offer individual therapy twice a week, MBT-F once a week, and MBT group therapy (MBT-G) twice a week (Bo et al. 2017; Rossouw 2018).

As is described in this chapter, MBT-A was developed for the treatment of adolescents who self-harm, both with and without symptoms of BPD. The treatment of these populations is highly pertinent to the management of suicidality in adolescence, as is evidenced by the associations between adolescent self-harm, depression, and suicidality (Wilkinson et al. 2011) and between adolescent BPD and suicidality (Fonagy et al. 2015b). MBT-A is designed to help patients improve their capacity to represent their own and others' feelings more accurately, particularly in the context of emotional challenges and interpersonal stressors, and has a strong focus on impulsivity and affect regulation. The MBT approach as a whole is primarily concerned with mental states in the here and now rather than with the unconscious processes driving these states or with cognitive-behavioral management strategies for behavioral symptoms.

Theoretical Model and Proposed Mechanism of Change

Mentalizing theory is strongly shaped by attachment thinking. We postulate that the capacity to mentalize is first developed in the context of early attachment relationships. The ability to mentalize is a constitutional human quality, but one that is highly subject to early environmental influence and genetic predisposition. A useful parallel is language: we all speak a language, but mother tongue and local idiom, personal expressiveness, and articulacy vary and shape how an individual uses language. The developmental model of mentalizing theory is that infants develop a sense of self, and what ultimately becomes a representation of their own mind, through a complex and ongoing process of interaction with their primary caregivers. Attachment theory has traditionally emphasized the importance of the contingent sensitivity of these interactions, postulating that the transmission of attachment occurs via the mechanism of parental sensitive caregiving (Bowlby 1969). We have argued that evolution has hijacked the attachment relationship in humans by adding a social cognitive role to contingent caregiving interactions. The attachment relationship serves as a pipeline for social communication that initially helps the infant construct a representation of their own mind and subsequently makes accurate communication and cooperative alignment with other minds possible (Fonagy et al. 2017a, 2017b).

That process is initiated in the attachment relationship through what has been described as marked mirroring (Fonagy et al. 2002; Gergely and Unoka 2008; Gergely and Watson 1996). In marked mirroring, the caregiver identifies the emotion that the infant is experiencing, and then reflects it back to the infant, while simultaneously communicating that the infant's own affective experience is being mirrored back *for* the infant, rather than the caregiver's own affect being directed *at* the infant. For example, if the infant is startled and then tearful, the caregiver may mimic a startled and then sad expression but in a softened, caricatured way while simultaneously seeking to reassure the infant physically. Thus, the infant's moment of fearfulness is identified and represented back to the child by mirroring at the same time as soothing and rendering it manageable. It is through the accretion of such interactions that the infant develops the capacity to mentalize. Mentalization begins with the recognition of the infant's selfhood and agency by the caregiver that marked mirroring provides, as in such interactions the caregiver is communicating their awareness of and interest in the infant's mind.

We would temper this account by adding that no caregiver accurately identifies and mirrors their infant's affect all the time; there will be many moments of misalignment, distraction, or inaccuracy in the mirroring interactions (Kim et al. 2014). This is in contrast to neglectful or abusive parenting experiences, in which the parent persistently fails to mirror at all (neglect) or has a grotesquely inaccurate or inappropriate response to the infant's affect experience (abuse). These experiences cause the child to feel isolated from the possibility of social support, whether through the outright absence or meaninglessness and incoherence of self that is created by hostility or grossly incongruous misrepresentations of needs. In the same way that philosophers have wondered about a tree falling in the forest with no one to hear it, an infant's mind (and, to a less urgent and immediate extent, adult minds too) needs other minds around to render their own meaningful and manageable.

As it emerges more fully across development, mentalizing is a multidimensional construct, with each dimension underpinned by distinct neurocognitive systems (Lieberman 2007). There are four distinct dimensions of mentalizing (Bateman and Fonagy 2016; Fonagy and Luyten 2009). These are 1) automatic versus controlled mentalizing (i.e., rapid and reflexive mentalizing versus more reflective, attentive mentalizing, which tends to be slower and more verbal and require more effortful control); 2) affective versus cognitive mentalizing (an emphasis on emotional cues versus rationalizing); 3) internally versus externally focused mentalizing (inferences about mental states made on the basis of internal states versus external features and perceptions); and 4) mentalizing of the self versus the other (a preoccupation with the mental states of the self versus another person). Effective mentalizing depends on the individual's capacity to access these different mentalizing poles as appropriate, changing one's position on each pole according to circumstances. For example, in light conversation with a friend we would largely be using automatic mentalizing; however, if our friend began to talk about a serious difficulty they were having, we would recruit a more reflective form of mentalizing, with a greater emphasis on the internal state of the other.

Mentalizing is a multifaceted and ever-ongoing, fluctuating process with complex implications for social cognitive functioning. It is inevitable that mistakes will be made and that at times the capacity for mentalizing will be weaker or undermined altogether, particularly in situations of interpersonal stress. Mentalizing, therefore, is subject to change, and individuals' strengths and weakness in the different mentalizing dimensions vary. Individuals with borderline traits often experience pronounced difficulties in maintaining robust and balanced mentalizing, particularly in the context of attachment relationships (Fonagy and Bateman 2008a, 2008b). There may well be a genetic component in individual variability in mentalizing and a strong gene and environment interaction (Fonagy and Luyten 2016).

The developmental stage of adolescence brings with it particular challenges to the capacity to maintain balanced mentalizing. Recent research (Crone and Dahl 2012; Dumontheil et al. 2010; Mills et al. 2014) has indicated that the brain still undergoes significant neurobiological change in adolescence, in ways that impact social cognition ability (Blakemore 2012). A growing body of literature on the ongoing development of the social brain across adolescence has led to the suggestion that this period should be regarded as a window of heightened developmental sensitivity in relation to social cognition (Blakemore and Mills 2014). Clinically, this research suggests that individuals who enter adolescence with a predisposed weakness in their capacity for mentalizing (for many different possible reasons, e.g., genetic, environmental, an interaction of the two) will be particularly vulnerable when faced with the considerable developmental challenges of this life stage. Given that aspects of neurobiological development related to mentalizing unfold quite late in adolescence, wider external systems that support controlled, cognitive mentalizing, particularly in the domains of affect regulation and in the face of challenges and stresses, may have an important role to play.

When mentalizing capacity is seriously disrupted, individuals can slip into what we have described as the nonmentalizing or ineffective mentalizing modes, also known as the prementalizing modes because they resemble the ways young children operate before their social cognitive capacities have developed. Because prementalizing involves partial rather than full mentalization, it is ineffective for constructively developing an understanding of oneself and others. There are three modes of prementalizing. In the *pretend mode*, thinking and affect are disengaged from reality. Individuals operating in this mode can talk about events and interactions without any meaningful contextualization tethered in objective reality. In more extreme cases, this mode can develop into dissociation. It can also manifest as hypermentalizing or pseudomentalizing, potentially resulting in a misleading and nonproductive therapeutic scenario in which interactions and events are discussed with apparently intense consideration but without being grounded in genuine meaning or interpersonal reality. For example, a hypermentalizing adolescent who is anxious to be accepted in his or her peer group may explain a social rejection in overly complex ways, such as "Jane did not ring me because she had been talking to Jill, who had seen me when I left school, although she pretended not to see me. So, Jill will have told her that I was talking to Peter, and I know that she does not like Peter. So, in the end they don't bother to ring me."

In the *psychic equivalence mode*, thinking and affect have a quality of excessively concrete and unchangeable reality. In this state of mind, it is very difficult for the individual to seriously entertain alternative perspectives. The experience of fear or sadness, for example, in psychic equivalence is particularly persecuting and distressing, as these feelings appear to be permanent and immoveable forces. In the *teleological mode*, thoughts and feelings are only regarded as believable and meaningful if they are associated with a tangible outcome, for example, affection with a caress (Bateman and Fonagy 2016) or anger with punishment. A patient may say that her boyfriend does not love her because she feels unloved and so is unloved as far as she is concerned. The lack of doubt and failure to question and consider this belief suggests that it is held in psychic equivalence mode. The clinician will naturally question the concern the patient has about her boyfriend only to find that the statement is repeated, "I know he doesn't." When asked for evidence, the patient says that he did not text her when she texted him. This failure of action in the physical world on the part of the boyfriend confirms her understanding of his mental state of not being loving or caring of her. Her psychic equivalent belief is further confirmed through teleological understanding of others' mental states.

It is possible for an individual whose mentalizing capacities are in a state of collapse to operate in more than one prementalizing mode at a time. In such moments, the clinical task is to attempt to establish which of these modes appears to be currently dominant. The presence of the teleological mode, which is associated with the need for physical action to bring relief to unbearable states of mind, is of particular concern when considering risk of self-harm or suicide.

In MBT, the alien self is a key concept used to understand suicidality and the impulse to engage in self-harm. When the capacity to mentalize collapses, in addition to experiencing the emergence of the nonmentalizing modes of functioning, individuals are also vulnerable to the overwhelming intrusion of the alien self. In accordance with the developmental model of mentalizing, constitutional vulnerabilities or exposure to consistently inaccurate or unmirrored responses from a caregiver can leave the child with a weakened representation of his or her own internal state, which is incompatible with a coherent self-representation. For example, if there is an absence of a response or a response in which the infant's frustration is met by the caregiver expressing anger *at* the child, a mismatched or inaccurate secondary representation of the infant is generated for him or her to internalize. The internalization of this noncontingent representation of the infant's state creates what we have termed the *alien self*. The representation of the child's mind by the caregiver is necessarily internalized by the infant to forge his or her sense of self, but the representation is not properly congruent with the infant's self-state, creating a discontinuity in the self-structure. Such discontinuity is an aversive experience, because it involves the uncomfortable sense of holding a feeling, belief, or wish that does not really feel like one's own. In cases where the alien self has resulted from caregiver abuse or neglect, it can be a particularly persecuting presence, and the need to externalize it may be intensely felt. This need can be manifested, for example, by provocatively irritating someone else if one is angry or by generating uncertainty in someone else if the alien affect is associated with vulnerability. It can also be externalized in relation to one's own body—in the need for punishment or relief in the form of self-harm or suicidality. Clinical experience with MBT-A has shown that the alien self can result in self-harm due to experiencing terrifying internal states in which the young person feels useless, like a failure, unlovable, hopeless, etc. As the capacity to mentalize in a protective, affect-regulating manner is lost, these feelings become unbearably painful; they are experienced as overwhelming and unchangeable truths.

The alien self can also generate experiences of incoherence and can undermine the individual's ability to represent internal states associated with emotional arousal, creating difficulties with affect regulation and mentalization. As a result, a vicious cycle can be activated in which the overwhelming presence of the alien self leads to further disruption to the mentalizing processes in moments of distress, making it even harder for the individual to makes sense either of his or her own or other people's minds and behavior. The substantial breakdown in mentalizing that can take place at such moments creates a vacuum in which one or more of the nonmentalizing modes come to direct social cognition, allowing for acts of violence against the body. The nonmentalizing modes can make acts of violence against the self (and indeed against others) possible via different cognitive mediators. In the case of psychic equivalence, distress and suffering become unbearably intensified; what is more, the distress is experienced as a fixed and inescapable reality, from which there is no conceivable way out other than perhaps through a punitive attack on the alien self. In pretend mode, the individual can enter a state of dissociation and meaninglessness: the whole self is alien and disconnected and attacking it does not possess the quality of realness or of substantively mattering. Finally, in the teleological mode the only solution to a crisis in relation to the overwhelming presence of the alien self, and the annihilation of agency this entails, might be a highly literal, physical one, of self-attack.

In the MBT model, the perspective on suicidality and self-harm, broadly speaking, is to regard it as a bid to maintain self-structure in the face of sudden destabilization and the unmanageable looming of the alien self. In the first instance, the suggested response is to attempt to manage the sensation of attachment loss and the primitive fear that accompanies that experience. Of course, we would not wish to be overly schematic about individual motivations, which are complex and unique; however, we suggest that often the need to take action arises when there is an overwhelming emptiness and perceived isolation from protective social support. The impact of MBT in reducing self-harm appears to be mediated by a reduction in avoidant attachment and an improvement in the capacity to mentalize (Rossouw and Fonagy 2012). The family component of MBT with adolescents may well be a critical component of its success. As Brent and colleagues (2013) noted in a review, the studies that have found the strongest effect size in reducing rates of adolescent self-harm were MBT and integrated cognitive-behavioral therapy (Esposito-Smythers et al. 2011), both of which have family components, as well as a large number of individual sessions. Given that reduction in attachment avoidance was found to be one of the mediators of change, the role of change within the family in reducing self-harm appears to be significant. To return to our developmental model of mentalizing, we would suggest that the creation of a more mentalizing social system around him or her is crucial for the young person who finds that the experience of interpersonal stressors and overwhelming affect have a powerfully disruptive effect on their capacity for balanced mentalizing. A family system that is able to respond to the young person's heightened affects and the emergence of nonmentalizing modes without triggering nonmentalizing in the rest of the system is critical. Without this containment, a vicious circle can emerge in which a difficult interaction/stimulus triggers nonmentalizing in the adolescent, which evokes a yet more negative social response from their surrounding family system, which causes an outright collapse in mentalizing and the emergence of prementalizing modes of functioning.

We suggest that adolescent self-harm often occurs in response to relationship stress, when the individual fails to represent the social experience in terms of mental states. When mentalizing is compromised, self-related negative cognitions are experienced with great intensity, leading to both intense psychological pain and an urgent need for distraction. Furthermore, when nonmentalizing engenders social isolation, engaging in manipulative behavior and self-harm may aid reconnection. When mentalization of social experience fails, impulsive (poorly regulated) behaviors and subjective states triggering self-harm become prominent. Supporting and working to improve mentalizing involves many significant and valuable experiences for the patient, but we argue that the mechanism of change in this process is not mentalizing per se; the mechanism of change is the experiences of social communication that are made possible by the interactions and improved interpersonal functioning that emerge as the result of more balanced mentalizing. This constructive social communication involves the development of *epistemic trust*, that is, trust in the authenticity and personal relevance of interpersonally transmitted knowledge. Epistemic trust enables social learning in an ever-changing social and cultural context and allows individuals to benefit from their (social) environment (Fonagy and Allison 2014; Fonagy et al. 2015a) and to access and engage with the mental states of others in a more benign and supportive manner.

Csibra and Gergely's *theory of natural pedagogy* (Csibra and Gergely 2009) is the foundation for the thinking on the relationship between epistemic trust and psychopathology. The starting point of the idea comes from the reality that humans are born into a world that is populated with objects, attributes, and customs whose function or use is *epistemically opaque* (i.e., not obvious from their appearance). Humans have evolved to both teach and learn new and relevant cultural information rapidly in order to transmit and build upon cultural knowledge. Human communication is specifically adapted for the transmission of epistemically opaque information that is enabled by an epistemically trusting relationship. Epistemic trust allows the recipient of the information being conveyed to relax their natural, *epistemic vigilance*—a vigilance that is self-protective and naturally occurring because, after all, it is not in our interest to believe everything indiscriminately. The relaxation of epistemic vigilance allows us to accept that what *we are being told matters to us.*

In terms of psychopathology, we suggest that the most significant implication of the developmental triad of attachment, mentalization, and epistemic trust lies in the consequences of a *breakdown in epistemic trust.* What we are suggesting here is that many, if not all, types of psychopathology might be characterized by temporary or permanent disruption of epistemic trust and the social learning process it enables.

An infant whose channels for learning about the social world have been disrupted—in other words, whose social experiences with caregivers have caused a breakdown in epistemic trust—is left in a quandary of uncertainty and permanent epistemic vigilance. Everybody seeks social knowledge, but when such reassurance and input is sought, the content of this communication may be rejected, its meaning may be confused, or it may be misinterpreted as having hostile intent. In that sense, many forms of mental disorder might be considered manifestations of failings in social communication arising from epistemic mistrust, hypervigilance, or outright *epistemic freezing,* a complete inability to trust others as a source of knowledge about the world, which may be characteristic of many individuals with marked trauma and personality problems. An individual who was traumatized in childhood, for instance, has little reason to trust others and will reject information that is inconsistent with their preexisting beliefs. As therapists, we may consider such people "hard to reach," yet they are simply showing an adaptation to a social environment where information from attachment figures was likely to be misleading. Put simply, we suggest that effective interventions specialize in generating epistemic trust in individuals who struggle to relax their epistemic vigilance in more ordinary social situations.

Review of Empirical Evidence

MBT has been found to be effective in reducing self-harm in adults. Bateman and Fonagy have examined the effectiveness of MBT for treating BPD in a series of randomized controlled trials, with patients receiving treatment as usual (TAU) in the community serving as comparison groups. The MBT day hospital program has been investigated in a series of outcome studies, culminating in an 8-year follow-up study (Bateman and Fonagy 2008) that is the longest follow-up of treatment for BPD conducted to date. In comparison with TAU, MBT decreased suicide attempts, emergency department visits, inpatient admissions, medication and outpatient treatment utilization, and impulsivity. Far fewer patients in the MBT group than in the comparison group met criteria for BPD at the follow-up point (13% vs. 87%). Moreover, in addition to symptomatic improvement, patients in the MBT group showed greater improvement in interpersonal and occupational functioning. Similarly, MBT delivered as an intensive outpatient program proved more effective than structured clinical management for BPD at the end of the 18-month treatment period (Bateman and Fonagy 2009), particularly for patients with more than two personality disorder diagnoses (Bateman and Fonagy 2013). This intensive treatment milieu for the delivery of MBT has been modified over two decades, and MBT is now delivered primarily in outpatient programs; in the United Kingdom, most patients with BPD and other personality disorders are now treated in outpatient programs, of which the best researched is an 18-month intensive outpatient treatment consisting of a weekly individual session of 50 minutes and a weekly group session of 75 minutes (Bateman and Fonagy 2009). Compared with TAU, the outpatient treatment resulted in lowered rates of suicidal behavior and nonsuicidal self-injury as well as fewer hospitalizations; in addition, the MBT group showed improved social adjustment coupled with diminished depression, symptom distress, and interpersonal distress.

In a randomized controlled trial of MBT-A, 80 adolescents presenting to mental health services who had self-harmed in the preceding month were randomly assigned to MBT or TAU; 97% received a diagnosis of depression, and 73% met the criteria for borderline personality disorder. Provided on an outpatient basis, the program provided weekly individual MBT-A sessions and monthly mentalization-based family therapy sessions; TAU was provided by community-based adolescent mental health services. At the end of 12 months of treatment, MBT-A was found to be more successful than TAU in reducing self-harm and symptoms of depression. By self-report, the recovery rate was 44% for MBT-A versus 17% for TAU, and by interview assessment, the rate was reported to be 57% versus 32%. A stronger reduction in depressive symptoms and BPD diagnoses and traits was also found in the MBT-A group (Rossouw and Fonagy 2012). Both groups showed significant reductions in both self-harm and risk-taking behavior, following both a linear and a quadratic pattern. The interaction term for group by time was also significant for both variables, indicating that the linear decrease in Risk-Taking and Self-Harm Inventory scores was significantly greater for the MBT-A group on both variables. At the 12-month point, self-harm scores were significantly lower for the MBT-A group (Rossouw and Fonagy 2012).

Treatment Components and Primary Intervention Strategies

MBT-A is usually delivered as a combination of individual MBT and MBT-F; some programs also incorporate group MBT for adolescents. Total treatment length is 12 months, divided into four phases.

The MBT-A four-phase structure is as follows:

- Assessment
    - Diagnostic
    - Cognitive
    - Mentalization

- Initial phase
    - Formulation
    - Contract
    - Crisis plan
    - Psychoeducation

- Middle phase
    - Enhance mentalization
    - Gain impulse control
    - Enhance awareness of mental states of others

- Final phase
  - Increase independence and responsibility
  - Consolidate stability
  - Develop follow-up plan
  - Understand and process the meanings of the ending with a focus on affective states associated with loss
  - Plan discharge and liaison with partner organizations

Assessment

The assessment phase involves the use of diagnostic, cognitive, and mentalizing measures such as the Reflective Function Questionnaire for youth (Sharp et al. 2009) (for a comprehensive description of the measures available for assessing mentalizing, see Luyten et al., in press). It also considers family functioning and the identification of the stressors that may disrupt parental mentalizing. The assessment phase typically lasts for 2 weeks and involves one or two sessions with individual therapists and one or two sessions with the family therapist. Ideally, the family therapist and the individual therapist are different individuals. Psychometric measures are conducted by research assistants.

Initial phase

The initial phase of the program normally covers 1 month.

Formulation

The initial phase of treatment begins with the patient receiving a written formulation that is discussed with him or her. The same process of providing and discussing a formulation takes place in the family component of treatment. Creating the family formulation frequently highlights and requires thought about the fact that different family members may well have quite different perspectives on the nature of the difficulties the family is facing. The formulation itself is a form of collaborative effort requiring acknowledgment and consideration of differences in views.

Contract

The contract is an agreement about the treatment plan, including duration of treatment and commitment required of all participants in the treatment, including the family.

Crisis Plan

A detailed crisis plan is included in the formulation. This plan seeks to highlight factors that might trigger emotion dysregulation and impulsive behavior and attempts to provide ways to prevent loss of mentalization and, if that fails, to set out alternative immediate solutions and courses of action rather than the dangerous ways forward that may otherwise present themselves. An example of a crisis plan might be the following.

> Trigger factors that you and I identified are times when you feel rejected, humiliated, or bad about yourself. As we have discussed, these feelings do not just arrive out of the blue, they are likely to have been triggered in a close relationship. When you have those feelings, you tend to rush into an action to take the feelings away. When you feel like that again, I would like you to try and stop the action by trying to delay it for 10 minutes. Use the 10 minutes to try and reflect on what was happening a few moments before you had the bad feeling. That might help you to understand more clearly what it is that you feel as well as what might have happened in a close relationship that may have contributed to the feeling. Once you have this more clear understanding, it may be easier to think about a solution or to see things from a different perspective. Once that has happened, you may not feel as if you need to rush into action anymore. If that fails and you still feel at risk to harm yourself, try to explore alternatives to self-harm, such as the following.
>
> 1. Do something physical and strenuous like going for a run, try and distract yourself or talk to a friend or someone you trust or try and think about a person you know who loves you and imagine what that person would feel and say to you if you were to talk to them.
> 2. Sometimes you harm yourself when you numb yourself emotionally. When you get into such a state of mind, try to remember that it is not a good state of mind for you to be in, and it is harmful to you. Try and bring yourself back to reality—do something to occupy yourself, like talking to someone, playing a game, writing a poem, painting, or watching something that can hold your attention on TV. Don't just sit and stare into space with your mind full of negative thoughts about yourself.
> 3. If all else fails, call the clinic and ask to speak to me, and I will call you back when I can.

Psychoeducation

The formulation session with the family is usually followed by a psycho-educational session. Its purpose is to introduce the underpinning idea of mentalizing therapy: that behavior has meaning, that feelings arise in a relational context, and that people have a powerful emotional impact on one another.

The format of this session can either be a multifamily group or an individual family. It is generally approached as a discussion with the family or families using examples from everyday life to illustrate the main principles. Particularly in a multifamily group context, it may be helpful to use games, role play, and video materials to assist the discussion.

To give a small example supporting the understanding of mentalizing and emotions—patients and families are asked to identify the most frequent feelings they have experienced over the past week, and a list of these is made with some identification of context for each emotion. This is an exercise in mentalizing self in emotional terms over time. Patients and family are then asked to consider their current feeling, which is an exercise in current mentalizing, that is, recognizing a current dominant and subdominant feeling and giving them contextual meaning. Most families talk about anger, anxiety, depression, and frustration but rarely suggest pleasurable feelings and never identify curiosity and genuine interest in the world as a feeling state. So, the clinician can identify this curiosity and interest as being a basic emotion that is required to form relationships that are constructive and pleasurable. It is a core component of mentalizing emotions of others. To form relationships, we all have to take an interest in how others feel, and this is a skill that families need to develop.

Middle Phase

The length of this phase is usually 9–10 months. In this stage of treatment, the overall purpose is to improve mentalizing skills in the patient and their family. MBT-A sessions are largely unstructured, which is necessary because the focus of each session is generally on the young person's current or recent interpersonal experiences and the mental states evoked by these experiences. A key component of this is helping both young person and family to gain better impulse control. Specific interventions are used to manage suicidal, parasuicidal, and other harmful or impulsive behaviors, such as substance use, threatening behavior, or binging and purging. We will describe specific interventions in more detail in the section "Primary Intervention Strategies."

Final Phase

The aim of the final phase, as with all psychotherapeutic treatments, is to develop the patient's independence. Crucial to this goal is building up relational stability and supporting the patient's sense of agency and autonomy within their relational networks. A coping plan is also created so both the patient and family know what to do should difficulties recur. In the outpatient program, the final phase usually lasts about 2 months, with the appointments becoming more widely spaced toward the end.

Primary Intervention Strategies

The Mentalizing Stance

Underpinning all MBT work is the concept of the mentalizing stance of the clinician. In the first instance, the therapist must seek to establish a therapeutic alliance with the young person with whom they are working. If the young person is struggling to mentalize, is emotionally dysregulated, and, in particular, appears to be operating in one or more of the nonmentalizing modes, the approach of the therapist should be to work to see the situation from the patient's point of view. For example, if the patient is in the grip of psychic equivalence, it may be impossible for him or her at that moment to imagine the current reality as anything other than how he or she is experiencing it. An example might be a young person who feels afraid that his or her romantic partner may be unfaithful but the next minute feels convinced that the partner has been unfaithful—the feeling of fear changes from a feeling to a concrete fact. In such a moment, pushing the patient to see it differently may feel like a grotesque and persecutory intrusion. Rather than conspicuously mentalizing "at" the patient, the therapist's task is instead to create an experience for the patient of having their agency and their subjectivity appreciated and recognized. This sounds straightforward but, in fact, may require considerable self-discipline and humility on the part of the therapist—because seeing the world from the patient's perspective may well involve seeing himself or herself from the patient's perspective, which may not be flattering. Experiencing empathy in this way, however, is an important start in learning about different ways of seeing the world for the patient whose mentalizing capacity is impaired. Only once the patient's own agency has been respected and recognized in this way, is it possible to introduce different ways of seeing the world.

The mentalizing stance involves the therapist keeping the state of mind of the patient as a primary concern throughout—attempting to continually adapt and reconstruct a sense of the patient's state of mind in order to help the patient comprehend what he or she is currently feeling and experiencing. As alluded to above, this process includes the therapist seeking to understand how he or she is being viewed in the mind of the patient. The clinician's primary interest is what is going on in the patient's mind in that very moment, even if they are discussing an event that happened in the past. But this focus on the patient's mind should not be assumed to be perfectly accurate; one of the fundamental principles of mentalizing is the acceptance of the difficult human truth that we can never really know what is happening inside someone else's mind with complete accuracy and certainty. The therapist, accordingly, needs to show appropriate humility and tentativeness about what they think may be going on in the patient's mind. Below, we list the elements that make up our definition of the mentalizing stance (Bateman and Fonagy 2016):

- Mentalizing in psychotherapy is a process of joint attention in which the patient's mental states are the object of attention.
- The clinician continually constructs and reconstructs an image of the patient to help the patient to comprehend what he or she feels.
- Neither clinician nor patient experiences interactions other than impressionistically.
- Differences are identified.
- Different perspectives are accepted.
- Active questioning is conducted.

The capacity of the clinician to acknowledge his or her own mentalizing failures and errors is a significant aspect of the approach. It is also important, when appropriate, for the clinician to own up to his or her own mentalizing mistakes. Being open about the fluctuating and imperfect process of mentalizing can reduce the feelings of blame and shame that the patient may experience in high-arousal interpersonal exchanges, and it also demonstrates the truth of the opacity of other people's minds and the need for tentativeness and lack of dogma with regard to other people's thoughts, feelings, and beliefs. This approach has been described as the "not-knowing stance."

The mentalizing stance also involves attempting to keep the focus of discussion on what is current. If a young person presents in a state of distress, the response is not to attempt to link it to a past or distant event. Rather, it is to try and understand what happened just before the distress was triggered. Focusing on the present this way is more likely to contribute to the young person's experience of being appreciated and recognized, as well as helping him or her to mentalize the moment when mentalizing may have broken down in a way that is more resonant and less abstract than the reconstruction of a past event might be. For similar reasons, highly complex and elaborate interpretations are not recommended. The mentalizing stance is, rather, more concerned with identifying affect and exploring emotional and defining context, with a fundamental empathic core, as illustrated below:

> Charlotte, a 16-year-old in our inpatient unit with a history of self-harm and anorexia, threatened to discharge herself, saying that she wanted to leave because she wanted to go home and kill herself. She seemed angry and upset, and she was not making eye contact with anyone, nor was she able to hear anything anyone was saying to her. She said over and over again, "Let me go, let me go, I need to go, I need to kill myself." Her state of agitation evoked anxiety and agitation in those around her, and very soon nonmentalizing cycles ensued in which all communication was reduced to communication about action: she was going to leave to kill herself, and the inpatient team was considering restraining her or sedating her to prevent her from leaving. The correct mentalizing technique would be to avoid jumping to action but rather to make empathic contact with her to try and understand what she is feeling, what happened, and within what interpersonal context her mentalizing abilities broke down.

> Therapist: Can I just try and understand what you are feeling?
> Patient: I want to leave, I want to die.
> Therapist: You seem very upset, what happened?
> Patient: Nothing, I just want to leave. I will not get better, and I've had enough. I want to die.
> Therapist: I hear that. You seem to feel very desperate.
> Patient: I have to die.
> Therapist: Why, what have you done, it sounds like a death sentence?
> Patient: I killed my mother.

Therapist: How do you think you killed your mother?

Patient: I gave her stress and that caused her cancer and that is why she is dead.

Therapist: It is also her cancer that caused you stress, and just as she did not deliberately have cancer to cause you stress, you did not deliberately have stress to cause her cancer. You must have felt very scared, perhaps like you are feeling now?

Patient: It was all my fault. I think I should call the police and tell them I killed my mother.

Therapist: Maybe sometimes, one should also be able to call the police to stop cancer taking one's mother away.

Patient: I really don't want to be alive. [cries]

Therapist: It is so, so sad to lose one's mom.

Patient: I don't know how to go on.

She became desperately sad and allowed herself to be consoled. She was no longer angry and threatening to kill herself. We moved from action mode to mentalizing mode in which feelings could be understood, shared, and contained.

Broadly speaking, the mentalizing response to self-harm or suicidality is in the first instance to use supportive and empathic interventions to establish the events around the act, including any interpersonal stressors. At this point, the therapist's response is simply validating and empathic. The next step is to address the patient's current state of mind. The therapist begins by asking the patient to provide a narrative outline of the buildup of events leading to self-harm or a suicidal act, which is necessary as a part of the process of risk assessment. Once this narrative has been established in adequate detail, the next stage is to get an account of the feelings leading up to the event. This requires asking the patient to go back in their narrative to the point at which they did not feel the compulsive need to self-harm (the rewind and explore process [see subsection below]). It may be difficult for the patient to feel that the desire to self-harm or thoughts of suicide are not ever present; the therapist should accept this but also seek to work back to identify when these thoughts changed into the compulsive need to act. This may be a matter of asking the patient when their thoughts changed and of trying to draw attention to the contrast in states of mind across time. We have labeled this process a mentalizing functional analysis (Bateman and Fonagy 2012, 2016), and its purpose is to reactivate mentalizing processes.

The mentalizing functional analysis works to explore the patient's state of mind in relation to an event and how states of mind changed through interaction with things that were happening. The patient may be reluctant to talk about an act of self-harm or may find the conversation highly anxiety provoking, in which case the therapist should respond sensitively, returning to the subject when the patient is better able to discuss it. It may also be the case that the patient finds it hard to remember the circumstances around the event, in which case it might be necessary for the therapist to "rewind and explore" further to the point at which the patient was less aroused and to attempt to work forward from there. This rewinding (often further than one might assume necessary) helps to explore and express the idea that states are not fixed and unchangeable and that they fluctuate in response to triggers and stimuli. The goal is to locate the *point of vulnerability*—the moment at which the patient's state of mind shifted toward the position where self-harm felt like a compulsion—and to work toward understanding the steps that led to the state that made any option other than harm impossible. Recognizing these moments of sensitivity that contribute to the ratcheting up of what might otherwise be background thoughts about the possibility of suicide or self-harm makes it possible to think about interrupting this cycle and preventing the collapse in mentalizing that accompanies the act of self-harm. The focus in these conversations should be on the conscious factors driving the act rather than on more complex psychological exploration. The therapist should avoid an emphasis on long-term personal history, unconscious processes, and manipulation, as they risk alienating the patient. Such accounts should only emerge within the course of treatment as more substantive evidence for them is developed and as the therapeutic alliance has developed as well. We will discuss in more detail the primary interventions in MBT below.

Clarification and Elaboration

The idea of clarification in MBT relates to an attempt to encourage the patient to construct a meaning around an incident (perhaps something that has caused recent distress and upset for the patient) that may be absent in an initial, nonmentalizing account. Clarification is not simply a request for the simple facts. Although facts may be needed for the story to be coherent, an extended, overelaborated factual account is not. Rather, actions need to be related to the feelings of the event. Clarification also does not refer to the therapist's clarification of the story for the patient; it is an interactive process in which patient and therapist work through the mental process of an incident in order to unpick moments in the account where mentalizing appears to have broken down and the situation (or the patient's reading of it) escalated into something distressing or dysfunctional. Asking open questions and focusing on the moment-to-moment states of mind in the account are strategies available in clarification.

Clarification is often a process that depends upon and involves affect elaboration. The complexity of emotions felt by a young person who has pronounced mentalizing difficulties may be difficult for them to identify and/or recognize. A young person who is in a state of distress and experiencing an overwhelming "attack" from the alien self may well feel hopeless, unlovable, angry, ashamed, and so on. The ferocity of feelings can be so intense that they are almost not recognizable as such: they have the quality of fact or an overwhelming force of reality. Clarifying and elaborating these affects can help to slow things down, making it possible to approach them in a more mentalizing way. Some of the techniques in which the clarification and elaboration of affect can be used are described below.

Rewind and Explore

The basic mentalizing technique of rewind and explore allows both the patient and therapist to pause and reconsider something in the session in order to better understand it. Such a moment might occur when it becomes apparent that the patient feels misunderstood or irritated by the clinician or when the patient appears to be reluctant to acknowledge the internal mental state of another person whom they are describing. The technique involves literally stopping the conversation and attempting to work back to the point at which mentalizing went offline. It can be a particularly useful technique in family work as well as individual sessions. In a family session, it provides the opportunity to explore different perspectives as to why an interaction has shifted in its mentalizing quality.

Challenge

This is another technique that can be used when mentalizing breaks down in a session; however, it is a technique that should be used with caution and gently because the aim is not confrontation but the introduction of an unexpected or unanticipated moment to the dialogue, so as to disrupt a nonmentalizing jag (Bateman and Fonagy 2012). The challenge could be a counterfactual comment and may contain an element of humor or self-deprecation. This can bring about a pause in a session and a change in thought processes that allow the clinician to redirect the conversation to what has been happening:

> An example of this technique is a session with a young person, Denise, who cut her face and neck prior to her mother picking her up for weekend leave. She was doing well in the week with no episodes of self-harm. She tends to see herself as an innocent victim in interpersonal interactions, and she has a constant mantra in her mind of herself as unlovable and a firm belief that others do not like her, despite clear evidence of the opposite. She constantly feels her mother does not understand her and that her mother is in the wrong for getting upset when she harms herself. Instead of seeing her mother's distress as a sign of her care, Denise sees it as evidence of her mother's lack of care.
>
> When her mother arrived to pick her up, she was confronted with Denise's face and neck looking like a road map. She was so distressed and shocked that she ran to the toilet and threw up. Denise innocently waited outside for her mother with a large piece of art in her hand with the words "I love you Mommy" written on it. In an emergency session, Denise was trying very hard to convince her mother that she cut herself because she hated herself. She could not elaborate on it or draw any links to anything that happened or any other feeling in her. She seemed unable to understand the impact of her behavior on her mother, and she mostly felt that her mother was being uncaring and selfish for being upset—could her mother not notice her love for her with the card she had made?

> Therapist: I think what your mom said is that she heard the message on your card that you love her, but I think she is battling at the moment with another message—she feels there is another message carved into your face, and she is struggling to understand it.
>
> Patient: But it has nothing to do with her. I did it because I hate myself, and when I do, I need to cut. It is the only way in which I can feel better.
>
> Therapist: I don't know, Denise. The whole week you did not cut, and then just before your mom comes, you cut yourself where she would be able to see it straight away. What did you think she was going to feel when she saw you?
>
> Patient: I knew she would be upset, but that is not why I did it. I hate myself. That is why I did it.

> Therapist: Do you want to ask your mom what she felt when she saw you?
>
> Patient: What did you feel?
>
> Mother: I felt angry, I felt devastated and upset, and I feel powerless. It so hurts me to see you in pain, and I do not know what to do to make it better.
>
> Patient: You are always angry with me and blaming me, but you don't understand, this is not my fault. I can't help it. I hate myself.
>
> Therapist: I did not think your mom was blaming you, Denise, but I think what it looks like is that things can now easily turn into an argument between the two of you. Is that right?
>
> Mother: Yes, at this stage we will start to accuse one another, and then we argue, and then Denise storms off, and I then worry about what she will do to herself.
>
> Therapist: Did you realize when you were cutting yourself this afternoon that it was creating a scenario that was going to lead to a fight?
>
> Patient: No, I just hated myself, and I did it.
>
> Therapist: It seems as if what you did set you and your mom up for a fight. That makes me wonder whether it may have been about any feelings you may have about going home?

In this example, the patient was in a concrete mentalizing mode in which behavior does not have meaning, and she was hanging on to a nonmentalizing filler by saying "I did it because I hate myself." She also didn't notice her impact on those around her and hoped that the concrete "I love you" message on the card would obscure the far scarier message. In the session, the challenge was used to try and turn mentalizing back on in the hope that the more difficult underlying feelings could be expressed and mentalized, which would de-escalate the nonmentalizing crescendo of acting out.

Transference Tracers

MBT does not use transference in the classical psychodynamic sense. In the context of MBT, we use "transference tracers" to draw a link between something happening in the session, or being described in the session, and a pattern of nonmentalizing that seems to reappear, either in the therapeutic relationship or in the patient's wider social world. An example of this is the following:

It seems that whenever you have to share your dad's attention with someone else, you feel angry, and then you feel he does not care. Perhaps that may mean that sometimes when you have to wait to speak to me, you may have similar feelings.

A transference tracer is always current: it relates an immediate event/preoccupation to a wider pattern. It can also be of value in signaling the relevance of the observation to therapy. So, to continue with the example above, it could be suggested that such feelings might have an impact on how the patient feels about working with the therapist.

Integrative Mentalizing

We have previously named this technique interpretive mentalizing—a label we have dropped for its classical connotations of seeking to interpret unconscious material. Rather, the emphasis in MBT is on drawing together a patient's narrative in a step beyond the clarification process. It is an intervention that should only be used when the session is not characterized by high arousal and dramatic swings in mentalizing, because it, in essence, challenges the patient to mentalize with greater complexity, drawing on other possible perspectives. This intervention might typically follow a process of clarification and affect elaboration. An example might be for the therapist to simply comment, following a discussion of the patient's feelings in relation to a difficult exchange with their mother, "I see that what you say about what you think about your mother's motives is a possibility, but I wonder if there may be other possibilities too."

Mentalizing the Transference

As is usual in MBT, the emphasis of transference in a mentalizing framework is on seeking to reflect upon the here and now of the interaction. The purpose is for the therapist and the patient to work together to make sense of how they are interacting: how they are affecting one another, what their different perspectives might be, and how and why they are seeing each other in certain ways. This process involves the therapist modeling their mentalizing and, critically, being open about his or her mistakes in mentalizing the patient. Such an intervention would only be used after the essential early steps of the basic process of MBT (beginning with validating the patient's experience and then working to clarify and elaborate the patient's feeling) have been taken. An example is provided below:

- Validate the feeling: "Gosh I can see that me frowning could make you feel that I am angry."
- Clarification and affect elaboration: "Could it be that I am not angry but that I may be feeling other feelings?"

> Patient responds: You don't believe me.
> Therapist: I am trying to understand what you are feeling at the moment, and I am trying to understand why you are feeling like that—I don't know if I am right, but you suddenly seem scared of me. Can we try and go back to when the feeling started? I want to see if I did or said something that made you feel like that.
> Patient: When I spoke about the abuse, you frowned, and it scared me because I thought you were angry with me and you did not believe me.
> Therapist: But my face showed that I was gripped by what you said, and I was affected by what you said—why on earth would I be angry?
> Patient: I don't know, maybe I am scared that I will shock and that you will feel disgusted.
> Therapist: I wonder if this is perhaps about a very painful and deep feeling of disgust inside you that was caused by the disgusting thing he did.
> Patient: I do feel such disgust.
> Therapist: And then it is hard to imagine that someone else may be feeling compassion and not disgust.

- Mentalize the transference and accept enactment (if any): "Yes I can see that I looked a bit angry. I think I did feel a bit frustrated when you said again and again that you were going to run away and kill yourself, and when I felt you did not want to allow any thinking or talking—I think I felt a bit pushed away by you and a bit helpless."

Mentalization-Based Treatment for Families

MBT-A incorporates family therapy as a key modality. Family work as part of MBT-A is based on MBT-F, which integrates systemic practice with attachment and mentalizing theory (Asen and Fonagy 2012a, 2012b, 2017a, 2017b). The aim of MBT-F is to develop mentalizing skills in family relationships and to reduce the appearance of impulsive enactments, coercion, affect storms, and nonmentalizing interactions. Asen and Fonagy, who developed MBT-F, describe the concept of the mentalizing "loop" (Asen and Fonagy 2012b). This loop involves working with the family to identify a nonmentalizing moment, which is then highlighted and named. Careful attention is given to the task of mentalizing that moment and making sense of what each participant experienced at that point, and the inner and external representations of the family in the mind of each family member can be explored. The emphasis is on thinking about feelings before planning any actions or attempting to think about how things might be done differently next time.

The "pause and review" technique, part of the mentalizing loop, has the effect of slowing down interactions, thereby gradually permitting each family member to resume effective mentalizing, in which emotion is integrated with cognition and the focus on self and others gets equal weight. The sequence of 1) action, 2) pause, and 3) reflection aims to restore balance to mentalizing. The rebalancing will be reflected in relevant commentary that implies 1) curiosity, 2) respect for the opacity of other minds, 3) awareness of the impact of affect on self and others, 4) perspective taking, 5) narrative continuity, and 6) a sense of agency and trust. There are various MBT-F techniques, often quite innovative and playful, which are intended to encourage family members to adopt new and different perspectives. The underpinning aim of the work is to focus on the states of mind of each person in the family and, through that process, each person's state of mind in relation to each other. This is not to set up circular, never-ending questions about family dynamics and family history but to achieve an awareness of how mental states affect people in the family. In particular, there is a focus on how the breakdown in mentalizing in response to heightened affect can undermine the capability of the family system to respond resiliently and supportively to the needs and challenges of family members.

Case Example

Background

Following admission to the inpatient unit, Sam, age 16 years, was anxious in the presence of others and initially preferred to spend her time in her bedroom. She reported feeling depressed and hopeless and certain that she would not be alive by the time she turned 17. Prior to admission, she had dropped out of school and lived a reclusive life with increasing social isolation to the point that a few weeks before admission she even stopped online contact with friends. She spoke of herself with extreme hatred, referring to herself and her body as horrible and ugly. She also expected hatred from those around her. She had an extensive history of self-harm, with a previous suicide attempt, mood fluctuations, and a lack of a sense of who she was and what she wanted from her life. Sam felt herself unable to perform academically but also expressed the wish to be a pediatrician one day. She was unable to travel on public transportation, describing every journey as an experience of being naked in front of a train full of people looking at her. Eating in front of others evoked similar horrors of mockery and ridicule; on further examination, this seemed to be linked to her experiencing a profound sense of shame when she was eating.

As we got to know Sam better, we noticed that she could be quick to criticize and to provide "supervision" to staff members about their interventions with other patients. She was sensitive about the way she was spoken to, and she frequently became very angry at staff members or her therapist for not using the right words or tone. Staff members increasingly felt as if they were "walking on eggshells" around her. Sam's parents separated when she was 3 years old. She and her four siblings grew up with their mother; there was little contact with her father, who resided abroad. Her mother had suffered from depression throughout her childhood and could at times be humiliating and dismissive of Sam. Sam's descriptions of childhood experiences were filled with feelings of loneliness and shame. She felt inferior to everyone at school and experienced herself as stupid and fat, even though she was in fact a very intelligent and beautiful young woman. She believed that she was monstrous and unlovable. Self-harm became the outward expression of her internal state. Very deep cuts to her arms at times revealed the underlying fat tissue, and although those around her showed strong aversive responses to her wounds, she would dismissively state that she did not feel anything and that the cuts were not deep enough.

The Therapeutic Intervention

The following clinical example is taken from Sam's third individual MBT-A session, which took place on the Monday after a weekend leave Sam spent at home with her mom. On Saturday, Sam had visited some old friends, and on Sunday she cut herself extensively. When she reported the self-harm in the session, the therapist tried to rewind to what happened before the self-harm in an attempt to try to identify the mental state and the unmentalized feelings underneath the self-harm.

Therapist: What happened before you cut yourself?

Patient: Nothing. I just wanted to cut myself.

Therapist: What was in your mind? What did you feel?

Patient: I just felt that I wanted to cut myself. I did not feel anything else. I just wanted to do some damage.

Therapist: Ah, but Sam, you know I believe that we always have deep feelings inside ourselves when we get desires like that.

Patient: I don't. I often just want to damage myself.

Therapist: You saw your friends the day before? When last did you see them?

Patient: Three months ago.

Therapist: What was it like to see them?

Patient: I could not connect to them. It gave me a lot of memories. [silence]

Therapist: What kind of memories?

Patient: I don't know, just memories from the time that I have very little memories. It is just kind of hazy.

Therapist: That sounds important. Could you try and take me there?

Patient: I don't know…I don't know.

Therapist: When you saw your friends, what feelings did you have?

Patient: I could not explain it. I don't have words for it. I get it sometimes that I have feelings that don't have a name. [This could be seen as a first indication of a flicker of improvement, as initially she indicated that she did not have feelings.]

Therapist: That is OK. I understand that. Could you describe them?

Patient: No, they are literally indescribable. They don't have names.

Therapist: Just listening to what you said, you said something about not feeling connected to them when you saw them? Maybe if I was in your shoes, I would have felt as if I did not fit in, but I don't know if that is how you felt.

Patient: She smiles. Yeah, but this is not even worth saying anymore. That is just a permanent feeling.

Therapist: No, I don't agree with you. If you feel it, it is worth saying, and even if you feel it all the time, then it is still worth saying. What you feel is important, and it is important to me. Was there anything in particular that made you feel like that?

Patient: I don't know if there are layers to it.

Therapist: If we draw a picture on this page, we can draw you, and then we draw your friends, and we put bubbles above their heads. Then if we write in the bubble what feelings we think they may have in their heads, what do you think they felt on Saturday evening?

Patient: I don't know. I don't know what people think. I cannot tell. I am too scared to think.

Therapist: For you to be scared what they think already means you have an expectation, doesn't it? What is your expectation?

Patient: That they look down on me.

Therapist: Shall we put that in the thought bubble?

Patient: Yes, and that I am not skinny and that I don't have the same clothes as them.

Therapist: OK, let's write that into the thought bubble as well. What should we write into your thought bubble?

Patient: I don't know. I feel bad about myself.

Therapist: Did they say or do anything that gave you the idea that they felt like that about you?

Patient: I don't know.

Therapist: Usually, the way we behave can give people an idea of how we feel inside. How did they behave when they saw you?

Patient: They were friendly, but they did not mean it.

Therapist: Is there any way that you could perhaps confuse what was in your mind with what they felt?

Patient: I don't know. [It is hard for her to imagine the mind of the other, and perhaps the way the question was phrased did not help. Although the statement provided an alternative perspective, it did not include the necessary affective attunement.]

Therapist: If a friend of mine becomes unwell and goes to hospital, I will feel caring feelings, I will feel concerned, and I will probably show that by being warm and friendly when I see the friend. I just wonder, you know I may be wrong, but you said they were friendly—is it possible that they were having caring feelings?

Patient: I don't know. I don't know what people feel.

Therapist: Hmm. I may be wrong, but I wonder if you don't perhaps make assumptions about what people feel? And you know when we make assumptions, we could be wrong.

Summary

The case material above clearly illustrates Sam's struggles with recognizing her own mental state and the mental states of those around her. The strength of the "alien self" in her mind, both subjectively and projected onto others, is clear, too. After Sam's description of self-harm, which can be seen as a manifestation of a collapse of mentalizing ability, the therapist rewinds to try to find the precipitating event that led to the unmentalized affective state; doing so allows it to be explored, understood, and ultimately mentalized. Because Sam's account of what was in her mind prior to the self-harm remains devoid of emotional content, the therapist uses techniques such as exploration of affect, clarification, and elaboration of affect by asking for more detail about the precipitating events. When Sam states that her feelings do not have words, the therapist uses herself to help with elaboration of affect, but the therapist poses this not as a statement of fact that Sam would feel the same but more as a question. This enables Sam to share the intensity of these feelings, albeit in a very dismissive manner.

Then the therapist switched to another set of techniques. She stated that she felt Sam's feelings were important, and that they were important to her. She shared her own thoughts and feelings; that is, she expressed her interest in Sam's mind and experiences and validated this as important to her despite it having been devalued and dismissed by Sam. This technique in particular may be of value for an individual with vulnerable narcissistic traits—characterized by a tendency to fluctuate between grandiosity and intense feelings of inadequacy and the use of self-harm to regulate internal storms (Rossouw 2015)—because they frequently expect criticism and coldness and are unable to accurately judge the intentions of others. Such young people may feel shame and humiliation in response to feeling misunderstood, which can lead to a collapse in their sense of self, which may lead to feelings of panic and abandonment. Declaring one's intentions explicitly and repeatedly provides the mentalizing scaffolding without which emotional closeness will not be possible. In addition, by stating, "What you feel is important to me," the therapist aims to provide a bridge of humanity for the patient as an escape from the cold, dehumanizing grip of the "alien self."

The clinical vignette also provides examples of thinking with psychic equivalence. This is demonstrated in Sam's descriptions of her conviction that the thoughts and feelings in her mind are exactly the same as those around her. The therapist uses active questioning and highlights alternative perspectives to help Sam see the difference between her mind and the minds of others and to facilitate her curiosity about the minds of others and to humanize others. The expectation is that the more Sam mentalizes, the more the world around her will become humanized and the more compassion she will have for herself. Ultimately, it is hoped this will lessen the grip of the humiliating and shaming alien self.

Outcome and Prognosis

As therapy with Sam progressed, the therapeutic relationship was filled with struggles that the therapist had to reflect on in order not to overreact or respond in an overly personalized fashion. As has been described, the therapist and other members of the team (and indeed Sam's family) had to walk a tightrope in terms of the views they expressed and the words they used. Carelessness in this regard could well lead to emotional injury. The therapist also had to battle against a strong sense of feeling useless or hopeless when every attempt to make emotional contact was rebuffed or devalued. Sam's dehumanizing approaches to herself when she was in the grip of rage driven by perfectionism could be relentless and served as another source of anxiety in the therapist.

For the therapist, the working-through phase of therapy with Sam was a slow process of managing strong countertransferential feelings while attempting to make emotional contact with Sam's feelings of anxiety, inadequacy, fears of rejection, and deep sense of shame. Nevertheless, as Sam became better able to tolerate emotional contact with those vulnerable states within her and better able to allow herself to feel close to her therapist, she was more able to see her therapist as separate from her and capable of warmth toward her. She also became more curious about the mental states of others, as well as her impact on others. She became more compassionate toward herself and expected a much less cold world around her, and her self-harm decreased. However, in meeting new people or forming new relationships, some of Sam's fragility reappeared, and she remained vulnerable to shying away from contact. Her perfectionism remained a problem but was toned down into a strong ambition for her future. Moreover, she was able to reengage in her education.

Recommendations for Clinicians Interested in Using This Treatment Approach

Adopting and Adapting the Treatment Across Various Practice Settings

The standard components of MBT-A vary somewhat depending on the program setting. The typical structure for outpatient treatment programs is weekly individual therapy and monthly or twice-monthly family therapy.

In an inpatient or day patient MBT-A program, family therapy takes place weekly, and there are additional twice-weekly group therapy sessions.

An adherence and competence manual for MBT-A has been developed, which researchers and clinicians can use to assess the fidelity of their treatment to the research-based MBT model. The adherence scale is available at www.annafreud.org/training/mentalization-based-treatment-training/mbt-adherence-scale/.

The scale is based on six core domains of MBT—sessional structure, not-knowing stance, mentalizing process, nonmentalizing modes, affect and interpersonal and significant events, and relational mentalizing. The clinician is rated on the frequency of interventions used within each domain, as well as the extensiveness of that work and skill level. Adherence to MBT requires the clinician to work in all domains flexibly. It is the unique combination of the interventions that makes MBT.

Most clinicians adapt formal models of psychotherapy to their own contexts and personal comfort zone of therapy. This is true for MBT. The adherence scale can identify which domains of therapy a clinician works in more frequently. For example, some clinicians focus primarily on affects related to significant events, which forms part of MBT, but when doing so, clinicians do not use a not-knowing stance but instead use a problem-solving approach. So, this is partial implementation of the model. In addition, it is arguable that a range of techniques other than those used in MBT target mentalizing.

Clinical Implementation

Improvement in mentalizing, we would argue, may be of value to any treatment modality (Bateman et al. 2017). In the case of BPD, for example, there is some evidence that improvements in reflective function are a mechanism of change in effective therapies (Levy et al. 2006) regardless of modality. MBT is explicit in its focus on mentalizing and its use of methods to support a more robust and balanced mentalizing capacity, but there are ways that any clinician can introduce a stronger emphasis on supporting mentalizing in treatment. Key to any attempt to do so is an understanding of the mentalizing stance (described above)—an attitude and approach to therapy that may be adopted by any practicing clinician. Similarly, rewinding to the point at which mentalizing collapsed and working to identify and revisit what each different player's thoughts and beliefs were at that moment can be a useful technique for any clinician seeking to encourage mentalizing. Key to the mentalizing approach, however, whatever the background of the clinician, is the idea that this is at its core an attitude rather than an imposition of mentalizing set pieces. Heavy-handed and overt mentalizing in relation to a patient who is not at that moment able to mentalize efficiently, particularly if he or she is in a state of heightened affect, is antithetical to the mentalizing approach. Rather, the mentalizing stance insists on a nondogmatic and respectful curiosity about the patient's current state. Elements of MBT that can be implemented in everyday practice are shown in Table 5–1.

TABLE 5-1. Elements of the treatment that can be easily implemented in everyday practice

---

- Integration of family and individual work
- Formulation and crisis planning to include mentalizing problems
- Not-knowing stance to explore patient experiences
- Empathic validation of the patient's internal states
- Contextualization of emotions
- Actively managing therapy process
- Identifying nonmentalizing modes

Conclusion

MBT-A has been evaluated in RCTs and found to be an effective treatment for borderline personality pathology in adolescence and has been shown to reduce self-harm and suicidality. MBT-A builds on neuroscientific research indicating that there are particular developmental vulnerabilities that compromise the capacity for balanced mentalizing in adolescents and postulates that young people who self-harm may benefit from particular support in relation to their mentalizing capacities. The MBT-A model understands the risk of self-harm and suicidality increases at moments of breakdown in mentalizing, in which the nonmentalizing modes emerge. In order to maintain some form of self coherence in the face of these difficulties, the alien self can arise, and it is at such moments that the individual is particularly vulnerable. As well as focusing on the young person's own capacity for mentalizing, the MBT-A approach is strongly informed by a relational perspective and the view that a mentalizing environment is crucial in helping to support and restore balanced mentalizing in a vulnerable young person. As a result, working with the family or system around the young person is a significant component of the approach.

Resource for Additional Training

Information on training in MBT-A can be found on the Anna Freud National Centre for Children and Families Web site: www.annafreud.org/training/ mentalization-based-treatment-training/mbt-a-training-programme/

Suggested Readings

Bateman AW, Fonagy P: Mentalization-Based Treatment for Personality Disorders: A Practical Guide. Oxford, UK, Oxford University Press, 2016

Fonagy P, Rossouw T, Sharp C, et al: Mentalization-based treatment for adolescents with borderline traits, in Handbook of Borderline Personality Disorder in Children and Adolescents. Edited by Sharp C, Tackett JL. New York, Springer, 2014, pp 313–332

References

Asen E, Fonagy P: Mentalization-based family therapy, in Handbook of Mentalizing in Mental Health Practice. Edited by Bateman AW, Fonagy P. Arlington, VA, American Psychiatric Publishing, 2012a, pp 107–128

Asen E, Fonagy P: Mentalization-based therapeutic interventions for families. J Fam Ther 34:347–370, 2012b

Asen E, Fonagy P: Mentalizing family violence part 1: conceptual framework. Fam Process 56(1):6–21, 2017a 27861799

Asen E, Fonagy P: Mentalizing family violence part 2: techniques and interventions. Fam Process 56(1):22–44, 2017b 28133724

Bateman A, Fonagy P: Effectiveness of partial hospitalization in the treatment of borderline personality disorder: a randomized controlled trial. Am J Psychiatry 156(10):1563–1569, 1999 10518167

Bateman A, Fonagy P: Treatment of borderline personality disorder with psychoanalytically oriented partial hospitalization: an 18-month follow-up. Am J Psychiatry 158(1):36–42, 2001 11136631

Bateman A, Fonagy P: 8-year follow-up of patients treated for borderline personality disorder: mentalization-based treatment versus treatment as usual. Am J Psychiatry 165(5):631–638, 2008 18347003

Bateman A, Fonagy P: Randomized controlled trial of outpatient mentalization-based treatment versus structured clinical management for borderline personality disorder. Am J Psychiatry 166(12):1355–1364, 2009 19833787

Bateman A, Fonagy P: Impact of clinical severity on outcomes of mentalisation-based treatment for borderline personality disorder. Br J Psychiatry 203(3):221–227, 2013 23887998

Bateman A, Fonagy P: Mentalization-Based Treatment for Personality Disorders: A Practical Guide. Oxford, UK, Oxford University Press, 2016

Bateman A, Campbell C, Luyten P, et al: A mentalization-based approach to common factors in the treatment of borderline personality disorder. Curr Opin Psychol 21:44–49, 2017 28985628

Bateman AW, Fonagy P (eds): Handbook of Mentalizing in Mental Health Practice. Washington, DC, American Psychiatric Publishing, 2012

Blakemore SJ: Development of the social brain in adolescence. J R Soc Med 105(3):111–116, 2012 22434810

Blakemore SJ, Mills KL: Is adolescence a sensitive period for sociocultural processing? Annu Rev Psychol 65:187–207, 2014 24016274

Bo S, Sharp C, Beck E, et al: First empirical evaluation of outcomes for mentalization-based group therapy for adolescents with BPD. Pers Disord 8(4):396–401, 2017 27845526

Bowlby J: Attachment and Loss, Vol 1: Attachment. London, Hogarth Press and Institute of Psycho-Analysis, 1969

Brent DA, McMakin DL, Kennard BD, et al: Protecting adolescents from self-harm: a critical review of intervention studies. J Am Acad Child Adolesc Psychiatry 52(12):1260–1271, 2013 24290459

Crone EA, Dahl RE: Understanding adolescence as a period of social-affective engagement and goal flexibility. Nat Rev Neurosci 13(9):636–650, 2012 22903221

Csibra G, Gergely G: Natural pedagogy. Trends Cogn Sci 13(4):148–153, 2009 19285912

Dumontheil I, Apperly IA, Blakemore SJ: Online usage of theory of mind continues to develop in late adolescence. Dev Sci 13(2):331–338, 2010 20136929

Esposito-Smythers C, Spirito A, Kahler CW, et al: Treatment of co-occurring substance abuse and suicidality among adolescents: a randomized trial. J Consult Clin Psychol 79(6):728–739, 2011 22004303

Fonagy P, Allison E: The role of mentalizing and epistemic trust in the therapeutic relationship. Psychotherapy (Chic) 51(3):372–380, 2014 24773092

Fonagy P, Bateman A: Attachment, mentalization, and borderline personality disorder. European Psychotherapy 8:35–47, 2008a

Fonagy P, Bateman A: The development of borderline personality disorder—a mentalizing model. J Pers Disord 22(1):4–21, 2008b 18312120

Fonagy P, Luyten P: A developmental, mentalization-based approach to the understanding and treatment of borderline personality disorder. Dev Psychopathol 21(4):1355–1381, 2009 19825272

Fonagy P, Luyten P: A multilevel perspective on the development of borderline personality disorder, in Developmental Psychopathology, Vol 3: Risk, Disorder, and Adaptation, 3rd Edition. Edited by Cicchetti D. New York, Wiley, 2016, pp 726–792

Fonagy P, Gergely G, Jurist E, et al: Affect Regulation, Mentalization, and the Development of the Self. New York, Other Press, 2002

Fonagy P, Rossouw T, Sharp C, et al: Mentalization-based treatment for adolescents with borderline traits, in Handbook of Borderline Personality Disorder in Children and Adolescents. Edited by Sharp C, Tackett JL. New York, Springer, 2014, pp 313–332

Fonagy P, Luyten P, Allison E: Epistemic petrification and the restoration of epistemic trust: a new conceptualization of borderline personality disorder and its psychosocial treatment. J Pers Disord 29(5):575–609, 2015a 26393477

Fonagy P, Speranza M, Luyten P, et al: ESCAP Expert Article: borderline personality disorder in adolescence: an expert research review with implications for clinical practice. Eur Child Adolesc Psychiatry 24(11):1307–1320, 2015b 26271454

Fonagy P, Luyten P, Allison E, et al: What we have changed our minds about: Part 1. Borderline personality disorder as a limitation of resilience. Borderline Personal Disorder Emotion Dysregul 4:11, 2017a 28413687

Fonagy P, Luyten P, Allison E, et al: What we have changed our minds about: Part 2. Borderline personality disorder, epistemic trust and the developmental significance of social communication. Borderline Personal Disorder Emotion Dysregul 4:9, 2017b 28405338

Gergely G, Unoka Z: Attachment and mentalization in humans: the development of the affective self, in Mind to Mind: Infant Research, Neuroscience, and Psychoanalysis. Edited by Jurist EL, Slade A, Bergner S. New York, Other Press, 2008, pp 50–87

Gergely G, Watson JS: The social biofeedback theory of parental affect-mirroring: the development of emotional self-awareness and self-control in infancy. Int J Psychoanal 77(Pt 6):1181–1212, 1996 9119582

Hutsebaut J, Bales DL, Busschbach JJ, et al: The implementation of mentalization-based treatment for adolescents: a case study from an organizational, team and therapist perspective. Int J Ment Health Syst 6(1):10, 2012 22818166

Kim S, Fonagy P, Allen J, et al: Mothers who are securely attached in pregnancy show more attuned infant mirroring 7 months postpartum. Infant Behav Dev 37(4):491–504, 2014 25020112

Laurenssen EM, Hutsebaut J, Feenstra DJ, et al: Feasibility of mentalization-based treatment for adolescents with borderline symptoms: a pilot study. Psychotherapy (Chic) 51(1):159–166, 2014 24059741

Levy KN, Meehan KB, Kelly KM, et al: Change in attachment patterns and reflective function in a randomized control trial of transference-focused psychotherapy for borderline personality disorder. J Consult Clin Psychol 74(6):1027–1040, 2006 17154733

Lieberman MD: Social cognitive neuroscience: a review of core processes. Annu Rev Psychol 58:259–289, 2007 17002553

Luyten P, Malcorps S, Fonagy P, Ensink K: Assessment of mentalizing, in Handbook of Mentalizing in Mental Health Practice, 2nd Edition. Edited by Bateman AW, Fonagy P. Washington, DC, American Psychiatric Association Publishing (in press)

Mills KL, Lalonde F, Clasen LS, et al: Developmental changes in the structure of the social brain in late childhood and adolescence. Soc Cogn Affect Neurosci 9(1):123–131, 2014 23051898

Rossouw TI: The use of mentalization-based treatment for adolescents (MBT-A) with a young woman with mixed personality disorder and tendencies to self-harm. J Clin Psychol 71(2):178–187, 2015 25604636

Rossouw T: Metalization-based therapy for adolescents: managing storms in youth presenting with self-harm and suicidal states, in Handbook of Attachment-Based Interventions. Edited by Steele H, Steele M. New York, Guilford, 2018, pp 419–440

Rossouw TI, Fonagy P: Mentalization-based treatment for self-harm in adolescents: a randomized controlled trial. J Am Acad Child Adolesc Psychiatry 51(12):1304–1313.e3, 2012 23200287

Sharp C, Williams LL, Ha C, et al: The development of a mentalization-based outcomes and research protocol for an adolescent inpatient unit. Bull Menninger Clin 73(4):311–338, 2009 20025427

Wilkinson P, Kelvin R, Roberts C, et al: Clinical and psychosocial predictors of suicide attempts and nonsuicidal self-injury in the Adolescent Depression Antidepressants and Psychotherapy Trial (ADAPT). Am J Psychiatry 168(5):495–501, 2011 21285141

Cognitive-Behavioral Therapy for Co-occurring Suicidal Behavior and Substance Use

Christianne Esposito-Smythers, Ph.D.
Anthony Spirito, Ph.D., ABPP
Jennifer Wolff, Ph.D.

Overview of Treatment Approach

Adolescent suicidal behavior and alcohol/other drug (AOD) use disorders both represent significant public health problems. It has been well documented that these behaviors co-occur at high rates among adolescent psychiatric populations (Esposito-Smythers and Spirito 2004; Esposito-Smythers et al. 2016), further increasing mortality risk. Moreover, the strength of this association increases as each problem grows in severity (Esposito-Smythers and Spirito 2004; Goldston 2004). These two behaviors are thought to be functionally interrelated, both temporally and distally (Bagge and Sher 2008). For some, the acute effects of intoxication may increase risk for a suicide attempt via heightened emotional distress, increased aggression, decreased inhibition, provision of perceived "courage" to make an attempt, and/or inability to employ adaptive coping strategies (Hufford 2001). These behaviors may also be distally related to negative consequences (social, academic, and legal), contribute to heightened stress, and trigger/worsen psychiatric symptoms, which, in turn, may increase risk for suicidal thoughts and behavior (STB; Hufford 2001). Thus, interventions that address both STB and AOD use disorders are needed.

Despite the high rates of co-occurrence between suicidal behavior and AODs, these problems are often treated independently by separate therapists. One therapist will address the suicidal behavior, and the other therapist will address the AOD. This approach may lead to suboptimal treatment outcomes resulting from conflicting treatment models, inconsistent treatment messages to families, and lack of coordination of care between providers (Hawkins 2009). It may also lead to a higher treatment burden for families and higher costs, which, in turn, may increase the likelihood of premature care termination (Hawkins 2009). An integrated treatment approach that addresses both STB and AOD use in one treatment protocol may offer greater promise. An integrated approach to care allows ongoing attention to and monitoring of both conditions, use of a consistent therapeutic model, and prioritization of treatment goals. This approach may be particularly useful given that these behaviors share many common precipitants as well as risk and maintaining factors (Goldston 2004).

Integrated cognitive-behavioral therapy (I-CBT) was designed to address adolescent STB *and* AOD use. I-CBT integrates cognitive and behavioral techniques to address adolescent STB and AOD use, as well as common co-occurring conditions that may negatively interfere with treatment of these conditions (e.g., depression, conduct disorder). In this sense, I-CBT is a transdiagnostic protocol; that is, it is designed to accommodate, rather than exclude, adolescents with comorbid psychiatric disorders. I-CBT also includes a motivational enhancement session, and motivational interviewing techniques intertwined throughout sessions, to improve motivation for change and treatment engagement as needed.

I-CBT is manualized and modular with a menu of sessions to choose from that allows for tailoring of the protocol to each adolescent and his or her family. I-CBT incorporates "core" adolescent skill modules to address skill deficits common to STB, AOD use, and common comorbid conditions. It also includes "supplemental" skill modules that are used, as needed, to address emergent crises and other less commonly presenting problems (e.g., grief over loss of loved one, impulsive aggression). Acknowledging that adolescents exist within multiple systems (family, peer, school) and that dysfunction within these systems prevents optimal treatment gains, this intervention contains modules for cognitive-behavioral individual therapy, cognitive-behavioral family therapy, and behavioral parent training. Coordination of services across providers (e.g., psychiatrists, pediatricians) and settings (e.g., schools) is also conducted.

Theoretical Model and Proposed Mechanism of Change

I-CBT primarily draws from social-cognitive learning theory (Bandura 1986, 1999). According to social-cognitive learning theory, human behavior is based in part on previous learning experiences, especially social and interpersonal behaviors (e.g., communication, problem solving) and central or core thoughts and beliefs (e.g., expectancies for control/competence, beliefs about oneself/others). Mental health problems, including STB and AOD use, are believed to result, in part, from faulty learning experiences and are reflected in maladaptive cognitions and behaviors. I-CBT combines cognitive processing and behavior change methods to modify clinical symptoms associated with adolescent STB, AOD use, and comorbid mental health conditions. Specifically, I-CBT targets common underlying vulnerabilities associated with STB, AOD use, and comorbid conditions, such as cognitive distortions, coping skills deficits, affect regulation deficits, and problematic social behaviors to remediate symptoms. Below is a brief review of the literature that links these vulnerabilities to both STB and AOD use.

Cognitive Distortions

Cognitive distortions have been found to underlie both AOD use and STB, although the content of these distortions may vary. Within the AOD literature, positive alcohol and drug expectancies (e.g., belief that alcohol or drugs are associated with enhancement of social behavior, sexual behavior, positive arousal, and/or relaxation) have been shown to contribute to the initiation, quantity, frequency, and relapse of AOD use as well as maintenance of social networks that are supportive of AOD use (Aas et al. 1998; Homish and Leonard 2008; Schafer and Brown 1991). With regard to STB, cognitive distortions in the form of cognitive processing errors (e.g., catastrophizing, personalization, selective abstraction, overgeneralization) and the tendency to exhibit a negative view of oneself have been linked to STB (Brent et al. 1990). A negative view of the future, or hopelessness, in particular, has been shown to have traitlike (i.e., stable or enduring) properties (Goldston et al. 2006) and to be predictive of repeat suicide attempts and eventual death by suicide (Brown et al. 2000; Goldston et al. 2001). Related to these cognitive distortions are negative automatic thoughts that tend to involve themes of personal loss and failure (Beck et al. 1987). Individuals who experience persistent thoughts of loss and failure may contemplate suicide as a means to escape their psychological distress. Psychoeducation and cognitive-restructuring skills may be a particularly helpful tool in remediating irrational and unhelpful beliefs that may drive STB and AOD use.

Coping Skills

Individuals with STB and AOD use also report poor coping skills (Galaif et al. 2007; Wills et al. 2001). Problem-focused coping (i.e., direct efforts to alter or remove a stressor) has been linked to lower levels of both AOD use and related problems (Wills et al. 1999, 2001) and suicidal behavior (Curry et al. 1992). In contrast, emotion-focused coping (i.e., managing negative emotion related to the problem) has been associated with higher levels of AOD-related problems (Wills et al. 1999, 2001) and STB (Spirito et al. 1989). Whereas emotion-focused coping may be helpful when managing short-term uncontrollable stressors, it is typically less effective for managing enduring controllable stressors (Wills et al. 1999). Individuals may indiscriminately use emotion-focused strategies without evaluating whether the stressor is controllable (Wills et al. 1999). AOD use and suicidal behavior may be used by some to relieve stress or escape distress resulting from the unsuccessful resolution of enduring stressors. Through problem-solving training, individuals may learn how to increase cognitive flexibility as well as identify and evaluate multiple options to deal with stressors.

Affect Dysregulation

Affect dysregulation has been defined as the inability to cope with heightened levels of emotion. Individuals who abuse substances (Brook et al.

1995) and/or engage in suicidal behavior (Esposito et al. 2003; Gonzalez et al. 2009) report a reduced capacity to regulate their internal states and may use healthy affect regulation skills less frequently relative to nonsymptomatic individuals. STB and AOD use may temporarily reduce intolerable emotional states (Colder and Stice 1998; Zlotnick et al. 1997). Teaching affect regulation skills, such as identification and monitoring of emotions, deep breathing, progressive muscle relaxation, and guided imagery, may all be helpful in this regard (Spirito and Esposito-Smythers 2012). Use of coping statements (as an extension of cognitive restructuring) may also be useful in helping adolescents calm themselves when distressed.

Social Behavior

Families of adolescents who engage in STB and use AODs report many of the same problems, including high parent-child/family conflict, low family cohesion, and poor family communication (Hufford 2001; Simons-Morton et al. 1999; Wagner et al. 2003; Windle and Davies 1999). The relationship between family dysfunction and mental health problems is likely reciprocal in nature. Although family dysfunction may initially serve as one trigger for STB and AOD use, it is likely maintained and/or worsened by the consequences (e.g., more conflict, loss of trust) of STB and AOD use (Trulsson and Hedin 2004). Therefore, interventions that incorporate family members can be beneficial when adolescents report a high degree of family dysfunction. Strong and supportive family relationships can play a significant role in recovery from both STB and AOD use (Brent et al. 2013; Williams and Chang 2000).

Having peers who use AODs has been linked to adolescent AOD use and predicts negative treatment outcome (Brook et al. 1995; Latimer et al. 2000). Low peer support, high peer rejection, and the interpersonal influence of suicidal friends has been associated with STB (Leslie et al. 2002; Prinstein et al. 2000). Therefore, helping youth who lack healthy peer relationships to develop prosocial peer support networks, spend time with prosocial peers, and manage unhealthy relationships can be an important part of intervention work. It can also help decrease social withdrawal commonly experienced by depressed and suicidal youth. Equally important is individual work with the parents of these adolescents, including psychoeducation about warning signs and ways to manage suspected AOD use and STB. Training in parental monitoring skills, problem solving, communication, and contingency management may be necessary to discourage adolescents from engaging in AOD use with peers.

Because many adolescents are not likely to view their alcohol and drug use as problematic and/or may be ambivalent about changing their use (Tevyaw and Monti 2004), I-CBT includes a one-session motivational enhancement interview that combines a collaborative, nonjudgmental, and empathic therapeutic style (Miller and Rollnick 2013) with personal feedback regarding drinking patterns and associated effects. In addition, short scripts containing motivational interviewing techniques targeting AOD use are interwoven into the beginning of treatment sessions and used as necessary by therapists. For example, if the therapist were planning to conduct a problem-solving session based on a manifesting problem in the prior session but at the check-in the adolescent reports AOD use, then the therapist elicits information on quantity/frequency of use, context of use, and consequences related to AOD use. Then, using a motivational interviewing style, the therapist encourages the adolescent to generate pros and cons associated with using AODs, especially with respect to risk for STB. If the adolescent is unable to generate cons, the therapist asks the adolescent for permission to share his or her concerns. The therapist also addresses actions that the adolescent could take if placed in a situation where AOD use is a possibility. Following is a sample script:

> So, tell me more about your alcohol/drug use this past week. What do you think about using alcohol/drugs while at increased suicide risk? What are some things that may not be so good about using alcohol/drugs while at risk for suicide? May I share some concerns that I have? How would you feel about spending a few minutes talking about things that you could do if faced with the same situation? Whether or not you use the strategies we discuss is completely up to you. It is your choice.

If this review seems effective, then the therapist can move on to the module that was going to be reviewed with the adolescent, in this case, problem solving. If AOD use remains a significant or unresolved issue, then the therapist may choose AOD use as the topic for discussion in the problem-solving module or may choose to replace problem solving with an AOD use–specific module, such as AOD refusal skills or the full motivational enhancement session.

Given the high rates of treatment dropout among families of youth with STB and AOD use alike (Crits-Christoph and Siqueland 1996;

Spirito et al. 2002) and poorer long-term outcomes associated with premature treatment termination (Moos and Moos 2003), I-CBT also includes a one-session parental motivational interview designed to improve treatment engagement. This session addresses motivational and practical obstacles (e.g., transportation, scheduling difficulties) that impede treatment adherence.

Review of Empirical Evidence

Comprehensive reviews of the adolescent treatment literature suggest that cognitive-behavioral approaches show promise in the treatment of youth suicidal behavior and AOD use disorders (Glenn et al. 2015; Hogue et al. 2014). I-CBT has been tested in one randomized clinical trial (Esposito-Smythers et al. 2011). Modified versions of the I-CBT protocol, with different inclusion criteria, have been tested in clinical trials with juvenile court, psychiatric inpatient, and home-based intensive outpatient samples, respectively. Analyses for these trials are underway. In our clinical trial (Esposito-Smythers et al. 2011), I-CBT was compared with enhanced standard care (ESC). Adolescents in both conditions received case management and medication management through study staff as needed. The same study child psychiatrist prescribed medications across both arms. Participants included 40 adolescents recruited from a psychiatric inpatient unit and a parent(s)/guardian(s) (herein referred to as parents). Inclusion criteria included clinically significant suicidal ideation in the prior month or a suicide attempt in the last 3 months and a co-occurring AOD use disorder (37% alcohol abuse, 28% alcohol dependence, 29% marijuana abuse, 54% marijuana dependence disorders). All adolescents reported suicidal ideation at baseline, and 75% reported a history of a suicide attempt (43% had multiple attempts). Adolescents also had multiple co-occurring psychiatric disorders (86% major depressive, 17% generalized anxiety, 34% social anxiety, 20% posttraumatic stress, and 34% conduct disorders).

Although adolescents in the I-CBT protocol received a greater dose of treatment, it did not have an effect on outcomes. The number of treatment sessions attended was not significantly associated with any dependent variable in study analyses. Adolescents in the I-CBT protocol who completed the equivalent of at least an adequate dose of outpatient treatment (24 adolescent sessions and 12 parent sessions) were defined as treatment completers. Approximately 74% of adolescents, 90% of parents, or 74% of families (mean $(M) = 34.3$ sessions, range $= 11$–48) in I-CBT were treatment completers. Using these same criteria, approximately 44% of adolescents, 25% of parents, or 19% of families $(M = 19.9$ sessions, range $= 0$–41) in ESC would be considered treatment completers.

I-CBT relative to ESC was associated with significantly fewer suicide attempts (5.3% vs. 35.3%), rehospitalizations (15.8% vs. 52.9%), and emergency department visits (15.8% vs. 58.8%) from baseline through 18 months. Moreover, three participants in ESC were placed in residential care compared with none in I-CBT. Those in I-CBT also reported significantly greater reductions in heavy drinking days (more than 50% reduction in the number of heavy drinking days), marijuana use days (more than 60% reduction in the number of marijuana use days), and marijuana-related problems over time relative to ESC. Adolescents across conditions showed comparable reductions in suicidal ideation, drinking days, and alcohol-related problems. In supplemental analyses, fewer adolescents in I-CBT relative to ESC retained an AOD use disorder by 18-month follow-up (26.7% vs. 76.5%). Furthermore, although not statistically significant due in part to the small sample size in subgroups analyses, adolescents receiving I-CBT relative to ESC had less mood (6.7% vs. 31.3%), disruptive behavior (0% vs. 40.0%), and anxiety (30.0% vs. 66.7%) disorders at 18 months, with medium to large effect sizes found.

Treatment Components and Primary Intervention Strategies

The I-CBT protocol contains modules for individual adolescent sessions, parent sessions, and family sessions. Two therapists are assigned to each case, one that conducts the individual adolescent sessions and one that conducts the parent training and family sessions (although the adolescent therapist also attends and participates in family sessions). As can be seen in Table 6–1, some adolescent sessions are "core" sessions (e.g., problem solving, cognitive restructuring, affect regulation) that all adolescents receive, and others are "supplemental" and only used as needed (e.g., chain analysis for dangerous behavior). Although there is no designation of core or supplemental parent and family sessions, most of the parent and family sessions listed in Table 6–1 are needed and used with families treated in this protocol. All sessions are 60 minutes in length, with the exception of the introduction to treatment and the motivational enhancement sessions, which are 90 minutes.

All sessions follow the same standard CBT format. They begin with a medication adherence check if applicable, followed by an assessment of mood, STB, and AOD use since the last session. Adolescents also complete the Beck Scale for Suicidal Ideation (Beck et al. 1997) at the start of every session, which allows the therapist to closely track severity of suicidal ideation over the course of treatment and adjust the treatment plan accordingly, consistent with a measurement-based care model (Shimokawa et al. 2010). The adolescent or parent/guardian is then asked to identify agenda items, homework from the prior session is reviewed, a new skill is introduced or a previously taught skill reviewed, the skill is practiced, and agenda items are discussed. The optimal goal of the session is to incorporate skills learned previously in treatment in order to address the designated problem. Worksheets and handouts for each skill are used to assist in the learning process. Individual sessions typically conclude with a brief conjoint meeting with the adolescent, parent(s), and both therapists. This check-in includes a review of the skills learned and positive praise for the hard work accomplished. Finally, the parent and adolescent are assigned a personalized homework assignment at the end of each session to facilitate practice of a particular skill.

If an adolescent comes to a therapy session and, by therapist observation, is considered to be under the influence of AODs, the session is rescheduled. Adolescents also receive a 10-panel urine drug screen at the start of every session to corroborate self-report of substance use and discourage substance substitution. Positive marijuana screens are not shared with parents during approximately the first month of treatment to allow time for marijuana to clear the system and for the adolescent to build motivation/skills to abstain. After that time, results are shared with parents in a therapeutic (nonpunitive) manner, and results of screens are integrated into treatment (e.g., via contingency management sessions). Positive screens for other drugs are shared (e.g., cocaine, heroin) to ensure the safety of the adolescent. This information is clearly stated in the consent forms as well as the introduction to treatment session so that all parties are fully aware of this procedure.

I-CBT includes a 6-month acute (adolescents attend weekly, parents weekly to biweekly), a 3-month continuation (adolescent attends biweekly,

TABLE 6-1. Overview of treatment modules in integrated cognitive-behavioral therapy (I-CBT)

Name of session	Type	Objective
Introduction to treatment	F	Introduce treatment program, enhance engagement, set goals, safety planning
Problem solving	A, P, F	Generate and evaluate options to problems and identify the most effective solution
Cognitive restructuring	A, P	Understand link between thoughts and feelings; identify and dispute untrue or unhelpful beliefs
Affect regulation	A, P	Learn triggers and signs of affect arousal and develop coping plan
Relaxation	A	Decrease stress through deep breathing and progressive muscle relaxation
Healthy pleasant events	A	Increase frequency of healthy non-substance-related pleasant activities
Increasing social support	A	Identify supporters and learn how to increase support/add new supporters
Assertiveness training	A	Understand communication styles and learn assertive communication skills
Skill practice	A, P, F	Practice applying previously learned skills to current problem
Motivational interview	A	Improve motivation for change around substance use via exploration and resolution of ambivalence
Coping with cravings	A	Become aware of triggers for urges to use substances and learn coping strategies
Refusal skills	A	Improve communication skills needed to effectively refuse offers to use substances
Planning for emergencies	A	Identify unanticipated situations that place teen at risk for poor decisions and develop a coping plan
Parental monitoring	P	Learn to monitor teen behaviors, activities, and friends to help prevent teen substance use
Positive attending	P	Learn to recognize and praise teen for good behaviors

TABLE 6-1. Overview of treatment modules in integrated cognitive-behavioral therapy (I-CBT) *(continued)*

Name of session	Type	Objective
Contingency management	P, F	Learn limit setting and how to set up rewards and consequences to help change teen problem behavior
Family communication	F	Learn and practice positive family communication skills
Positive family interactions	F	Identify strengths in each family member and the family as a whole to improve family attachment
Progress/skill review	A	Practice applying multiple previously learned skills to current problem and review treatment progress
Relapse prevention	F	Review treatment progress, recommendations, prevention plan, and conclude treatment
Guided imagery	*A	Decrease stress and improve relaxation via use of guided imagery
Chain analysis	*A	Identify and address sequence of thoughts, feelings, and behaviors that precede suicidal behavior
Grief	*A	Learn normal grief symptoms, share narrative, and dispute beliefs that prevent healing
Managing aggression I	*A	Address affective arousal that precedes aggressive behavior
Managing aggression II	*A	Address thoughts and behaviors that precede aggressive behavior

Note.   *A=supplemental adolescent session used as needed; A=adolescent session; F=family session; P=parent session.

parents biweekly to monthly), and a 3-month maintenance (adolescent and parents attend monthly) treatment phase. Frequency of sessions may be increased for purposes of stabilization. During the acute phase of treatment, core skills are taught and practiced. The treatment introduction session for adolescents and parents, as described below, sets the stage for the I-CBT protocol. The next few adolescent sessions are primarily geared toward addressing triggers for STB to stabilize adolescents upon entrance into treatment. More specifically, these sessions teach adolescents the skills needed to control emotional outbursts, improve decision-making skills, and clarify thought processes so that they are less likely to engage in suicidal and other high-risk behaviors, including AOD use. AOD-specific sessions can be interjected into this sequence as clinically indicated, particularly when adolescents become suicidal under the influence of substances or are using substances in ways that endanger their safety (e.g., binge drinking, blackouts, high-risk behavior when intoxicated). A motivational enhancement interview is typically the first AOD-specific session that is administered to improve readiness to change AOD use. During this interview, adolescents are educated about the association between AOD use and STB as well as other negative effects of AOD use on treatment outcome.

Parent sessions typically begin with a motivational enhancement interview around treatment adherence. Consistent with literature and our collective clinical experience, this session is necessary for parents to fully understand the gravity of their adolescent's clinical condition and the importance of their active involvement in their adolescent's care (e.g., safety planning, monitoring, treatment attendance).

The sequence of other core sessions during the acute phase of treatment for adolescents and parents is flexible, allowing for tailoring of the treatment protocol to each family. "Skill practice" sessions are also included; this allows the therapist to practice any previously learned skills with the adolescent, parent(s), and family at any point in the protocol. These sessions provide therapists with the flexibility to repeat skills as needed and manage crises while staying "in protocol." Please see the "Objective" column in Table 6–1 for the main content covered in each adolescent, parent, and family session. Notably, although there are many sessions included in the I-CBT protocol, most integrate use of the same core skills (e.g., problem solving, cognitive restructuring, affect regulation) to address various problem areas. For example, in the "Increasing social support" session, adolescents use problem solving to help generate options for increasing their support network. Problem solving is also deliberately taught and employed across adolescent, parent, and family sessions in order to provide a common language and skill set for adolescents and parents, allow parents to better support their adolescent in the use of skills, facilitate skill acquisition and generalization, improve ease of training for study therapists, and increase the likelihood of dissemination. In the continuation phase of treatment, existing skills are practiced, and new supplemental sessions may be used as needed. In the maintenance phase, sessions are focused on generalization of skills and relapse prevention.

Consistent with our theoretical model, I-CBT places a particular emphasis on the use of problem-solving, cognitive-restructuring, and affect regulation skills. These core skills are taught to both adolescents and parents, although they are used to improve parenting skills when administered to parents. They are augmented with other skills selected by the therapist to best address the needs of each unique family. Safety planning is another key technique for reducing risk, primarily for suicidal behavior (Brent et al. 2009), but in the I–CBT protocol, it is also used to reduce risky AOD use.

Overview Session and Safety Plan

The first session is devoted to rapport building, safety planning, an overview of the treatment approach, and initial goal setting. During the first 45 minutes, adolescents and parents meet alone with their respective therapists to allow time for rapport building, "sharing their story," and expressing their feelings in a safe place. Some time is then spent conducting a safety check-in and on safety planning. After the safety check-in in the adolescent session, the therapist works with the adolescent to develop a reasons-to-live list. Specifically, the adolescent is asked to generate at least five reasons to live (e.g., family, friends, long-term goals, enjoyable activities) and write them on a worksheet. Then the adolescent completes a safety plan template that includes components of those developed by Brent and Poling (2011) and Stanley and Brown (2012). The adolescent begins by identifying warning signs of distress including physiological signs and behaviors (e.g., physical tension, isolating, irritable responses) that signal the need to use the safety plan. Adaptive coping strategies for decreasing distress are listed (e.g., listen to music, go for a walk, talk with a friend), and support persons are identified. The safety plan also lists trusted adults to ask for help and numbers to contact in an emergency. Safety plans are written out and regularly revisited and updated throughout therapy.

In the parent session, parents also complete a safety check-in with regard to their adolescent's behavior. The therapist then discusses how to make the home environment safe, including removing access to lethal means (e.g., medications, firearms, sharp objects, alcohol, drugs), monitoring the adolescent to promote safety, obtaining needed services in case of an emergency, and providing a stable and supportive home environment (e.g., avoid heated arguments).

The adolescent, parent, and both therapists then come together for the second half of the introductory session. The safety plans are reviewed together, and introductory material is presented. This material includes an overview of the treatment protocol, compliance enhancement procedures (e.g., review of expectations for treatment, problem solving around any barriers to treatment attendance), and a discussion about CBT and how it works. Each family member is then asked to identify individual, family, school/work, peer, and any other goals they would like to address in therapy. Each family member shares their goals, and the therapist helps identify how they might be addressed using skills in the I-CBT protocol.

Problem Solving

Often adolescents who are suicidal and use AODs evidence deficits in problem solving, such as limited flexibility, difficulty generating alternative solutions, and limited ability to identify positive consequences of potential solutions. The therapist begins the problem-solving module by helping the adolescent generate a list of problems (typically two to five) that trigger the targeted maladaptive behavior (e.g., suicide attempt, AOD use). Next, the therapist teaches the adolescent a problem-solving skill that can be used to help address these problems. Our protocol uses the acronym "SOLVE" to cover the basic steps in problem solving. Each letter in the word SOLVE stands for a different step of the problem-solving process: S stands for "select a problem," O for "generate options," L for rate the "likely outcome" of each option, V for choose the "very best option," and E stands for "evaluate" how well each option worked.

The adolescent and therapist go methodically through the SOLVE system together in relation to the identified problem (e.g., breakup with a boyfriend/girlfriend). Problems that trigger STBs are targeted first, although often the same problems also trigger AOD use. Adolescents are taught how to clearly define the problem in a manner that can be effectively addressed (e.g., "how to" cope with a breakup). The therapist then helps the adolescent brainstorm all possible options he or she can think of to address the problem. Notably, a suicide attempt and AOD use may be listed along with other options the adolescent has tried in the past. Next, the adolescent and therapist evaluate the pros and cons of each option. High-risk behaviors (such as suicide attempts and AOD use) should be fleshed out in detail to ensure that the adolescent thinks through the pros and cons of these options, guiding the adolescent to see how the cons outweigh the pros for these behaviors. Openly discussing these pros and cons helps the therapist to understand some of the factors that contributed to the selection of these options in the past. It is important to note the differences between short- and long-term pros and cons. For example, cutting or using substances may provide some temporary relief, but in the long term, there may be additional consequences to these behaviors that should be discussed. Based on these pros and cons, the adolescent should pick the very best option (or combination of options) for solving the problem. After the adolescent evaluates how well the solution(s) will work, the therapist may need to do additional problem solving or troubleshooting to help the adolescent address any barriers to the solution.

At the end of the session, the therapist reframes suicidal behavior as a failure in problem solving. The therapist explains that people often feel "stuck" if they do not have helpful and safe options for resolving difficult problems, and thus they may choose unsafe options, such as suicide attempts or AOD use.

Cognitive Restructuring

The goal of the cognitive-restructuring session is to help adolescents identify negative automatic thoughts and generate alternative rational and helpful thoughts. We use the ABCDE acronym to help adolescents remember the steps in our cognitive-restructuring method. We introduce this method as a skill that helps adolescents deal with negative beliefs or thoughts that may arise when they experience problems. The experience of negative thoughts is normalized for the adolescent, but it is noted that these thoughts become problematic when they occur too frequently. This is typically what happens when suicidal thoughts or urges to drink/use substances emerge. Adolescents are guided to address and change irrational and/or unhelpful thoughts through the "ABCDE method." "A" represents the activating event or trigger. For an adolescent with a history of a suicide attempt, this would be the event that primarily triggered the attempt. "B" stands for beliefs or thoughts that automatically come into the adolescent's mind after the triggering event. "C" stands for the consequences or emotions that follow the beliefs (e.g., sad, guilty, angry). "D" stands for dispute. In this step, the adolescent generates alternative statements that they can say to themselves. Finally, "E" stands for the effect of using this skill, which is typically that the adolescent feels somewhat better.

After explaining the rationale for the skill and the steps involved in disputing negative automatic thoughts, the therapist helps the adolescent practice using the skill. In the first cognitive-restructuring session, the therapist practices the ABCDE method using the primary suicide attempt precipitant as the activating event (the same one used in the former problem-solving session). The adolescent lists the beliefs and feelings associated with this event, and the therapist helps him or her to dispute irrational and unhelpful beliefs. When teaching the adolescent to dispute, we ask the adolescent to begin by asking himself or herself two simple questions regarding beliefs surrounding a negative activating event: 1) "Is this belief true?" And if it is true, 2) "Is this belief helpful?" The adolescent is also presented with a list of cognitive distortions (e.g., black/white thinking, predicting the worst, missing the positive, misconstruing feelings as facts, jumping to conclusions, expecting perfection; Beck et al. 1979), which we have adapted to include simpler language and call "thinking mistakes." We ask the adolescent if he or she can identify any thinking mistakes in his or her beliefs that can aid in the development of disputes. After the adolescent generates a list of disputes, the therapist helps the adolescent evaluate the effect or outcome of creating disputes for the irrational and/or unhelpful automatic beliefs originally identified. It is acknowledged that the adolescent will never feel "happy" about the fact that the negative activating event occurred. However, by viewing the event in a more rational and helpful way, the adolescent may experience some relief from distress and negative emotion. Time is also spent discussing the possibility that the automatic thoughts that the adolescent experienced around the negative activating event played a role in the decision to make a suicide attempt.

Thus, learning the ABCDE method helps decrease future risk for suicidal behavior.

Affect Regulation

The affect regulation session helps adolescents recognize the warning signs for intense negative emotions and develop a list of coping statements and strategies to feel better. First, the adolescent identifies the negative emotion that he or she would like to address. In the first affect regulation session, this is typically the emotion most strongly associated with suicidal behavior that was identified in the cognitive-restructuring session. The therapist then helps the adolescent to identify the physical sensations and behaviors or "body talk" that accompany that emotion (aided by a worksheet that lists common physiological sensations and behaviors that occur when one is upset). Automatic thoughts associated with worsening of the emotion are also identified. The therapist then presents a "feelings thermometer" that labels the targeted emotion and offers an intensity rating (with open lines by each rating) on a 1–10 scale. The adolescent assigns each physiological and behavioral symptom previously identified, as well as negative automatic thoughts, to the numbers indicating increasing intensities of the thermometer. Next, the adolescent is asked to indicate his or her personal "danger zone" on the thermometer, or the point where his or her body spirals so far out of control that he or she is at risk for unsafe or suicidal behavior. The importance of recognizing "early" body talk and working on decreasing it before it escalates to the danger zone is discussed. Finally, the adolescent is asked to create a "stay cool" plan to use when he or she begins to notice early body talk and negative beliefs. This includes various self-soothing behaviors and positive self-statements. Finally, the parents are brought into the adolescent's session and briefed on the session content so that they can support the adolescent's coping plan.

Note that although the skills discussed above are typically first taught in relation to problems and emotions associated with STB, this is not mandatory. If the adolescent reports becoming suicidal when drinking/using or drinking/using in a way that seriously endangers his or her life and/or the severity of the adolescent's AOD use problem is much greater than that of his or her current STB, the therapist may choose to teach one or more of these skills in relation to AOD use first. For example, problem solving and cognitive restructuring may be used in relation to a problem that triggers binge drinking. However, as noted above, the problems identified typically trigger both STB and AOD use and thus help address both problems simultaneously. Moreover, repeated practice of these skills leads to skill generalization and thus helps to address a range of mental health problems and high-risk behaviors.

When problem solving, cognitive restructuring, and affect regulation are taught to parents, they are practiced in relation to parenting decisions and behavior. For example, parents may use problem solving to generate solutions for helping their adolescent improve his or her sleep, take prescribed medication, develop relationships with prosocial peers, or decrease arguments at home. Cognitive restructuring is used to address beliefs that get in the way of effective parenting, such as "My adolescent should know what to do," "My adolescent is purposely doing this to hurt me," "I have tried everything—there is nothing more that I can do," or "If I were a better parent, my adolescent would never have attempted suicide." A parent who holds such beliefs may be more apt to lose his or her temper, engage in heated arguments, give up on parenting, or choose not to discipline his or her adolescent. Helping parents identify such beliefs and learn to develop more rational and helpful beliefs can lead to improvements in parenting.

Similarly, when affect regulation is taught to parents, it is designed to help them manage strong emotions that get in the way of effective parenting and/or providing needed support to their adolescent. These sessions begin with psychoeducation on adolescent development so that parents better understand typical adolescent behavior (e.g., questioning parental decisions, choosing time with friends over family). They are also taught how to best manage challenging situations with their adolescent (e.g., giving choices rather than making demands, allowing the adolescent to participate in decision making when appropriate) as well as techniques to control strong emotions (e.g., taking time away to cool down before responding, deep breathing). The session concludes with a brief review of tips for communicating in a way that will decrease conflict and avoid causing emotional harm to the adolescent (e.g., focus only on the current incident, show disapproval of the adolescent's behavior and not the adolescent).

As in individual and parent sessions, problem solving is also commonly practiced in the context of family sessions to address multiple types of problems that negatively affect the adolescent and/or family unit. Family sessions help shift the focus away from the adolescent. They show the adolescent that all members of the family can benefit from learning skills, and they demonstrate commitment on the part of the parents. Moreover, family sessions provide the opportunity for therapists to provide feedback as families practice skills in session, thus increasing the likelihood of success outside of session. With the integration of other skills (e.g., family communication, increasing positive family interactions, contingency management), family sessions can help to address conflictual issues that may have contributed to the adolescent's STB and/or AOD use, modify negative communication patterns and interactions among family members, improve family support and relationships, and provide a safe and structured home environment.

Case Example

Jack is a 16-year-old white male who was hospitalized on an adolescent psychiatric inpatient unit for a suicide attempt. He was diagnosed with major depressive disorder (1-year history) and an alcohol use disorder (severe). He started drinking when he was 14 years old after joining a new peer group. He reportedly drank with his friends about 3–4 days a week. This was Jack's first suicide attempt and first time receiving mental health services.

Jack's parents are married, and he is an only child. They are both college educated and own a restaurant in town. As a result, they work very long and late hours. With regard to family mental health history, Jack's dad reported that he was a "partier" as a teenager and young adult, and he drank a lot back then. Although Jack's father denied drinking regularly anymore, Jack shared that his father came home intoxicated at least one night per week. Jack's mom stated that she had a difficult upbringing and experienced periods of depression throughout her life. She reported currently taking antidepressants, which she said are effective.

With regard to family relationships, Jack stated that although he got along with his parents, he was not as close to them as he used to be. He rarely spent time with them anymore because they were always working. They were often sleeping when he left for school and at work when he got home. When he was younger, his mom spent more time at home. However, when he turned 14, the family business started to suffer, so his parents let some staff go, and his mom picked up their shifts at work. Jack's parents felt that he was capable of managing on his own.

Jack used to be a very strong student. However, when his mom was no longer home to monitor his work, he began to let his work go, and his grades dropped. Jack's parents were upset with him for letting his grades drop and grounded him, but they were never home to enforce the grounding. Jack also used to play organized basketball after school with his good friends, but his mother was no longer available to transport him, and finances were tight, so he stopped playing. Instead, he started hanging out with a group of peers from the neighborhood after school. They would hang out at one of their houses, play video games, and drink or smoke pot. Jack dated one of the girls in the group with whom he grew very close over the prior year. When he got into what he called his "down" periods, she helped him through them. He did have suicidal thoughts on occasion, primarily when drinking, but said he would not hurt himself because of her.

Jack was intoxicated at the time of his suicide attempt. The trigger was a fight and breakup with his girlfriend that occurred after she found out that he had cheated on her while intoxicated. Jack went home, drank whiskey that was in his parent's liquor cabinet, and took his mother's antidepressants. His parents found him unconscious on the couch when they arrived home from work and called an ambulance. Jack was medically treated and then admitted to a psychiatric inpatient unit for treatment.

Brief Case Conceptualization

Consistent with social-cognitive learning theory, Jack exhibited maladaptive thought and behavior patterns, which in large part drove his STB, depression, and alcohol use. Specifically, Jack evidenced cognitive distortions, coping skills deficits, affect regulation deficits, and problematic social behaviors. Notably, Jack learned many of these patterns through his familial and peer experiences, via modeling and reinforcement of maladaptive behaviors.

A primary source of Jack's maladaptive behaviors was ineffective parenting. Jack's parents prematurely stopped providing for Jack's needs, rarely engaged in any positive family activities, and failed to communicate with him. When they did, it was often to reprimand him for his poor grades and other mistakes that he made, rather than to provide any form of praise. Although Jack "intellectually" understood that his parents needed to work long hours to maintain the family business, he still felt abandoned by them. He believed that they chose money over him, which left him thinking that he was worthless. He did not communicate these feelings to his parents because he did not know how. As Jack noted, he did not have the "type of family that sat down and talked about their problems." He also assumed that his parents should know how he was feeling. Jack felt "stuck." His cognitive distortions and lack of effective coping skills left him feeling hopeless and fueled his depression. As a result, he turned to alcohol to help temporarily stop or cope with his negative thoughts and affect. Jack held positive alcohol expectancies and believed that alcohol would reduce his stress and negative affect.

Jack's parents also failed to follow through with any stated consequences for misbehavior (e.g., grounding) and did not monitor Jack's whereabouts, friends, or behaviors. Lack of effective parenting helped shape and reinforce Jack's problem behavior. It was easy for Jack to miss school, fail to do homework, hang out with deviant peers, and use alcohol. Jack was also careful to hide his alcohol use from his parents. Moreover, his parents were not available to provide positive protective factors against deviant behavior and AOD use. They allowed him to drop his one positive prosocial activity (basketball), which he did with prosocial peers. They also failed to provide positive family activities. In addition, Jack was well aware of his father's drinking, so his father served as a model for drinking and intoxication. He also believed his dad would be a hypocrite if he punished him for drinking.

Jack's peers also offered a maladaptive learning environment that promoted and modeled deviance, poor school engagement, and AOD use. They provided Jack with alcohol, reinforced his alcohol use via attention and positive statements, and on occasion pressured him to binge drink with them. Having lost his prosocial peers over time, he did not have any other friends to whom to turn. In addition, his girlfriend was part of this peer group, and he feared that if he left the group, he would lose her. Jack knew that he was compromising his ability to get into a good college, which had always been a dream of his, but he did not see a way out. Nor did he think that anyone other than his girlfriend really cared about him. Jack described himself as "a total failure." When Jack lost his one primary reason for living (his girlfriend) and his ability to inhibit his suicidal impulses due to intoxication, he made a suicide attempt to end what he perceived to be a meaningless and painful life.

Application of Cognitive-Behavioral Treatment Protocol

As is evident, Jack presented with cognitive distortions, coping skills deficits, poor affect regulation, and multiple maladaptive behaviors, including STB and alcohol misuse. Jack also had a home and peer environment that shaped his maladaptive thoughts and modeled negative behaviors. Below, we present an example of how the I-CBT protocol was used to address Jack's case, with a focus on core skills.

Session 1: Introduction to Treatment

Jack and his parents attended the first session, which included rapport building, safety planning, discussion about treatment compliance (i.e., expectations for treatment and resolution of obstacles to treatment attendance), an overview of CBT (including how it will be used to address STBs and AOD use), and the creation of treatment goals in the areas of mental health, AOD use, school, and family/peer relationships.

Session 2: Problem Solving

Jack was asked to list potential triggers for his suicide attempt, and then learned the "SOLVE" problem-solving method to help generate and evaluate alternative options to suicidal behavior and alcohol use. Jack selected "how to cope with the loss of his girlfriend" as the problem to be solved because it was the primary trigger for his attempt. Jack was able to come up with alternative options to self-harm and drinking and added them to the safety plan he developed in the first session.

In Jack's parents' session, the therapist conducted a motivational interview to enhance parental treatment engagement. Jack's parents were provided with a feedback form that contained information about their son's diagnoses, symptom severity, coping skills, and affect regulation strategies. It also included information about their degree of parental monitoring, family functioning, parental alcohol use, and parental distress/mental health based on assessments that they completed. To create this feedback form, the therapist added diagnoses and scores from assessment measures completed at intake into a feedback template created for this protocol. The template included the name of each measure administered, the name of scales included in each measure, and the clinical cutoff for denoting whether scores were clinically significant for each scale. Therapists explained information contained in the feedback form and answered any questions. As Jack's parents processed this information, they shared that they did not know that their son was struggling to this degree nor the severity of the effect that their work decisions were having on Jack. Time was spent discussing what the future potentially held for Jack and their family if changes were or were not made. Jack's parents developed family goals for treatment (e.g., decrease time at work, improve family relationships, improve monitoring) and selected relevant skills from the I-CBT treatment menu (e.g., problem solving, increasing positive family interactions, parental monitoring) to aid in accomplishing these goals. The therapist then helped Jack's parents to "problem solve" obstacles to their goals and elicited/supported self-efficacy statements to improve their likelihood of success.

Session 3: Motivational Interview for Alcohol Use

During check-in, Jack reported that he drank with his friends this past week. He stated that he could control his drinking so there was nothing to worry about. Given that Jack reinitiated drinking and did not understand associated risks, such as a greater likelihood of a repeat attempt, the motivational enhancement interview was conducted. First, Jack created a list of the pros (e.g., fun to do with friends, takes away stress) and cons (e.g., do things I regret, act on suicidal thoughts) of drinking. Next, he was given a feedback form that included three types of information about his AOD use. He was then provided with information about his AOD use rates relative to same sex and aged peers across the United States:

> In the month prior to beginning the study, you drank 5 or more drinks within a couple of hours more often than 61% of boys your age, you were drunk more often than 76% of boys your age, your use of marijuana occurred more often than 0% of boys/girls your age (you did not use).

Next, he was provided with his highest and average blood alcohol levels in the 3 months prior to treatment and the effects of an elevated blood alcohol level on the body. Last, he was provided with information about emotional/behavioral problems associated with his AOD use:

> Your answers to some of our questions show that you use alcohol to cope with unpleasant feelings more often than 90% of boys your age. Your answers to our questions about what happens when you drink suggest that you get in trouble when you drink more than 86% of boys your age.

This was followed by a list of the problems that Jack endorsed as associated with his drinking on the Adolescent Drinking Index (Harrell and Wirtz 1989). To create this feedback form, the therapist added scores from assessment measures completed at intake into a feedback template created for this protocol. This includes AOD questions from the national Monitoring the Future (Johnston et al. 2017) and Youth Suicide Risk Behavior Surveillance surveys (Kann et al. 2016), which provide accompanying norms; questions needed to calculate blood alcohol level using an online calculator; and results from the Adolescent Drinking Index to assess emotional and behavioral difficulties associated with alcohol use.

After processing his feedback report, Jack generated a list of things that could happen if he chose to change (e.g., get into a good college) or not change (e.g., end up back in the hospital) his drinking. Jack then generated alcohol-related goals (e.g., try to avoid drinking with friends), formulated strategies for achieving his goals (e.g., tell friends parents are checking him for alcohol/drugs), used problem-solving to identify obstacles to achieving his goals (e.g., peers who drink), and generated self-efficacy statements (e.g., "I am still smart and can do this").

In the parent session, Jack's parents learned parental monitoring skills around AOD use. These skills included how to identify signs of AOD use, how to monitor for AOD use and Jack's whereabouts, and what to do if they found Jack intoxicated. They also brainstormed rewards for abstinence and consequences for use.

Sessions 4 and 5: Contingency Management

Jack and his parents worked together to create a behavioral contract to address Jack's alcohol use and academic failure, two primary triggers for his cognitive distortions and suicidal thinking. They discussed house rules around alcohol use (e.g., abstinence) and academic work (e.g., attend class, no tardies, complete homework) and then chose rewards and consequences for adhering to the rules. With parental permission, Jack's therapist also contacted his school to gather information on his attendance and academic performance, develop a reasonable plan for making up missed work, and discuss how to best communicate with Jack's parents about his academic progress and attendance. This information was shared with Jack's parents so that they could regularly communicate with Jack's school. This contract not only encouraged good decision making but also helped decrease Jack's hopelessness about his future and challenged his belief that he was not loved or important.

Session 6: Cognitive Restructuring

Jack shared that he got drunk with his friends over the prior weekend. His mother caught him when he tried to sneak into the house but did not enforce any consequences. Jack stated that he found out that his ex-girlfriend had a new boyfriend and all he wanted to do was get drunk to forget. He also reported an increase in suicidal thoughts while drinking but did not act on them. Jack was praised for not attempting suicide, a suicide risk assessment was performed, and Jack's reasons for living and a safety plan were reviewed. Jack was not deemed to be at imminent suicide risk so the rest of the session was spent teaching and practicing cognitive restructuring to help Jack identify and dispute irrational and unhelpful thoughts. The trigger selected was "finding out my ex-girlfriend has a new boyfriend." Jack was able to identify irrational and unhelpful thoughts associated with his sadness and urge to drink (e.g., "She never cared about me," "I am a complete screwup," "I can't handle the pain"), and with the therapist's guidance, Jack developed more rational and helpful thoughts (e.g., "She did care but chose to move on," "I made a mistake and won't make the same one again," "I can learn skills in therapy to help me"). Time was also spent helping Jack develop a coping plan to use when he had urges to drink, which was added to his safety plan.

The parent session was spent addressing beliefs that interfere with effective parenting, using the same cognitive-restructuring model used with Jack. With therapist guidance, Jack's parents identified irrational or unhelpful thoughts that interfered with following through with the contract (e.g., "It is our fault he is this ill," "We will push him further away," "It will just hurt him more") and were able to develop disputes with therapist guidance and provision of education (e.g., "We would have been home more if we knew he needed us," "Following through on the contract will show him that we do care," and "We could lose him to suicide or alcohol poisoning if we don't"). The therapist shared that although Jack was not trying to be rebellious in this particular circumstance, structure and consistency bring safety and stability. Moreover, consequences can be delivered in a nonpunitive manner that shows how much you care (e.g., "We know this is hard for you, but we love you too much not to follow through").

Jack's dad also expressed guilt and admitted that he drinks heavily at times. The therapist asked if he would be willing to change his drinking behavior to provide a more positive role model for Jack and if he might need help to do so. Jack's father agreed to decrease his drinking and accepted referrals from the therapist. The therapist also confirmed that Jack's parents were still following their safety plan for the home, checking in with Jack, and monitoring for both suicidal thinking and alcohol use.

Sessions 7, 8, and 9: Affect Regulation, Relaxation, Coping With Cravings

Over the next few sessions, Jack was taught additional skills to help him manage negative affect and urges to drink. These skills included how to recognize signs of arousal (physiological, behavioral, cognitive) associated with negative affect and urges to drink and how to respond with adaptive coping techniques (e.g., self-soothing activities). He was also taught new relaxation techniques to include in his coping plan (i.e., deep breathing, progressive muscle relaxation) and other skills were reviewed/ practiced when addressing agenda items (i.e., problem solving, cognitive restructuring).

Jack's parents were taught how to "catch" and praise Jack for positive effort and good decision making (e.g., no signs of alcohol use, homework and chore completion, kind acts) in order to improve Jack's self-esteem, provide positive reinforcement for good behavior, and improve family relationships. They were also taught how to use problem solving to generate good options when faced with obstacles to effective parenting (e.g., lack of time to monitor) and parenting decisions (e.g., how to modify the home contract to improve Jack's homework compliance). In addition, they were provided with strategies to help decrease anxiety around parenting (e.g., deep breathing, positive self-talk).

Session 10: Assertive Communication Training

Jack primarily used a passive communication style with his parents, rarely sharing his feelings with them, which left him feeling hurt and isolated. In preparation for family work, Jack learned and practiced assertive communication skills. At the end of the session, in preparation for the next session, Jack role-played sharing his feelings with his parents around issues that still bothered him. Owing to scheduling conflicts, Jack's parents did not attend a session this week but did check in over the phone with their therapist.

Sessions 11 and 12: Family Communication

Jack and his parents spent two sessions learning and practicing general principles of good communication and reflective listening skills. The therapists modeled these skills via role plays and then asked Jack and his parents to practice. During practice, Jack shared that he felt alone and hurt when both parents worked late and he had to stop playing on the basketball team with his friends. Jack's parents reflected Jack's thoughts and feelings and then shared their regret over their decisions, noting that they did not realize how they were affecting him. After talking through these issues, they all agreed to try to communicate better and share quality time together. This session also helped Jack further challenge his belief that he was not loved or important.

Sessions 13+

The first 12 sessions were primarily spent on improving engagement in treatment and teaching Jack and his family core skills centered around maintaining Jack's safety, improving Jack's mood, fostering abstinence, improving family relationships, and creating a supportive and structured home environment. By the end of this sequence of sessions, Jack did not report suicidal thoughts but did still binge drank on occasion when out with his friends. As a result, many of the subsequent sessions during the acute treatment phase were spent revising the home contract to better reinforce abstinence as well as learning new skills to address alcohol use. Because peer pressure was still a trigger for alcohol use, Jack learned skills to help him build new relationships with prosocial peers and reconnect with his old peers (increasing social support module); identify healthy alternatives/activities to drinking, including re-engaging in basketball (increasing healthy, pleasant events module); address peer pressure to use (alcohol/drug refusal skills module); and restructure thoughts that promoted drinking behavior (e.g., "There is nothing else fun to do with my friends"). Other sessions were spent practicing skills in response to agenda items brought to the session (e.g., problem solving around how to further improve Jack's grades); further strengthening family relationships, support, and functioning (e.g., increasing positive family interactions module, problem solving, communication); and identifying and planning for unanticipated stressors that could place Jack at heightened risk for future suicidal behavior and escalation in drinking (e.g., another breakup, failure in a course).

The sessions during the continuation and maintenance phases of treatment were spent practicing acquired skills (skill practice module) and discussing skill acquisition and progress over the course of treatment (treatment progress and skill review module), as well as ways to prevent relapse of both suicidal behavior and old drinking patterns (relapse prevention module). The association between Jack's prior drinking and suicidal behavior was highlighted. By the end of treatment, Jack did not report suicidal thoughts or depressive symptoms, no longer engaged in binge drinking (and rarely drank at all), brought up his grades, resumed playing on the school basketball team, began spending time with his old school friends, and was communicating much better with his parents.

Recommendations for Clinicians Interested in Using This Treatment Approach

Adopting and Adapting the Treatment Across Various Practice Settings

I-CBT lends itself well to clinical practice as one manual can be used to address multiple types of mental health problems and high-risk behaviors (rather than using multiple, nonintegrated manuals). It also offers multiple modes of intervention (cognitive-behavioral individual therapy, cognitive-behavioral family therapy, and behavioral parent training) to address the multitude of problems that often exist within and across the systems (family, peer, school) in which high-risk youth are involved.

As an example of the flexibility of the protocol, we are currently using a variation of I-CBT in a study taking place in a community mental health clinic intensive outpatient program (IOP) for adolescents with co-occurring substance use and psychiatric disorders. This population has a relatively higher proportion of externalizing disorders and lower proportion of internalizing disorders than our initial trial with adolescents discharged from a psychiatric inpatient unit. Approximately half of the sample are in state custody or involved in the juvenile justice system. This study, implemented in a resource-constrained environment, with typically trained clinicians, is meant to mimic usual care in community-based agencies. Therapists have typically completed requirements for a Mental Health Counselor degree but are usually not licensed and use their job to accrue hours toward licensure. In addition, care is being delivered within the constraints of the session limits of a family's insurance plan. The myriad of different insurance plans can make it challenging to plan a treatment course with complex patients.

Our work in this community clinic has shown that therapists with relatively little clinical experience can be trained in the protocol, and some have become quite skilled. Nonetheless, therapist training and supervision must be a priority with inexperienced therapists in such agencies. Staffing issues are a major concern in community agencies, and we have had periods when one therapist has had to conduct the protocol. Although not ideal with such complex cases, it is possible for a single therapist to use the protocol effectively. Under such conditions, supervision is very important. With regard to session preparation, the therapist will need time to prepare a preplanned new module (mainly during acute treatment) as well as worksheets from previously learned skills in the event that an adolescent and/or parent bring in pressing agenda items that call for practice of existing skills. It takes some time and practice for a therapist to feel comfortable with the range of modules available in the protocol and to effectively deliver these types of modules, which are rarely used by therapists in standard practice settings.

Staff turnover is a major problem in community agencies; this makes training in the I-CBT model challenging. Staff turnover also poses a problem in client care. The most severe cases may require *chronic care*, or medical care that addresses long-term illness, as opposed to *acute care*, which accommodates severe illnesses of brief duration. A model of care that offers evidence-based practices and services as adolescents and families progress through the course of chronic illness may accommodate the myriad of challenges faced by these families. Notably, staff turnover makes such long-term care more challenging. We have videotaped exemplar sessions to assist with training new staff and to use when retraining experienced staff in a module when there is drift from the protocol. Systematic, ongoing supervision is important to successful implementation of this protocol with these very high risk clients, and taping sessions is critical to monitoring both fidelity and competency when delivered in usual care, not just clinical research studies.

Clinical Implementation

There are multiple elements of the I-CBT protocol that can be readily implemented in everyday practice. See Table 6–2 for a list of these elements.

TABLE 6-2. Elements of the treatment that can be easily implemented in everyday practice

---

- Include parents in treatment.
- Offer skills-based adolescent sessions, parent training sessions, and family sessions.
- Assess for suicidal ideation, suicidal behavior, and alcohol/drug use at every session.
- Create a safety plan with adolescents *and* parents.
- Use motivational enhancement language and motivational interviewing sessions to increase engagement in target behaviors and improve readiness to change.
- Teach problem-solving skills to improve cognitive flexibility and decision making.
- Teach cognitive-restructuring skills to address irrational and untrue beliefs.
- Teach affect regulation skills to manage strong emotions.
- Teach relaxation skills to help keep daily levels of stress and anxiety low.
- Identify and encourage engagement in healthy, pleasant events to improve mood and number of activities that do not involve alcohol or drugs.
- Teach how to increase social support to decrease social isolation and foster relationships with prosocial peers.
- Teach communication skills as a tool for solving problems and improving relationships.
- Teach skills for managing alcohol/drug cravings and effectively refusing offers to use.
- Teach parents how to attend to positive behaviors when the focus of parent-child interactions has been on negative behaviors.
- Use strategies to help increase positive family interactions as needed.
- Teach families how to create and use a behavioral contract to effectively address adolescent problem behaviors.
- Work with the adolescent to understand and process grief when a loss is experienced.
- Review treatment progress and relapse prevention strategies before discharge.

Conclusion

I-CBT incorporates core modules to address underlying skill deficits that cut across numerous psychiatric disorders and high-risk behaviors. This protocol also includes supplemental skill modules that are used as needed to address problems unique to various co-occurring conditions. Therapists are taught how to apply skill modules to address STB, AOD use, and other comorbid mental health problems. Use of a modular protocol provides a structured approach to tailoring treatment to each client's needs, thus offering a "personalized" approach to care (Ng and Weisz 2016). Moreover, approaches such as I-CBT, which simultaneously address psychopathology and substance use, include family sessions, and incorporate motivation enhancement techniques, have shown considerable promise (Brent et al. 2013). However, clinical research on this topic is very limited. Additional clinical research on how to best address the needs of adolescents with co-occurring presentations is warranted. It will also be important to obtain a better understanding of the relative importance of and need for a broad range of treatment modules if we are to determine the most efficient protocol for complex cases (such as a stepped-care delivery model) that is sensitive to staffing and service demands of community agencies. Advancing the adoption of evidence-based treatments in the community setting also remains a challenging task worthy of future dissemination and implementation studies.

Resource for Additional Training

Please contact the first author (C.E-S.) for information on potential trainings (cesposi1@gmu.edu).

Suggested Readings

Esposito-Smythers C, Perloe A, Machell K, et al: Suicidal and non-suicidal self-harm behaviors and substance use disorders, in Youth Substance Abuse and Co-Occurring Disorders. Edited by Kaminer Y. Arlington, VA, American Psychiatric Association Publishing, 2016, pp 227–252

Spirito A, Esposito-Smythers C: Addressing adolescent suicidal behavior: cognitive-behavioral strategies, in Child and Adolescent Therapy: Cognitive-Behavioral Procedures, 4th Edition. Edited by Kendall PC. New York, Guilford, 2012, pp 234–258

Spirito A, Esposito-Smythers C, Wolff J: Developing and testing interventions for adolescent suicidal and non-suicidal self-injury, in Evidence-Based Psychotherapies for Children and Adolescents. Edited by Weisz JR, Kazdin AE. New York, Guilford, 2017, pp 235–252

Wolff J, Frazier E, Davis S, et al: Cognitive-behavioral therapy for depression and suicidality in children and adolescents, in Clinical Handbook of Psychological Disorders in Children and Adolescents: A Step-By-Step Treatment Manual. Edited by Flessner CA, Piacentini J. New York, Guilford, 2017, pp 55–93

References

Aas HN, Leigh BC, Anderssen N, et al: Two-year longitudinal study of alcohol expectancies and drinking among Norwegian adolescents. Addiction 93(3):373–384, 1998 10328045

Bagge CL, Sher KJ: Adolescent alcohol involvement and suicide attempts: toward the development of a conceptual framework. Clin Psychol Rev 28(8):1283–1296, 2008 18676078

Bandura A: Social Foundations of Thought and Action: A Social Cognitive Theory. Saddle River, NJ, Prentice Hall, 1986

Bandura A, Pastorelli C, Barbaranelli C, Caprara GV: Self-efficacy pathways to childhood depression. J Pers Soc Psychol 76(2):258–269, 1999 10074708

Beck AT, Rush AJ, Shaw BF, Emery G: Cognitive Therapy of Depression. New York, Guilford, 1979

Beck AT, Brown G, Steer RA, et al: Differentiating anxiety and depression: a test of the cognitive content-specificity hypothesis. J Abnorm Psychol 96(3):179–183, 1987 3680754

Beck AT, Brown GK, Steer RA: Psychometric characteristics of the Scale for Suicide Ideation with psychiatric outpatients. Behav Res Ther 35(11):1039–1046, 1997 9431735

Brent DA, Poling KD: Getting started, in Treating Depressed and Suicidal Adolescents. Edited by Brent, DA, Poling KM, New York, Guilford, 2011, pp 99–125

Brent DA, Kolko DJ, Allan MJ, Brown RV: Suicidality in affectively disordered adolescent inpatients. J Am Acad Child Adolesc Psychiatry 29(4):586–593, 1990 2387793

Brent DA, Greenhill LL, Compton S, et al: The Treatment of Adolescent Suicide Attempters study (TASA): predictors of suicidal events in an open treatment trial. J Am Acad Child Adolesc Psychiatry 48(10):987–996, 2009 19730274

Brent DA, McMakin DL, Kennard BD, et al: Protecting adolescents from self-harm: a critical review of intervention studies. J Am Acad Child Adolesc Psychiatry 52(12):1260–1271, 2013 24290459

Brook JS, Whiteman M, Cohen P, et al: Longitudinally predicting late adolescent and young adult drug use: childhood and adolescent precursors. J Am Acad Child Adolesc Psychiatry 34(9):1230–1238, 1995 7559319

Brown GK, Beck AT, Steer RA, et al: Risk factors for suicide in psychiatric outpatients: a 20-year prospective study. J Consult Clin Psychol 68(3):371–377, 2000 10883553

Colder CR, Stice E: A longitudinal study of the interactive effects of impulsivity and anger on adolescent problem behavior. J Youth Adolesc 27:255–274, 1998

Crits-Christoph P, Siqueland L: Psychosocial treatment for drug abuse: selected review and recommendations for national health care. Arch Gen Psychiatry 53(8):749–756, 1996 8694688

Curry JF, Miller Y, Waugh S, et al: Coping responses in depressed, socially maladjusted, and suicidal adolescents. Psychol Rep 71(1):80–82, 1992 1529081

Esposito C, Spirito A, Boergers J, et al: Affective, behavioral, and cognitive functioning in adolescents with multiple suicide attempts. Suicide Life Threat Behav 33(4):389–399, 2003 14695054

Esposito-Smythers C, Spirito A: Adolescent substance use and suicidal behavior: a review with implications for treatment research. Alcohol Clin Exp Res 28(5)(suppl):77S–88S, 2004 15166639

Esposito-Smythers C, Spirito A, Kahler CW, et al: Treatment of co-occurring substance abuse and suicidality among adolescents: a randomized trial. J Consult Clin Psychol 79(6):728–739, 2011 22004303

Esposito-Smythers C, Perloe A, Machell K, et al: Suicidal and non-suicidal self-harm behaviors and substance use disorders, in Youth Substance Abuse and Co-Occurring Disorders. Edited by Kaminer Y. Arlington, VA, American Psychiatric Association Publishing, 2016, pp 227–252

Galaif ER, Sussman S, Newcomb MD, et al: Suicidality, depression, and alcohol use among adolescents: a review of empirical findings. Int J Adolesc Med Health 19(1):27–35, 2007 17458321

Glenn CR, Franklin JC, Nock MK: Evidence-based psychosocial treatments for self-injurious thoughts and behaviors in youth. J Clin Child Adolesc Psychol 44(1):1–29, 2015 25256034

Goldston DB: Conceptual issues in understanding the relationship between suicidal behavior and substance use during adolescence. Drug Alcohol Depend 76(Suppl):S79–S91, 2004 15555819

Goldston DB, Daniel SS, Reboussin BA, et al: Cognitive risk factors and suicide attempts among formerly hospitalized adolescents: a prospective naturalistic study. J Am Acad Child Adolesc Psychiatry 40(1):91–99, 2001 11195570

Goldston DB, Reboussin BA, Daniel SS: Predictors of suicide attempts: state and trait components. J Abnorm Psychol 115(4):842–849, 2006 17100542

Gonzalez V, Bradizza C, Collins R: Drinking to cope as a statistical mediator in the relationship between suicidal ideation and alcohol outcomes among underage college drinkers. Psychol Addict Behav 23:443–451, 2009

Harrell A, Wirtz PW: Adolescent Drinking Index: Professional Manual. Odessa, FL, Psychological Assessment Resources, 1989

Hawkins EH: A tale of two systems: co-occurring mental health and substance abuse disorders treatment for adolescents. Annu Rev Psychol 60:197–227, 2009 19035824

Hogue A, Henderson CE, Ozechowski TJ, et al: Evidence base on outpatient behavioral treatments for adolescent substance use: updates and recommendations 2007–2013. J Clin Child Adolesc Psychol 43(5):695–720, 2014 24926870

Homish GG, Leonard KE: The social network and alcohol use. J Stud Alcohol Drugs 69(6):906–914, 2008 18925349

Hufford MR: Alcohol and suicidal behavior. Clin Psychol Rev 21(5):797–811, 2001 11434231

Johnston LD, O'Malley PM, Miech RA, et al: Monitoring the Future National Survey Results on Drug Use, 1975–2016: Overview, Key Findings on Adolescent Drug Use. Ann Arbor, MI, Institute for Social Research at the University of Michigan, 2017, pp 76–79

Kann L, McManus T, Harris WA, et al: Youth Risk Behavior Surveillance—United States, 2015. MMWR Surveill Summ 65(6)(No. SS-6):1–174, 2016 27280474

Latimer WW, Newcomb M, Winters KC, et al: Adolescent substance abuse treatment outcome: the role of substance abuse problem severity, psychosocial, and treatment factors. J Consult Clin Psychol 68(4):684–696, 2000 10965643

Leslie MB, Stein JA, Rotheram-Borus MJ: Sex-specific predictors of suicidality among runaway youth. J Clin Child Adolesc Psychol 31(1):27–40, 2002 11845647

Miller WR, Rollnick S: Motivational Interviewing: Helping People Change, 3rd Edition, New York, Guilford, 2013

Moos RH, Moos BS: Long-term influence of duration and intensity of treatment on previously untreated individuals with alcohol use disorders. Addiction 98(3):325–337, 2003 12603232

Ng MY, Weisz JR: Annual Research Review: Building a science of personalized intervention for youth mental health. J Child Psychol Psychiatry 57(3):216–236, 2016 26467325

Prinstein M, Boergers J, Spirito A, et al: Peer and family models of suicide ide-ation severity among adolescent inpatients. J Clin Child Adolesc Psychol 29(3):392–405, 2000 10969423

Schafer J, Brown SA: Marijuana and cocaine effect expectancies and drug use patterns. J Consult Clin Psychol 59(4):558–565, 1991 1918560

Shimokawa K, Lambert MJ, Smart DW: Enhancing treatment outcome of pa-tients at risk of treatment failure: meta-analytic and mega-analytic review of a psychotherapy quality assurance system. J Consult Clin Psychol 78(3):298–311, 2010 20515206

Simons-Morton B, Haynie DL, Crump AD, et al: Expectancies and other psy-chosocial factors associated with alcohol use among early adolescent boys and girls. Addict Behav 24(2):229–238, 1999 10336104

Spirito A, Esposito-Smythers C: Addressing adolescent suicidal behavior: cognitive-behavioral strategies, in Child and Adolescent Therapy: Cognitive-Behavioral Procedures, 4th Edition. Edited by Kendall PC. New York, Guilford, 2012, pp 234–258

Spirito A, Overholser J, Stark LJ: Common problems and coping strategies. II: findings with adolescent suicide attempters. J Abnorm Child Psychol 17(2):213–221, 1989 2745901

Spirito A, Stanton C, Donaldson D, et al: Treatment-as-usual for adolescent sui-cide attempters: implications for the choice of comparison groups in psy-chotherapy research. J Clin Child Adolesc Psychol 31(1):41–47, 2002 11845649

Stanley B, Brown GK: Safety planning intervention: A brief intervention to mit-igate suicide risk. Cogn Behav Pract 19:256–264, 2012

Tevyaw TO, Monti PM: Motivational enhancement and other brief interven-tions for adolescent substance abuse: foundations, applications and evalua-tions. Addiction 99 (Suppl 2):63–75, 2004 15488106

Trulsson K, Hedin UC: The role of social support when giving up drug abuse: a female perspective. Int J Soc Welf 13:145–157, 2004

Wagner BM, Silverman MAC, Martin CE: Family factors in youth suicidal be-haviors. Am Behav Sci 46:1171–1191, 2003

Williams RJ, Chang SY: A comprehensive and comparative review of adolescent substance abuse treatment outcome. Clin Psychol Sci Pract 7:138–166, 2000

Wills TA, Sandy JM, Shinar O, Yaeger A: Contributions of positive and negative affect to adolescent substance use: Test of a bidimensional model in a longi-tudinal study. Psychol Addict Behav 13(4):327–338 1999

Wills TA, Sandy JM, Yaeger AM, et al: Coping dimensions, life stress, and ado-lescent substance use: a latent growth analysis. J Abnorm Psychol 110(2):309–323, 2001 11358025

Windle M, Davies PT: Depression and heavy alcohol use among adolescents: concurrent and prospective relations. Dev Psychopathol 11(4):823–844, 1999 10624728

Zlotnick C, Donaldson D, Spirito A, et al: Affect regulation and suicide attempts in adolescent inpatients. J Am Acad Child Adolesc Psychiatry 36(6):793–798, 1997 9183134

A Psychiatric Adaptation of Multisystemic Therapy for Suicidal Youth

Melisa D. Rowland, M.D.

Overview of Treatment Approach

Multisystemic therapy with psychiatric supports (MST-Psychiatric) is an adaptation of multisystemic therapy (MST; a trademarked intervention). MST-Psychiatric was created to address the treatment needs of youth at risk of out of home placement due to serious psychiatric symptoms. Grounded in MST, a treatment model with well-established effectiveness in treating adolescent substance use and conduct disorder, MST-Psychiatric is specifically designed to identify and address adolescent high-risk mental health symptoms including suicidal, self-injurious, and aggressive behav-

Author Disclosure Note: Dr. Rowland is a board member and stockholder of MST Services LLC, the Medical University of South Carolina–licensed organization that provides training in multisystemic therapy (MST).

iors. This adaptation of MST has primarily been used to serve youth at risk of out of home placement in correctional or mental health facilities due to serious behavioral problems or drug use/abuse with co-occurring mental health symptoms such as thought disorder, bipolar disorder, depression, anxiety, and/or suicidal behaviors.

MST-Psychiatric was initially evaluated as an evidence-based alternative to psychiatric hospitalization in a National Institute of Mental Health–funded randomized clinical trial (RO1MH51852, Principal Investigator: Scott W. Henggeler) conducted from 1994 to 1999 and has subsequently been assessed as a component of continuum of care treatment programs in Honolulu, Philadelphia, and New York City. To enhance the generalizability of research findings, these studies have focused on providing services in real-world settings with community-based clinicians. As a result, MST-Psychiatric has evolved from randomized efficacy studies to randomized effectiveness studies to careful transport in community settings over the last 20 years. Published outcomes from these evaluations support the capacity of MST-Psychiatric to reduce suicidal (Huey et al. 2004) behaviors in high-risk adolescents. Yet, to date, this treatment has primarily been utilized to target a broad heterogeneous population of youth demonstrating behaviors that place them at imminent risk of out of home placement rather than narrowly focusing on suicidal behaviors. As a result, this model may differ from other treatments described in this book in that it targets youth who present with multiple serious problems in settings that convey high risk (e.g., poverty, comorbid substance use, criminal/externalizing behaviors).

MST-Psychiatric has well-established training materials and an intensive, empirically validated quality assurance protocol (Schoenwald et al. 2003, 2008, 2009). It is recognized as an evidence-based practice by the Substance Abuse and Mental Health Services Administration (SAMHSA), National Registry of Evidence-based Programs and Practices (NREPP; https://nrepp.samhsa.gov/Legacy/ViewIntervention.aspx?id=17), and the National Institute of Justice's Crime Solutions program (www.crimesolutions.gov/ProgramDetails.aspx?ID=176). MST-Psychiatric is an intensive treatment model that is most appropriate for children and adolescents presenting with complex, multifaceted, and challenging mental health and behavioral problems that are costly to service systems.

Theoretical Model and Proposed Mechanism of Change

Like MST, MST-Psychiatric is first and foremost a family therapy model of treatment. Grounded in Bronfenbrenner's (1979) theory of social ecology and informed by social-ecological family therapy models (Haley 1987), MST-Psychiatric is a community-based, family-centered treatment. Consistent with Bronfenbrenner's theory, a primary assumption of the MST theory of change is that adolescent problem behavior is driven by the interplay of risk factors across, within, and between the multiple systems in which the youth and family are embedded. Hence, to be optimally effective, interventions need to have the capacity to address a comprehensive array of risk factors and be tailored to meet the individual needs of families. Another important assumption underlying MST is that caregivers are considered the key avenue through which sustainable change occurs. Thus, MST therapists strive to improve caregiver and family functioning. Working with the caregivers to leverage strengths in the systems, MST therapists help the family impact the school, community, peer, and individual risk factors that are sustaining the identified problems (Henggeler et al. 2009b; MST Logic Model www.episcenter.psu.edu/sites/default/files/ebp/MST%20Logic%20Model%20FINAL%201-13-11.pdf).

The MST theory of change emphasizes the central role of improved parental functioning in reducing youth risk behaviors. The capacity of MST to impact youth problem behavior through improved family functioning (i.e., improved cohesion and parental monitoring) is supported by both quantitative (Deković et al. 2012; Henggeler et al. 2009a; Huey et al. 2000) and qualitative (Kaur et al. 2015; Paradisopoulos et al. 2015; Tighe et al. 2012) research. Although these investigations have been conducted primarily with MST studies of youth presenting with antisocial behavior, there is reason to believe that similar mechanisms of change are in effect for youth presenting with internalizing disorders, including suicidal behaviors. For instance, there are numerous risk factors across the school, family, and peer systems that increase the odds of youth experiencing internalizing problems in general, as well as suicidal thoughts, feelings, and behaviors specifically. Some examples of common factors that place youth at risk for suicidal behaviors include the following: access to firearms in the home and community; use of alcohol or drugs; youth and/or family member psychopathology; family conflict, rejection, or neglect; harsh discipline; low parental responsiveness; peer rejection; bullying; exposure to peer suicide; and exposure to contagion effect through social media (Wagner 1997, 2009; Wagner et al. 2003). The MST-Psychiatric model is well fitted to address the problem of youth suicidality as it allows for an in-depth, systemic evaluation of the underlying causes of the suicidal behavior and the creation of empirically driven, ecologically valid interventions, implemented with families to block or diminish the specific risk factors that are driving the behavior for a particular youth (Henggeler et al. 2002).

Review of Empirical Evidence

The MST-Psychiatric model is grounded in MST, an internationally recognized program with over 30 years of research demonstrating positive outcomes with chronic juvenile offenders and youth who present with other serious antisocial behavior. Currently, there are 16 outcome studies of MST with serious juvenile offenders (11 randomized trials, 7 independent studies, 2 international studies) and 16 outcome studies of MST with adolescents experiencing serious conduct problems (6 randomized trials, 13 independent studies, 6 international studies) as well as 2 randomized clinical trials with substance-abusing or dependent juvenile offenders. Across these studies of youth with serious antisocial behavior, research supports the model's ability to diminish re-arrest rates, reduce out of home placement, improve family functioning, improve peer relations, decrease substance use and externalizing symptoms, and improve mental health symptoms for youth while obtaining high levels of client satisfaction and demonstrating considerable cost savings (http://mstservices.com/files/outcomestudies.pdf).

Building on the success of MST with youth who present with antisocial behavior, the MST-Psychiatric adaptation was developed to serve the needs of families with youth at risk of out of home placement due to serious mental health problems. It was evaluated in a randomized clinical trial conducted from 1994 to 1999 that included 156 Medicaid or crisis-funded families with youth accepted for inpatient admission into a university psychiatric hospital. Half of these youth received MST, and half were admitted to the psychiatric hospital and received routine care after discharge. Note that inclusion in the study required that youth be in psychiatric crisis and meet American Academy of Child and Adolescent Psychiatry Criteria for emergent psychiatric hospitalization (level of care placement criteria for psychiatric illness, American Academy of Child and Adolescent Psychiatry 1996). Hence all participants in the study were deemed to be suicidal (38%), homicidal (17%), psychotic (8%), or a threat of harm to self or others (37%) as a primary reason for hospitalization by intake staff not affiliated with the study.

Findings From NIMH-Funded Randomized Clinical Trial, Efficacy Study

Analyses of data collected at 4 months (Henggeler et al. 1999; Schoenwald et al. 2000) revealed the following significant findings for MST relative to comparison youth and families, based on both youth and caregiver reports: improved youth externalizing symptoms, improved family cohesion and structure, and higher consumer satisfaction. MST youth also spent significantly more days in school and fewer days in the psychiatric hospital (72%) and demonstrated a 49% reduction in nonhospital out of home placements relative to their counterparts. A trend toward MST youth reporting less alcohol use was also noted. One of the most important findings for the trial came approximately 16 months after intake at 1-year follow-up (Huey et al. 2004) when youth who had received MST reported a significant reduction in suicide attempts relative to youth in the control condition. Outcomes from this trial led to further validation.

Findings From Hawaii Randomized Clinical Trial, Effectiveness Study

Funded by the Hawaii Department of Health and Adolescent Mental Health Division, the Annie E. Casey Foundation, and the National Institute on Drug Abuse, the Hawaii randomized clinical trial was designed to determine if an MST-based continuum of mental health treatments spanning from home-based to foster care and inpatient services would be more effective than routine services provided in Hawaii's newly created continuum of care (Rowland et al. 2005). MST-Psychiatric was the model of MST utilized for this project, which served families with youth ages 9–17 years at imminent risk of out of home placement due to comorbid serious mental health and behavioral problems. Data from the 31 youth and families completing treatment and 6-month follow-up measures revealed several significant findings favoring youth in the MST condition over youth in the control condition: improved youth internalizing and externalizing symptoms; decreased youth self-reported minor delinquency; decreased days (68%) in out of home placement; increased days (42%) in regular school settings; and marginally significant improvements in caregiver satisfaction with social supports. Experience with this effectiveness study led to a third validation study of MST-Psychiatric, again in a community-based setting serving youth within a continuum of care.

Findings From Philadelphia Randomized Clinical Trial, Effectiveness Study

Funded by the City of Philadelphia's Department of Public Health and Behavioral Health System and the Annie E. Casey Foundation, the Philadelphia randomized clinical trial was designed to evaluate the effectiveness of an MST continuum of services in treating juvenile offenders ages 10–16 years with a comorbid mental health disorder and at imminent risk of out of home placement. All youth in the comparison condition were admitted to a residential treatment center, and the majority of these were still in placement at 6 and 12 months postintake. Sixty-three youth reached 6-month follow-up, and 44 reached 12-month follow-up before funding sources for the project ended. Although results of this trial have not been published in a peer-reviewed journal, findings are outlined in a final report submitted to the Annie E. Casey Foundation (author communication, S.K. Schoenwald, "MST-based Continuum of Care in Philadelphia," 2004). In this study, statistically significant findings favoring MST at 6 months postrecruitment $(n=63)$ included decreased internalizing symptoms by youth and caregiver report; decreased caregiver self-report of alcohol use; increased family cohesion by youth report; and increased days in community-based placements (home- and MST-based therapeutic foster care). Meanwhile, youth in the usual services condition spent significantly more days in residential placement. Additionally, studies of the relationship between adherence to the MST treatment protocol and clinical indicators at 6 and 12 months revealed significant findings. Specifically, caregiver report of therapist adherence on the MST Therapist Adherence Measure (TAM) predicted improved caregiver discipline at 6 and 12 months and a trend toward improved family cohesion at 12 months. Importantly, independent observer ratings of MST adherence on audiotaped sessions predicted decreased caregiver self-reported psychiatric symptoms at 12 months.

On the basis of the outcomes of these trials, MST-Psychiatric is now being implemented in several community-based settings. One of these projects, the Arrow Program, has been providing services to at-risk youth and families in New York City for 8 years.

Findings From a Transportability Project, the Arrow Program

Funded by the Robin Hood Foundation, the Arrow Program, housed within the New York Foundling Agency, is designed to provide MST-Psychiatric treatment across three boroughs (Manhattan, Queens, and Brooklyn) for families served by the New York City Administration for Children's Services (ACS), Juvenile Justice Initiative (JJI), and Family Assessment Program (FAP). These programs have access to an array of evidence-based practices, and MST-Psychiatric is utilized when the youth or caregivers have psychiatric service needs that are too intense for standard MST or the other evidence-based models funded by these initiatives. JJI youth are designated delinquents court-ordered to out of home placement due to criminal behavior. The FAP program serves families that have filed with ACS to have their children removed from the home because of unruly or unmanageable behavior. This project does not have an experimental design, yet substantial data are collected pretreatment and posttreatment for all families served. From the project's inception in March 2010 through December 2016, intake and discharge data were collected on 148 families. Highlights of these outcomes are described in an annual report provided to the Robin Hood Foundation in 2017 (M. Rowland, Multisystemic therapy psychiatric adaptation program: the New York Foundling's final report to the Robin Hood Foundation, 2017). Statistically significant findings for MST-Psychiatric families based on data collected pretreatment and posttreatment (4–7 months) are 1) caregiver reports of reduction of total number of youth problem behaviors (both externalizing and internalizing); 2) caregiver self-reports of improved levels of psychological distress, interpersonal sensitivity, depression, anxiety, paranoid ideation, psychoticism, and hostility and fewer overall symptoms; and 3) a reduction in youth affiliation with deviant peers, based

on youth and caregiver reports. In summary, the Arrow Program is an example of a stand-alone MST-Psychiatric team working effectively with children
and families that represent some of the highest-end users of child welfare
(ACS) and juvenile justice resources in New York City.

Treatment Components and Primary Intervention Strategies

MST-Psychiatric is grounded in the MST treatment model and subsumes
all aspects of routine MST, including the treatment manuals, training materials, clinical protocols, and detailed supervisory, administrative, and
quality assurance processes. These quality assurance protocols allow MST-
Psychiatric to leverage the strongly established effectiveness of routine
MST in treating youth externalizing disorders, supplemented with an additional layer of training materials and quality assurance protocols designed
to serve youth with serious co-morbid internalizing disorders and psychiatric symptoms.

MST-Psychiatric therapists are master-level clinicians and work in teams
of 3–4 therapists supported by a clinically experienced MST-Psychiatric
supervisor. A child psychiatrist (1 day a week per team) and a bachelor's-
level crisis caseworker are integrated into the team to provide additional clinical supports. Services are delivered in the home and community two times
per week (or more as needed) for 4–7 months by therapists with a caseload
of 3–4 families. Team members are on call for MST families 24 hours a day,
7 days a week and respond directly in the community to crisis situations
(e.g., meeting families at home or in the emergency department if a youth
becomes suicidal). MST-Psychiatric supervisors work full-time in the model
and are closely involved with treatment, providing clinical oversight and in-
struction as well as direct therapeutic assistance in the field for therapists. All
MST-Psychiatric clinicians, including the team child psychiatrist, receive
standard MST training and ongoing quality assurance support as well as supplemental trainings.

Each MST team is assigned an expert MST consultant. This person is
a doctoral-level or experienced master's-level MST expert whose roles are
to support clinician implementation of MST; promote clinical competence of the therapists, crisis caseworkers, and supervisor; and help the
team address organizational and systemic threats to model fidelity. The

expert MST consultant provides weekly consultations to the team and quarterly booster trainings.

In MST-Psychiatric, an additional layer of consultation supports is provided to assist the team in managing clinical issues or concerns that pertain to psychiatric problems. A child and adolescent psychiatrist who is also an expert in the MST treatment model is available to support the team on a weekly basis. Support from the MST expert psychiatrist includes a weekly hour-long meeting with the MST expert consultant, team supervisor, and team administrator to cover urgent psychiatric or programmatic/administrative concerns; ongoing monitoring of cases with serious psychiatric issues in youth and/or their caregivers; interfacing with the team psychiatrist as indicated; and assistance with the development of boosters and trainings that pertain to medical and/or psychiatric issues.

Standard MST program development and ongoing organizational support is quite extensive and includes the items outlined in Table 7–1. These supports are provided by MST Services or one of 24 network partner organizations. MST Services is a technology transfer organization licensed through the Medical University of South Carolina, created in 1996 to provide training, support, and consultation for community-based MST teams. Network partner organizations are state, university, or nonprofit agencies with a strong track record in implementing MST effectively and that have developed their own internal capacity to provide MST quality assurance services. Network partner organizations remain linked with MST Services to ensure the ongoing interchange of knowledge and information.

MST interventions draw from research-based treatment techniques and include behavioral therapy, parent management training, cognitive-behavioral therapy (CBT), and pragmatic family therapies (Henggeler et al. 2009b). The MST-Psychiatric teams receive supplemental trainings in the following: assessing safety risks associated with suicidal, homicidal, and psychotic behaviors in youth; the treatment of adolescent and caregiver substance use/abuse using contingency management (Henggeler et al. 2012); and the evidence-based assessment and treatment of youth and caregiver mental illness. The specific interventions utilized vary from family to family depending on need. A careful protocol, termed the MST Analytical Process, is used to assess each family and determine which interventions should be utilized and when. The case example described in the next section helps to highlight this approach.

TABLE 7-1.   Multisystemic therapy (MST) program development supports

Organizational support

    Assistance to community stakeholders and provider agencies at start-up. Development of process to allow the funding organization and provider agency to track key outcomes

    Ongoing organizational support—includes semiannual outcomes-based program reviews, problem solving of organizational and stakeholder barriers to implementation, and support for program directors

Implementation measurement and reporting: the following measures are collected and input into a centralized MST database

    Measures of therapist adherence collected from caregivers of each family monthly

    Measures of supervisor adherence collected from therapists every other month

    Measures of consultant adherence collected from teams every other month

    Youth outcome measures agreed upon by stakeholders at program start-up

Training

    Initial 5-day orientation training to MST

    Quarterly booster trainings

    Weekly on-site supervision by the supervisor

    Weekly consultation with an MST expert and MST psychiatrist expert

MST-Psychiatric teams also receive the following supplemental trainings

    Training in safety risks associated with suicidal, homicidal, and psychotic behaviors in youth and interventions to address these risks

    Training in the treatment of adolescent and caregiver substance use/abuse utilizing an evidence-based treatment, contingency management

    Training in the evaluation, diagnosis, and evidence-based treatment of psychiatric symptoms in youth and adults

Case Example

A case example is provided to better describe the process by which MST is implemented, the tools and interventions that are used, and how these are selected and carried out by the team.

Background Information

Camila Martinez, a 16-year-old female of Puerto Rican and Mexican descent, was referred to an MST-Psychiatric team based in New York City from a Queens psychiatric emergency department for suicidal behavior. Camila had locked herself in her bedroom after a family argument the night before and taken a handful of aripiprazole (Abilify). She had a history of two past psychiatric hospitalizations for similar incidents 5 and 9 months prior and carried a diagnosis of bipolar disorder for which she was prescribed aripiprazole by a psychiatrist at a local community mental health center. Camila and her family were referred to an intensive outpatient therapy after her first hospitalization, but they discontinued treatment after a few visits. Camila saw her current therapist and psychiatrist, accessed after the second suicide attempt, about twice a month. Camila had been diagnosed with attention-deficit/hyperactivity disorder (ADHD) at an earlier age but was not receiving treatment for this problem at the time of referral. She was also struggling with truancy and academic problems, routinely smoked marijuana, and had been arrested with peers for shoplifting 3 months earlier but was released and not charged.

Engagement

Engagement and alignment are essential ingredients in all MST interventions and are often the focus of trainings, weekly supervision, and consultation. Early in treatment, MST therapists use several strategies to enhance engagement. These include meeting with all key family members in their homes at convenient times to discover their perspectives on the manifesting problems and opinions concerning the strengths and barriers found in their ecology. Substantial time is spent assessing these systems, developing a shared understanding of the manifesting problems, and setting overarching goals for the family. Some of the materials collected by MST-Psychiatric therapists on all families during their initial assessment phase include a genogram; a description of the frequency, intensity, and duration of referral behaviors; a list of the desired outcomes of each family member and key stakeholder; a description of the strengths and needs of each system; and finally, the development of overarching goals for treatment.

The MST therapist met the family in their home three times during the first week and collected the following information.

Genogram

Genograms are used by the therapist to easily convey information about the family and their indigenous social supports to other team members. Some strengths noted on this genogram (Figure 7–1), which the therapist will use to help the family leverage change, include the strong bonds between the parents and between Camila and her Aunt Angelia.

Frequency, Intensity, and Duration Chart of Referral Behaviors

The frequency, intensity, and duration (FID) chart, often referred to as the FID assessment, helps to anchor the family and team in a clear behavioral assessment of the problems (see Table 7–2). The FID assessment is used to reach a consensus on the behaviors that are most concerning and to clarify their extent and duration. This provides a concise summary of the key problems and helps the team track symptom improvement over time.

Desired Outcomes

Early in treatment, MST therapists ascertain the desired outcomes of each family member as well as other family supports and stakeholders (e.g., probation officers, guidance counselors) who may play an important role in helping the family establish and maintain outcomes. Therapists try to capture the goals in each person's words. These will play a key role at the end of the assessment period when the therapist and family work to generate the *overarching goals of treatment*. The *desired outcomes* (Table 7–3) help to guide treatment and serve as useful reference points for the team when engagement or alignment issues develop during treatment.

Strengths and Needs Assessment

Therapists collect the strengths and needs assessment both by observing and interviewing family members (Table 7–4). This assessment is a living

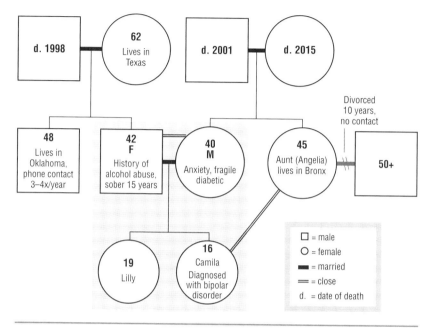

FIGURE 7-1.   **Martinez family genogram.**

document and is updated throughout treatment. This tool helps therapists identify barriers or risk factors that may need to be changed and strengths that can be leveraged to promote such change.

Safety Checklist and Tools

MST-Psychiatric therapists complete a *safety checklist* with every family during the initial assessment. This is a semistructured interview done in the family's home with the caregivers and focuses on the assessment of youth and family safety risks as well as the restriction of lethal means. During this interview, the therapist asks the family about the availability of guns and other weapons in the home. The therapist also creates a list of all medications and alcohol in the home and helps the parents perform a safety check of the home and the youth's room for potential weapons, drugs, or objects that put the youth or family at risk. This information along with sequences and fit assessments (see below) of high-risk behaviors (e.g., suicidal, aggressive) are used to help the family generate a formalized *safety plan* when indicated. If therapists uncover weapons, alcohol, or potentially dangerous medications, an immediate plan is developed to

TABLE 7-2.   Referral behaviors

Behavior	Frequency	Intensity	Duration
Suicide attempts	Three known attempts	Took handful (5–6 pills) of aripiprazole (Abilify) behind locked door after fight with parents.	Recent attempt 2 days before intake.
		Took a partial bottle of acetaminophen (Tylenol) about 15 pills after fight with sister. Camila called her father immediately afterward and was taken to ED, admitted to hospital for a day, then to a psychiatric ward for a week.	Second attempt 5 months ago.
		Tried to take bottle of diphenhydramine (Benadryl) after fight with mother, swallowed approximately 5 pills before mother grabbed bottle. Admitted to psychiatric hospital for 9 days.	First attempt 9 months ago.
Truancy	Every Tuesday and Thursday this semester	Skips after lunch, missing math and physical education	Skipped classes off and on starting in the ninth grade (last year). This school year (tenth grade) has skipped 2 times/week most of fall semester.
Marijuana use	Smokes about once/ week per youth report	Shares blunt with friends	Started to smoke approximately 15 months ago, at start of ninth grade

TABLE 7-2. Referral behaviors *(continued)*

Behavior	Frequency	Intensity	Duration
Shoplifting/arrest	Reports shoplifting only once, being arrested only once	Attempted to take sunglasses and an energy drink with peers	9 months ago, prior to last hospitalization, reports this was a one-time incident. Mom thinks she may have shoplifted before with same friends.
Verbal aggression	2–3 times/week	Youth screams, slams doors, cries, and shouts	Has always been temperamental, tantrums as a child. Current level since early ninth grade.

Note. ED = emergency department.

TABLE 7-3.   Desired outcomes of treatment with multisystemic therapy

Participant	Goal
Father	For Camila to stay safe, not harm herself, stop fighting with the family, stay in school
Mother	For Camila to be happy and stop trying to hurt herself, go to school, start to do something useful with her free time
Camila	To feel better, for everyone to stay off my case and stop bothering me
Lilly (sister)	For the family to stop fighting so much, for Camila to grow up and stop giving Mom and Dad such a hard time
Angelia (aunt)	For Camila to stay in school and get healthy, realize her potential

mitigate the risk. This often involves securing or removing alcoholic beverages and locking medications and knives in lock boxes provided by the team. The protocol also requires that all firearms be removed from the home.

Finding the Fit

MST is based on nine treatment principles (Henggeler et al. 2009b). The first principle states, "the primary purpose of MST assessment is to understand the 'fit' between the identified problems and their broader systemic context" (p. 15). Therapists use a tool to help them adhere to this process, termed a *fit assessment* or *fit circle*. This is completed by first identifying a behavior that is the target of treatment, defining it clearly in behavioral terms, and placing that label in the middle of a circle (see Figures 7–2 and 7–3). Therapists then create hypotheses, also termed *fit factors* about potential drivers of the problem. These are listed around the circle with arrows pointing to the target behavior as a visual aid. Therapists attempt to assess causes from each of the systems in which the youth is embedded and to focus on factors that are present focused, are clearly linked to the problem, and can be changed. Often therapists will introduce the fit assessment to families early in treatment as a way to teach them the therapeutic process, hence starting early to generalize their gains.

TABLE 7-4. Multisystemic therapy (MST) strengths and needs assessment

Systemic strengths	Systemic weaknesses/needs
Individual	
Artistic, enjoys drawing cartoons, creative	Diagnosed with ADHD as a child, no medications
Is physically healthy	Diagnosed with bipolar disorder
ED and MST intake drug screens negative for all substances except marijuana	Hospitalized 9 months ago for suicide attempt
Sense of humor	Hospitalized 5 months ago for suicide attempt
Was compliant with Abilify most days the month before intake	Recent suicide attempt
Interested in art classes, art-related professions	No current prosocial activities
Likes to be spontaneous	Impulsive by parent report
Can engage well with adults she likes	ED and MST intake drug screens positive for marijuana
Reports not being sexually active	
Family	
Mom and Dad have been together 20 years.	Dad has a history of alcohol abuse, sober for 15 years.
Mom and Dad both try to parent together.	Family had child protective services involvement 16 years ago, related to Father's alcohol use.
Older sister graduated from high school, works in sales at a nearby mall.	Mom struggles with anxiety and depression.

TABLE 7-4.   Multisystemic therapy (MST) strengths and needs assessment *(continued)*

Systemic strengths	Systemic weaknesses/needs
Family *(continued)*	
Aunt (Mom's sister) lives nearby and is close to Camila and a support for Mom.	Mom struggles with type 1 diabetes, insulin dependent.
No known physical altercations or violence occur during family arguments.	Mom tries to set rules but often gives in.
Parents seem to have positive affective bonds with one another and both girls.	Father is at times rigid with rules.
Family tries to eat dinner together 2 times/week.	Parents and sister tend to get into arguments with Camila, which become loud and lead to Camila screaming, shouting, and slamming doors.
Some shared family activity takes place—movie night once or twice a month.	Parents are not accessing social supports, e.g., aunt.
Dad works in apartment building as superintendent/handyman.	Mom cannot work full time due to diabetes.
Mom works part-time as a nurse's aide at local hospital.	Camila has a short temper with Mom and sister Lilly.
Camila is more easy going, less easily angered with her father.	
	School
Located in safe neighborhood	Large school, with large class sizes
Has automatic call line to notify parents of truancy	Impersonal setting
Offers a large variety of courses and extracurricular activities	Youth and caregivers not connected to school
Camila is in regular classes.	No IEP or 504 plan despite past diagnosis of ADHD and recent diagnosis of bipolar disorder
Camila has not failed a grade.	Guidance counselor seems overwhelmed.
Older sister graduated from this school.	

TABLE 7–4. Multisystemic therapy (MST) strengths and needs assessment *(continued)*

Systemic strengths	Systemic weaknesses/needs
Peers	
Camila has two long-standing friends, Jasmine and Nicole whom mom approves of and considers prosocial.	Began hanging out with three girls in ninth grade—Shaniqua, Maria, and Cindy—who get into trouble (e.g., shoplifting, marijuana use)
Mom knows the mothers of Jasmine and Nicole and can communicate with them.	One of these girls (Cindy) has been psychiatrically hospitalized before, self-harms, and has dropped out of school.
Camila has a couple of friends who are boys but not romantically involved with anyone at this time.	Camila does not hang out with Jasmine and Nicole much now.
Community	
Relatively safe neighborhood, community police station near housing complex	Unsafe areas on the way to school
Close to school, shopping	Negative peers (Shaniqua, Maria, and Cindy) frequently hang out in nearby park.
Close to park, public transport	Gunfire in park 1 month ago after midnight, apparently related to drug deal
Positive peers (Jasmine and Nicole) live nearby, same housing complex.	

Note. ADHD=attention-deficit/hyperactivity disorder; ED=emergency department; IEP=individualized education program.

The therapist for the Martinez family completed a fit circle for each of the youth's five referral behaviors (e.g., suicide attempts, truancy, marijuana use, shoplifting/arrest, verbal aggression). The fit assessment for Camila's suicide attempts is provided in section "Behavioral Sequence of Suicide Attempts" to highlight this process. To help elucidate precursors to the event, the therapist also obtained a *behavioral sequence* of each of Camila's three suicide attempts before completing the fit assessment.

Behavioral Sequence of Suicide Attempts

When sequencing the three suicide attempts, the therapist found several recurring patterns. In all three instances, Camila experienced a significant psychosocial stressor several hours before the event. Her first attempt occurred the same day that she was arrested for shoplifting and subsequently released to her mother. On the day of the second attempt, her sister caught her smoking marijuana in the park during school hours and threatened to call their mother. The argument between the sisters escalated, and Camila accidentally broke a mirror that fell from the wall in the family room when she slammed her bedroom door. On the day of her third attempt, Camila had received a notice from the school of a failing grade on a report card and a request to schedule a family conference. In all three instances, she was involved in a verbally aggressive argument with her mother and/or sister over these events. Mom reported strong feelings of hopelessness during these arguments and substantial "all or none" thinking such as "Camila is going to end up in jail for the rest of her life," or "be a total failure." In one instance, Camila's father stepped in to back up her mother, and in the other two circumstances, her sister either stepped in to back up their mother or threatened to call her. In each instance, as the arguments escalated, Camila began to feel overwhelmed, ganged up on, and hopeless as well as angry. Each time she grabbed a nearby bottle of medication and attempted to swallow the pills either immediately or after running into her room and locking the door. These sequences helped the therapist and family establish the following fit assessment of Camila's suicide attempts (Figure 7–2).

Agreement on the Overarching Goals of Therapy

The final step in the MST intake assessment process is to help the family develop *overarching goals for treatment* (Table 7–5). These will serve as

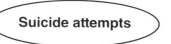

Potential causes or drivers of the problem
Family conflict
■ Academic failure, difficulties in school, or truancy underlie conflicts in all 3 attempts.
■ Affiliation with negative peers is source of conflict in all 3 attempts.
Youth is impulsive, has poor emotional regulation, is diagnosed with ADHD and bipolar disorder.
Youth has easy access to method of self-harm, medications.
Parents lack knowledge and skills to de-escalate and manage conflict.
Parents allow sister to take on a parenting role.
Peer (Cindy) has modeled this behavior and may encourage it directly or indirectly.
Youth is irritable, may have a mood disorder, is diagnosed with bipolar disorder, has depressive symptoms.
Marijuana use: youth was positive for marijuana on urine drug screen after each attempt.

FIGURE 7-2. Fit assessment of Camila's suicide attempts.

ADHD = attention-deficit/hyperactivity disorder.

the anchor points for MST, as all clinical decisions focus on reaching these targets. The overarching goals of treatment are created by the therapist, with input from the family and clinical team. Ideally, meeting these goals will diminish the referral behaviors, achieve the desired outcomes of key participants, and help to establish clear discharge criteria.

TABLE 7-5. Overarching goals of treatment

Camila will refrain from self-injurious behaviors such as taking pills, as evidenced by self and family report.

Family will learn to use effective problem solving and communication strategies, as evidenced by therapist observation and family report, utilizing family interaction tracking chart.

Camila will reduce truancy from school by obtaining a 90% attendance record for all classes over the next 3 months.

Camila will increase association with prosocial peers, as evidenced by involvement in at least one prosocial activity and confirmed by parent report.

Camila will stop smoking marijuana, as evidenced by clean urine drug screens.

Developing and Implementing Interventions

MST therapists follow a specific procedure called the *analytic process* by which they develop hypotheses concerning the most powerful proximal drivers to the identified problem and select therapeutic steps to target these drivers. Care is taken to keep family members aligned with interventions, which is facilitated by their active involvement in the assessment process and participation in the development of fit assessments and the case conceptualization. When choosing interventions, priority is placed on using evidence-based empirically validated approaches whenever possible. Once a decision is made to try an intervention (e.g., teach family problem-solving and communication strategies), the concept is proposed to the supervisor and consultant in weekly supervision and consultation meetings. Then, when given approval, therapists will break down the process into smaller steps and report to the team concerning the accomplishment of these steps weekly (e.g., intermediate goal for this week: have Mother and Father reenact a recent dispute, practice identifying trigger points, and brainstorm alternative steps at each juncture). Therapists are constantly tracking outcomes from various perspectives. When sticking points develop, they bring these barriers up in supervision and consultation meetings to receive feedback and develop new strategies for overcoming the barriers. A brief overview of some of the interventions implemented with the Martinez family is described next.

Interventions to Enhance Safety

Soon after obtaining the safety checklist, sequence, and fit assessment of the youth's suicidal behavior, the therapist worked with the family to clean out the medicine cabinet. The mother threw out old unused prescriptions and locked up the remaining medications in a lockbox provided by the team. The parents put away or locked up other potential weapons or sharp objects, such as kitchen knives, as well, helping to decrease the risk of the youth harming herself or family members during an impulsive outburst. The family also confirmed that they did not keep alcohol or guns in the home. A safety plan was developed, outlining clear pragmatic steps for each individual to take if another family conflict or incident involving verbal aggression were to arise. This plan encouraged the family to call the therapist or MST on-call team during a crisis, and the plan was then practiced during a family therapy session. The aunt was engaged later in treatment and noted on this safety plan as a resource for the youth or Ms. Martinez to access if they were struggling to calm down or feeling suicidal or distressed. The safety plan was a living document, updated throughout treatment to reflect the evolving nature of the family's needs.

Interventions to Improve Family Communication

Once the immediate risk factors were alleviated, the team decided that *family conflict* was a powerful and proximal driver of the safety concerns and needed to be better managed for treatment to progress. Interventions included sessions tailored to improve each parent's knowledge and skill set and to provide the opportunity for them to practice communicating with each other and their daughters in ways that reduced conflict. As the parents were learning the skills, the therapist or crisis caseworker would go to the home during potentially difficult times (e.g., during scheduled room safety checks) to observe and provide in vivo feedback. As work with this family advanced, it quickly became apparent that the mother's anxiety made it difficult for her to remain calm and rational during family arguments. As a result, the family interventions were modified to put the father in the lead parenting role during stressful interactions. The sister was also encouraged to take a less confrontational role in family discussions and to better support Camila in deescalating when Mr. Martinez was not present. Camila worked with the therapist and crisis caseworker to develop stress management skills and practiced using them in vivo with support from the therapist. To help the family generalize their gains, the aunt was recruited to fill in the roles initially provided by the therapist or caseworker in supporting Camila as she de-escalated either in person or by phone.

Interventions to Improve Mom's Mental Health Symptoms

As treatment progressed, it became increasingly apparent that Ms. Martinez's symptoms of anxiety and depression were impacting her functioning at both home and work. As a result, a fit assessment of these symptoms was completed. Through this process, the therapist discovered that Mom was a "fragile diabetic" and low or high blood sugars seemed to be a powerful driver of her anxiety symptoms. As a result, the MST psychiatrist and team helped Ms. Martinez connect to a diabetes clinic near her home that provided substantial hands on assistance with insulin monitoring and advice concerning medications. Ultimately, Ms. Martinez received an insulin pump, and this greatly improved her ability to maintain adequate serum glucose levels and, secondarily, diminished her anxiety. Other interventions targeting Ms. Martinez's anxiety and depression included an evaluation by the MST team psychiatrist, who prescribed an antidepressant to target mood symptoms and assisted the team in monitoring her progress and establishing follow-up services. The therapist employed CBT with Ms. Martinez to help her better identify faulty cognitions and beliefs that were driving her symptoms and to develop strategies for overcoming these. Mr. Martinez participated in some of these sessions so that he could better support his wife as she learned new skills. By discharge from MST-Psychiatric, approximately 6 months after intake, Ms. Martinez was receiving antidepressants from her physician in the diabetic clinic and was attending a weekly support group there as well. She was also connected with the clinic's social worker, with a clear plan in place for accessing further mental health treatment should problems arise.

Interventions to Improve Camila's Mental Health Symptoms

Assessment of Camila's mental health began at intake, with the parents and youth completing a Child Behavior Checklist (Achenbach 1991). This, along with a thorough clinical evaluation and subsequent teacher reports, suggested that Camila continued to struggle with symptoms of ADHD as well as with the signs of depression, including irritable mood and sleep disturbance. She did not, however, demonstrate symptoms specific to bipolar disorder either on clinical evaluation or based on measures obtained from the youth or her parents on the Young Mania Rating Scale (Gracious et al. 2002). Once these assessments were complete, at approximately 3 weeks into treatment, the MST team psychiatrist evaluated Camila with her mother and the therapist attending the session. On the basis of this interview, past hospitalization records, and the assessment provided by MST team colleagues, the psychiatrist decided that the diagnosis of bipolar disorder was not warranted. Rather, the diagnoses of depression with comorbid ADHD and marijuana abuse seemed most appropriate. In light of this analysis, the psychiatrist worked with the team and family to discontinue the aripiprazole and begin monotherapy with a selective serotonin reuptake inhibitor (SSRI) as recommended by evidence-based treatment guidelines (Hughes et al. 2007; Pliszka et al. 2006). A decision was made to target Camila's depression first because these symptoms were considered to be more proximal drivers of her suicidal behaviors.

The therapist and parents developed a plan to give Camila the medication each day and track compliance and sleep patterns with weekly pill counts and sleep charts. Symptom response was monitored at 2 and 4 weeks with a Revised Children's Anxiety and Depression Scale (Chorpita et al. 2011; www.childfirst.ucla.edu/resources), which was completed by the parents and youth to track depression/anxiety. Therapists also tracked Camila's suicidal thoughts to ensure the SSRI was not having unintended consequences. By 4 weeks, Camila's depressive symptoms, in particular her sleep pattern and irritability were improved, yet as expected, she continued to struggle with ADHD symptoms. As a result, the MST psychiatrist saw the family again and added a stimulant to her medication regimen. This resulted in an improvement in Camila's ADHD symptoms based on both caregiver and teacher report on a standardized measure (Conners 1989). As a result, Camila was ultimately treated with a low-dose long-acting stimulant and a routine dose of an SSRI. At discharge from MST-Psychiatric, both sets of symptoms were improved based on clinical assessment and objective measures. The family was linked with the nearby community mental health center a month before discharge, and the MST therapist attended the first session with Camila's future providers to ensure adequate follow-up services. The MST psychiatrist wrote a note to the receiving psychiatrist detailing treatment recommendations. In terms of psychotherapeutic interventions, the MST therapist attempted to provide CBT strategies to assist Camila with symptoms of anxiety and depression. The youth had little patience for this process, yet she responded well to the therapist's attempts early in treatment to teach and help her develop coping strategies for managing her irritability and anger that were practiced routinely with the crisis caseworker. Toward the end of treatment, the therapist taught Camila's father and aunt how to help her access these coping skills, so that they could continue to be generalized.

School Interventions

Assessment of Camila's school situation began with the therapist helping the family set up and prepare for a meeting with the guidance counselor and teachers. The goals of this meeting were to help the team and family better understand Camila's strengths and needs in each class and the factors within the school and peer subsystems in the school that sustained or improved her functioning. A secondary purpose of the meeting was to assess each parent's ability to interact productively with school personnel and to facilitate improved caregiver and school relations. The team found that Camilla was failing math and physical education (PE) and was generally considered a troublemaker by those two teachers. She frequently skipped these classes with her friends Maria and Shaniqua. On the other hand, she was passing her other classes with a B or C and seemed to be unnoticed and somewhat neglected by those teachers. A fit assessment of poor school performance revealed the drivers shown in Figure 7–3.

A series of interventions ensued over the next 5 months to address these barriers to better school performance. In summary, the MST Team advocated that an Individual Educational Evaluation (IEE) be conducted to determine if Camila qualified for an Individualized Education Program (IEP) or 504 Plan. Although the school was at first reluctant, a call and written request from the MST team psychiatrist helped speed this process along. More pragmatic immediate steps included a decision by the family and school to pull Camila out of the two classes she was failing. With the encouragement of the guidance counselor, she was enrolled in an art class taught by a teacher that had a strong track record of engaging youth like Camila. Her math class was replaced by a closely monitored math study hall designed to help remediate students and better prepare them for future math classes. These changes resulted in Camila being placed on a different lunch schedule, which served to diminish her contact with negative peers and placed her at lunch with one of her previous prosocial friends (Nicole). Importantly, the guidance counselor worked with the family to enroll Camila in a new program that contained a more vocational focus and included a track for youth interested in art. Camila was able to begin this new program after winter break, approximately 3 months into MST treatment. These interventions combined with the ongoing work to stabilize her medications resulted in greatly improved school attendance. The family also worked with the therapist on the home-school link, creating a

Poor school performance in PE & Math

- ■ Maria and Shaniqua, labeled as negative peers by the family and school, are in these classes.
- ■ Camila enjoys leaving with Maria and Shaniqua to get high instead of attending class.
- ■ Classes occur after lunch; low school monitoring during lunch makes it easy to sneak off campus.
- ■ Camila feels disengaged from the school academically.
- ■ Camila has lost connection with her prosocial peers who do well in school.
- ■ Camilla is not involved in a prosocial or extracurricular activity in the school.
- ■ Camila struggles with inattention and impulse control, untreated ADHD.
- ■ Parent-school link is poor, teachers and parents do not routinely communicate, and parents are unaware of their role in advocating for their daughter's needs or how to carry that role out.
- ■ Camila struggles with math, does not understand material.
- ■ Camila does not have a positive relationship or close link to an adult in the school.
- ■ There is no IEP or 504 Plan in place to address Camila's needs related to ADHD and depression.

FIGURE 7-3. **Fit assessment of Camila's poor school performance.**

ADHD=attention-deficit/hyperactivity disorder; IEP=Individualized Education Program; PE=physical education.

process to monitor her homework completion and attendance and provide rewards and consequences for these behaviors.

Substance Use and Peer Interventions

Substance use and peer interventions in MST are often interwoven because hanging out with substance-using peers is the single most powerful predictor of adolescent substance use and abuse (Henggeler 1991; Jenkins 1996; Kosterman et al. 2000). Hence interventions to reduce drug use must address peer influence to be successful.

In Camila's case, the use of marijuana was problematic as it was linked to all three suicide attempts and to the antisocial behaviors of truancy and shoplifting. Although initially Camila reported that she only smoked marijuana about once a week, further evaluation revealed that she was smoking 3–4 times a week. She smoked primarily with Shaniqua, Maria, and

Cindy either in the context of skipping classes on Tuesdays and Thursdays or on the weekends when the girls would often meet in the nearby park and smoke. During these times, they would sometimes go into local bodegas and shoplift small food items or trinkets. Camila had only been caught once, but Maria and Shaniqua were both on juvenile probation for shoplifting, and Cindy, who was 17, had been locked up for 6 months on Rikers Island on robbery and assault charges.

All MST-Psychiatric therapists are trained in *contingency management (CM) for adolescent substance abuse* (Henggeler et al. 2012). This is an evidence-based intervention designed to work with adolescents and their families to reduce teen substance use or abuse. There is also substantial evidence supporting the effectiveness of MST alone (Henggeler et al. 2009b) in reducing adolescent substance use. Thus MST-Psychiatric therapists often combine the more individually focused cognitive and behavioral treatment tactics of CM (e.g., functional analysis of drug use, drug refusal skill training, self-management plans) with the systemic family interventions of MST (e.g., increased parental monitoring and supervision, increased parental awareness of and involvement in peer systems) to reduce youth substance use.

The usual MST approach of sequencing and obtaining a fit assessment of Camila's drug use, combined with the CM work of obtaining a functional analysis, led the MST team to believe that the best course of action to help Camilla stop drug use was to help her parents cut off her access to the drug-using peers and get her involved in prosocial activities. Interventions to address Camila's ADHD and depressive symptoms were also considered important as were strategies to increase academic success. Given the central role that family conflict played in driving the high-risk referral behaviors of suicide attempt and verbal aggression, the team prioritized implementing the family interventions first. Once the therapist felt comfortable with the parent's ability to manage difficult situations, the problem of the youth's marijuana use was reintroduced.

By this time, some progress was being made with the school interventions, and the parents were beginning to understand the central role played by peers in their child's antisocial behaviors. A behavioral plan was already in place, and the family had experienced some success in using the plan to decrease truancy, increase homework completion, and improve sibling interactions. The parents had also been taught to search the youth's room and backpack for marijuana/drugs and to dispose of any drugs or drug paraphernalia early in treatment as part of the safety checklist and safety-planning process. The parents had experienced mixed success, up to this point, in impacting Camila's affiliation with problematic peers. She continued to sneak away from the house after school or on weekends to meet up with the drug-using friends. Her parents felt that she was still using marijuana and in danger of being arrested again.

With this foundation, the team facilitated the following interventions to impact peers and substance use:

- Introduced contingency management to the youth and caregivers and completed a functional analysis of Camila's marijuana use
- Taught the mother (first with the therapist supporting her, then with the father doing so) to collect urine drug screens using a home test kit provided by the team
- Developed an in-depth understanding, with the mother in session, of the triggers of the youth's drug use—which often involved peers
- Worked with the family to create a reward menu with behavioral incentives for the youth to stay clean
- Helped the family stick to their plan, implementing rewards when the youth tested clean

As might be expected, the family became a bit overwhelmed at some point and struggled to follow through with this somewhat intense protocol. The youth continued to test positive for marijuana and began to sneak out of the house and hang out with her substance-using friends more as the behavioral plan fell apart.

At this point, Camila's friend Maria was arrested again for shoplifting and held in detention. Apparently, Camila narrowly escaped being caught as well. This event seemed to motivate the family and helped the therapist engage everyone in taking a renewed look at their strengths and struggles in impacting Camila's drug use and peers. On the basis of a fit assessment, the team decided to back off some of the cognitive-behavioral aspects of the CM treatment, as they seemed to be overwhelming the family, and to focus on simplifying the behavioral plan and helping the parents access prosocial peers and activities. Ms. Martinez also agreed to pull her sister into treatment more, specifically to help her monitor and reward Camila.

As a result, the parents tied one important reward, the youth's cell phone, to testing clean. Camila was tested once a week at random times, and if she tested clean, she was allowed to have the phone until the next test. If she refused to test, the test was considered "dirty," and the parents held her phone until she tested clean again. The team helped the family follow through with this plan in a manner that minimized conflict. As a result, Camila lost access to her phone for several weeks and became more invested in getting clean.

To increase prosocial peer activities, the parents encouraged and rewarded Camila for participating in an after-school activity with her art class, painting sets for the high school play. This helped keep Camila occupied during after-school hours, and she began to make new friends among the high school art crowd while increasing her links with the art teacher.

A family session was held at Aunt Angelia's home with the parents and therapist. In this session, it was decided that Angelia would help Camila and one of her prosocial peers (Jasmine) enroll in and attend a weekend teen program at a nearby art museum. Aunt Angelia also agreed to have Camila come to her house after school on Wednesdays for dinner, to fill in a gap in the family monitoring plan.

Slowly, with the family's and school's support and reinforcement of prosocial peers and positive activities, Camila disconnected from her drug-using peers and began to routinely test clean from marijuana. At the end of treatment, the family was left with a clear and simple behavioral plan designed to promote sobriety. This plan provided guidelines to help the family continue to drug test periodically with screens purchased from a local pharmacy and to withhold the cell phone if the drug screen was dirty. The family also continued to routinely check Camila's room for drugs and to strongly enforce positive peer experiences, while limiting interface with negative peers as much as possible.

Closure

As described in the subsection "Finding the Fit," MST is based on nine treatment principles (Henggeler et al. 2009b). The ninth principle is as follows: "interventions should be designed to promote treatment generalization and long-term maintenance of therapeutic change by empowering caregivers to address family members' needs across multiple systemic contexts" (p. 15). Some of the processes in MST specifically designed to foster generalization include the following: the home-based model of service delivery; the continuous attention to engagement and alignment throughout treatment; the focus on placing caregivers front and center in both the assessment and intervention process; and the emphasis on systemic strengths and the use of indigenous resources to facilitate and maintain change. One outcome of this process, which sets MST apart from most conventional treatments, is that therapists spend substantially more time with caregivers than adolescents and do not routinely meet with the youth alone. Rather, consistent with the research supporting the mechanisms of change underlying MST, caregivers are directly involved in most youth therapy sessions. This builds the caregiver's capacity to help their child, a role they will likely need to continue to fill for many years.

For instance, the entire Martinez family learned and practiced coping skills with Camila at some point in treatment. Ms. Martinez participated in CM interventions with the therapist. As a result, she was aware of the triggers of Camila's drug use and was able to obtain a fit assessment and functional analysis of such use. Ms. Martinez also learned to help her daughter develop self-management plans to avoid drug use and practice drug refusal skills. Substantial time was spent with the parents, helping them work together to develop and practice strategies for dealing with common problems such as Camila's suicidal behaviors, truancy, and verbal aggression. By developing these plans and practicing, with the therapist providing frequent assistance early on, the parents experienced success and learned to modify the behavioral plans and intervene with less assistance over time. Similarly, the parents learned to communicate routinely with the school and more closely monitor and advocate for Camila's needs with the guidance counselor and teachers. Ideally, these gains will generalize, and the family will be better suited to manage the problems that will certainly arise over time.

To further promote generalization, MST therapists will often have families prepare for treatment termination by reviewing the overarching goals of treatment and completing a fit assessment on the gains made. This helps the family better understand how they have reached their goals and participate in designing strategies to sustain these gains.

For instance, in the case of the Martinez family, the parents listed each achievement and then created a set of steps they planned to take to sustain each treatment gain. Care was taken to ensure that each of these steps was an extension of tasks already successfully undertaken by the family, and, thus, they were sustainable in the natural ecology. Table 7–6 is similar to the one created by this family and placed in a central location in their home at discharge.

The last day of treatment occurred close to Ms. Martinez's birthday. Capitalizing on this opportunity, the therapist brought a small birthday cake along to celebrate the family's accomplishments and help to formalize the closure. A research assistant met with the family a few days later to collect outcome measures, closing the loop in the team's analytic process.

Recommendations for Clinicians Interested in Using This Treatment Approach

Adopting and Adapting the Treatment Across Various Practice Settings

As depicted in this case example, MST-Psychiatric is an intensive intervention implemented by a team of trained clinicians providing home-based services while following a well-researched (Schoenwald et al. 2003), carefully specified, quality assurance protocol. As such, clinicians are not individually certified in the model; rather teams of therapists embedded in licensed agencies are qualified to provide MST and MST-Psychiatric. These agencies are often part of private service provider organizations contracted to provide services by public juvenile justice, child welfare, or mental health authorities (Sheidow et al. 2007). To date, MST-Psychiatric has been funded by federal research grants, foundations, and juvenile justice or mental health service system initiatives. By design, it targets the families of children and adolescents presenting complex, multifaceted, and challenging mental health and behavioral problems that are costly to service systems. Hence, it is most salient for agencies or organizations that wish to provide evidence-based effective services for youth that are not responding to routine clinical care or are at risk of out of home placement.

Clinical Implementation

At this time, there are no adaptations to the MST model for use by individual therapists or those providing office rather than home-based services. This is largely because research strongly supports the need for high

TABLE 7-6. Martinez family achievement maintenance plan

Improved family communication

Parents to continue to discuss problems and plan together before acting

Parents to continue to maintain behavioral plan that rewards Camila for curfew compliance, attending school, and completing homework on time

Camila to continue new anger management/coping skills and reach out to Aunt or Father or Lilly if skills are not working

Ms. Martinez to continue to use her new anxiety management skills and reach out to her husband or sister if skills are not working

All family members to take a break and initiate a time out if conflict starts

Family to reach out to Aunt, Mom's social worker, or Camila's therapist if they need advice

Medication compliance for Camila

Medications to remain in lock box, dispensed by Mr. Martinez daily to ensure compliance, key to box to remain in parents' possession at all times

Camila to continue to see therapist and psychiatrist at local mental health center for refills monthly. Ms. Martinez to ensure this happens

Ms. Martinez's improved anxiety symptoms

Continue medications for anxiety/depression and diabetes

Continue to reach out to diabetes clinic, doctor, and social worker as needed

Continue to practice coping techniques

Mr. Martinez to help as needed

Camila staying abstinent from marijuana

Parents will continue to do urine drug screens periodically at random or if Camila seems high.

Parents will continue to make clean screens a requirement for having the phone.

Family will continue to help Camila pursue after-school and art activities.

Aunt to help with weekend art activity and stay involved.

Ms. Martinez will continue to call and stay in touch with parents of friends to monitor.

School: attendance and grades improved

Ms. Martinez will continue to touch base with the guidance counselor once a week by email.

Parents will meet with the guidance counselor and teachers twice a semester or more as needed.

Parents will continue to stay in touch with art teacher, facilitate prosocial activities.

levels of quality assurance to ensure treatment fidelity and promote strong clinical outcomes (Schoenwald et al. 2008). Hence, MST is best carried out by therapists nested in peer, supervisory, and organizational structures that support and maintain fidelity to the model. These needs, in turn, are best met by the home-based, team-oriented model of service delivery that has been utilized for over 30 years and evaluated in 62 outcome, implementation, and benchmarking studies (http://mstservices.com/files/outcomestudies.pdf).

Therapists interested in taking a more MST-like approach to treatment may want to consider utilizing social-ecological principles to frame assessment and treatment (Bronfenbrenner 1979; Cicchetti and Toth 1998). To do this, the youth's suicidal behavior should be understood within the context of the youth's level of development as well as the family, school, peer, and neighborhood systems within which the behavior was created. To better comprehend these drivers and to create effective interventions, it is important to obtain the perspectives of caregivers and supportive adults, siblings, and peers in the youth's ecology. Once these perspectives are obtained, it is essential to keep caregivers actively engaged in treatment so that improvements can be generalized to the home environment. For youth who have attempted suicide or who are reporting significant levels of suicide ideation, credible steps should be taken to limit access to means, with special attention given to firearms and the availability of alcohol or other drugs that might synergistically increase risk (Brent et al. 1987). Therapists should address identified risk factors with evidence-based interventions whenever possible and strive to keep caregivers engaged and actively involved throughout treatment. Table 7–7 lists the treatment elements that can be implemented in everyday practice. Ideally, caregivers should be present and active in every treatment session as they are ultimately responsible for helping their child obtain and sustain clinical gains.

Resources for Additional Training and Suggested Readings

As noted previously, MST-Psychiatric is recognized as an evidence-based practice by the Substance Abuse and Mental Health Services Administration (SAMHSA) National Registry of Evidence-based Programs and Practices

TABLE 7-7.	Elements of the treatment that can be easily implemented in everyday practice

- Assess the drivers of the presenting problems across multiple systems (e.g., family, school, peer, community) and from multiple perspectives (e.g., youth, family members, teachers).
- Involve the family and stay strength focused; try to leverage each person's strengths to help the family move toward positive gains.
- Identify potential means of self-harm, evaluate access to means, and create clear action-oriented goals to reduce access to means. Assess that these goals are met and sustained throughout treatment.
- Utilize evidence-based interventions and therapeutic techniques to treat the identified drivers of manifesting problems.
- Prioritize caregiver engagement and involvement in treatment.
- Teach caregivers to assess and intervene with their child to increase safety.
- Be prepared to treat or find effective services for family members.

(NREPP; http://www.nrepp.samhsa.gov/viewintervention.aspx?id=17) and the National Institute of Justice's Crime Solutions Program (https://www.crimesolutions.gov/ProgramDetails.aspx?ID=176). More information about the model can be found on these websites and the home webpage for MST Services (MSTServices.com), an organization designed to assist agencies and the larger systems in which they are embedded in implementing MST and MST-Psychiatric with fidelity.

A book describing the treatment model has also been written and is published by Guilford Press (Henggeler et al. 2002) and can be found at www.guilford.com/books/Serious-Emotional-Disturbance-in-Children-and-Adolescents/Henggeler-Schoenwald-Rowland-Cunningham/9781572307803.

References

Achenbach TM: Manual for the Child Behavior Checklist and 1991 Profile. Burlington, Vermont, University of Vermont Department of Psychiatry, 1991

American Academy of Child and Adolescent Psychiatry: Level of Care Placement Criteria for Psychiatric Illness. Washington DC, American Academy of Child and Adolescent Psychiatry, 1996

Brent DA, Perper JA, Allman CJ: Alcohol, firearms, and suicide among youth: temporal trends in Allegheny County, Pennsylvania, 1960 to 1983. JAMA 257(24):3369–3372, 1987 3586265

Bronfenbrenner U: The Ecology of Human Development: Experiments by Design and Nature. Cambridge, MA, Harvard University Press 1979

Chorpita BF, Ebesutani C, Spence SH: Revised Children's Anxiety and Depression Scale. 2011. Available at: https://www.childfirst.ucla.edu/wp-content/uploads/sites/163/2018/03/RCADSUsersGuide20150701.pdf. Accessed December 3, 2018.

Cicchetti D, Toth SL: The development of depression in children and adolescents. Am Psychol 53(2):221–241, 1998 9491749

Conners CK: Manual for the Conners Teacher Rating Scales (CTRS) and Conners Parent Rating Scales (CPRS). Toronto, ON, Canada, Multi-Health Systems 1989

Deković M, Asscher JJ, Manders WA, et al: Within-intervention change: mediators of intervention effects during multisystemic therapy. J Consult Clin Psychol 80(4):574–587, 2012 22563638

Gracious BL, Youngstrom EA, Findling RL, et al: Discriminative validity of a parent version of the Young Mania Rating Scale. J Am Acad Child Adolesc Psychiatry 41(11):1350–1359, 2002 12410078

Haley J: The Jossey-Bass Social and Behavioral Science Series: Problem-Solving Therapy, 2nd Edition. San Francisco, CA, Jossey-Bass, 1987

Henggeler SW: Multidimensional causal models of delinquent behavior and their implications for treatment, in Context and Development. Edited by Cohen R, Siegel AW. Hillsdale, NJ, Erlbaum, 1991, pp 211–231

Henggeler SW, Rowland MD, Randall J, et al: Home-based multisystemic therapy as an alternative to the hospitalization of youths in psychiatric crisis: clinical outcomes. J Am Acad Child Adolesc Psychiatry 38(11):1331–1339, 1999 10560218

Henggeler SW, Schoenwald SK, Rowland MD, Cunningham PB: Serious Emotional Disturbance in Children and Adolescents: Multisystemic Therapy. New York, Guilford, 2002

Henggeler SW, Letourneau EJ, Chapman JE, et al: Mediators of change for multisystemic therapy with juvenile sexual offenders. J Consult Clin Psychol 77(3):451–462, 2009a 19485587

Henggeler SW, Schoenwald SK, Borduin CM, et al: Multisystemic Therapy for Antisocial Behavior in Children and Adolescents, 2nd Edition. New York, Guilford, 2009b

Henggeler SW, Cunningham PB, Rowland MD, et al: Contingency Management for Adolescent Substance Abuse: A Practitioner's Guide. New York, Guilford, 2012

Huey SJ Jr, Henggeler SW, Brondino MJ, et al: Mechanisms of change in multisystemic therapy: reducing delinquent behavior through therapist adherence and improved family and peer functioning. J Consult Clin Psychol 68(3):451–467, 2000 10883562

Huey SJ Jr, Henggeler SW, Rowland MD, et al: Multisystemic therapy effects on attempted suicide by youths presenting psychiatric emergencies. J Am Acad Child Adolesc Psychiatry 43(2):183–190, 2004 14726725

Hughes CW, Emslie GJ, Crismon ML, et al: Texas Children's Medication Algorithm Project: update from Texas Consensus Conference Panel on Medication Treatment of Childhood Major Depressive Disorder. J Am Acad Child Adolesc Psychiatry 46(6):667–686, 2007 17513980

Jenkins JE: The influence of peer affiliation and student activities on adolescent drug involvement. Adolescence 31(122):297–306, 1996 8726891

Kaur P, Pote H, Fox S, et al: Sustaining change following multisystemic therapy: caregiver's perspectives. J Fam Ther 39:264–283, 2015

Kosterman R, Hawkins JD, Guo J, et al: The dynamics of alcohol and marijuana initiation: patterns and predictors of first use in adolescence. Am J Public Health 90(3):360–366, 2000 10705852

Paradisopoulos D, Pote H, Fox S, et al: Developing a model of sustained change following multisystemic therapy: young people's perspectives. J Fam Ther 37:471–491, 2015

Pliszka SR, Crismon ML, Hughes CW, et al; Texas Consensus Conference Panel on Pharmacotherapy of Childhood Attention Deficit Hyperactivity Disorder: The Texas Children's Medication Algorithm Project: revision of the algorithm for pharmacotherapy of attention-deficit/hyperactivity disorder. J Am Acad Child Adolesc Psychiatry 45(6):642–657, 2006 16721314

Rowland MD, Halliday-Boykins CA, Henggeler SW, et al: A randomized trial of multisystemic therapy with Hawaii's Felix Class Youths. J Emot Behav Disord 13(1):13–23, 2005

Schoenwald SK, Ward DM, Henggeler SW, et al: Multisystemic therapy versus hospitalization for crisis stabilization of youth: placement outcomes 4 months postreferral. Ment Health Serv Res 2:3–12, 2000 11254068

Schoenwald SK, Sheidow AJ, Letourneau EJ, et al: Transportability of multisystemic therapy: evidence for multilevel influences. Ment Health Serv Res 5(4):223–239, 2003 14672501

Schoenwald SK, Carter RE, Chapman JE, et al: Therapist adherence and organizational effects on change in youth behavior problems one year after multisystemic therapy. Adm Policy Ment Health 35(5):379–394, 2008 18561019

Schoenwald SK, Chapman JE, Sheidow AJ, et al: Long-term youth criminal outcomes in MST transport: the impact of therapist adherence and organizational climate and structure. J Clin Child Adolesc Psychol 38(1):91–105, 2009 19130360

Sheidow AJ, Schoenwald SK, Wagner HR, et al: Predictors of workforce turnover in a transported treatment program. Adm Policy Ment Health 34(1):45–56, 2007 16767507

Tighe A, Pistrang N, Casdagli L, et al: Multisystemic therapy for young offenders: families' experiences of therapeutic processes and outcomes. J Fam Psychol 26(2):187–197, 2012 22329390

Wagner BM: Family risk factors for child and adolescent suicidal behavior. Psychol Bull 121(2):246–298, 1997 9100488

Wagner BM: Suicidal Behavior in Children and Adolescents. New Haven, CT, Yale University Press 2009

Wagner BM, Silverman AC, Martin CE: Family factors in youth suicidal behaviors. Am Behav Sci 46(9):1171–1191, 2003

Attachment-Based Family Therapy for Suicidal Youth and Young Adults

Guy S. Diamond, Ph.D.
Quintin A. Hunt, Ph.D.
Bora Jin, Ph.D.
Suzanne A. Levy, Ph.D.

Overview of Treatment Approach

Attachment-based family therapy (ABFT; Diamond et al. 2014) rests on the assumption that secure attachment relationships between parents and adolescents provide both a foundation for direct, supportive communication and a buffer against the stressors that lead to suicide (Bowlby 1988). This relationship, however, is not only a safe haven from stress; it is also the context within which adolescents develop perspective taking, emotion regulation, and other developmental competencies that protect against depression and suicide (Kobak et al. 2006). Secure attachment thus helps to solidify an internal capacity to resolve conflicts cooperatively with caregivers, peers, and romantic partners.

In addition to theory, a growing body of research has established a link between negative family processes (parental control, parental criticism, emotional unresponsiveness, lack of support, lack of care, or experienced rejection) and suicide ideation and/or attempts (Wagner et al. 2003). Suicide attempts and ideations occur more frequently in families with higher levels of conflict and lower levels of cohesion (Beautrais et al. 1996). In addition, insecure attachment to parents can intensify the symptoms of depression or suicide (Restifo and Bögels 2009; Sheeber et al. 2001; Sheftall et al. 2013).

Whereas negative family factors can be a risk factor for suicide, positive family factors can be a protective factor. Family cohesion is associated with lower depression and fewer suicide-related thoughts and behaviors (McKeown et al. 1998; Rubenstein et al. 1998). Adolescents that report high levels of shared interests with their parents and describe their parents as involved and emotionally supportive are three to five times less likely to be suicidal than their peers from less supportive families (Rubenstein et al. 1998). Parental monitoring (rather than control) and supportive parent-child relationships have been associated with decreased depression and suicidal thinking and behaviors and better overall functioning (Rushton et al. 2002; Summerville et al. 1996). On the basis of this body of research, recommendations to include family in the treatment of suicidal thoughts and behaviors in youth have increased (Asarnow and Miranda 2014; Brent et al. 2013; Frey and Hunt 2018). ABFT aims to reduce negative family processes and increase positive or protective family factors.

Theoretical Model and Proposed Mechanism of Change

Fundamental Considerations

Attachment-based family therapy is a brief, family-based therapy grounded in attachment theory (Bowlby 1988). Attachment theory proposes that children are "hardwired" to seek support and comfort from their parents when distressed. When children experience their parents as responsive and available in the face of distress, they feel that 1) the world is a safe place and 2) they are worthy of being protected (and loved). Over time, these experiences of protection are internalized as working models (or expectations) of relationships. If children are treated well, then as adolescents they seek out relationships in which they will be treated well. If children are treated poorly, they internalize expectations that relationships will be unresponsive, if not hurtful. As a result of these untrustworthy relationships, children develop attachment (interpersonal) strategies to protect themselves from emotional harm. The *avoidant attached child* begins to stop wanting or expecting parental responsiveness. The *ambivalent attached child* keeps hoping for responsiveness but constantly expects to be rejected and so acts in ways that ensure that he or she *will* be rejected. The *disorganized attached child* has no effective relational strategies and often finds himself or herself confused and unable to protect himself or herself. Disorganized attached children are usually those with histories of more severe trauma (e.g., sexual or physical abuse).

In ABFT, the therapist does not "diagnose" a patient's attachment style. However, the therapist does try to reach below or behind the defensive mask of protection to resuscitate the adolescent's desire and hope for a better relationship with his or her parents. To accomplish this goal, the therapist works with parents to try to improve their natural caregiving instinct. Many parents have given up on their "problem" child, feel like they do not know how to be helpful, or lack the psychological stability to be available to their adolescent. Many also have their own histories of attachment ruptures and/or struggles with depression, substance abuse, or trauma. As with the adolescent, therefore, the therapist has to find a way to get beneath their pain or distrust and reactivate their caregiving instincts. Once this is accomplished, it is easier to promote the parents' capacity for reflective functioning and ability to comfort the adolescent by entering empathically into the adolescent's inner world.

Resuscitating the desire for attachment and caregiving sets the foundation for the remainder of the therapy. The central action of the treatment is facilitating parent-adolescent conversations about interpersonal failures that have ruptured the attachment bond. These stories usually pertain to the adolescent's experience of being ignored, uncared for, or overcriticized or a larger trauma such as abuse. Therapists do not blame the parents, rather they help the parents to listen to the adolescent express his or her feelings about these events. In this way, the adolescent has to put their anger, resentment, or sadness into words rather than keep it to himself or herself or engage in self-injury. These conversations are therefore exercises in interpersonal problem solving and emotion regulation. They also help revise the adolescent's internal working model ("Oh, maybe my parents can be there for me when I need them") as well as the parent's internal working model of their child ("My child has legitimate concerns and can express them in a regulated way"). As trust begins to reemerge, therapists focus on helping parents promote the adolescent's autonomy and competence while maintaining an age-appropriate, trustworthy, and mutually satisfying relationship.

Foundational Influences on ABFT

The ABFT treatment model integrates principles and techniques from several therapy traditions: structural family therapy (Minuchin 1974), multidimensional family therapy (Liddle et al. 2001), emotion focused/ experiential therapy (Greenberg 2011; Johnson 2004), and contextual family therapy (Böszörményi-Nagy and Spark 1973).

Perhaps the biggest impact of the structural family therapy tradition on ABFT is the belief that effective parenting is essential for healthy child and adolescent development. Although Minuchin (1974) focused mainly on the need for parents to provide boundaries and hierarchy, ABFT focuses on the need for parents to provide a secure base of support and safety as the foundation for behavioral control. The concept of enactment also plays an important role in ABFT. Minuchin believed that in-session, in vivo experiences of good family functioning were essential to solidifying change in relationships. Whereas structural therapy promotes behavioral change episodes in the session (e.g., putting parents in charge), ABFT facilitates deeply emotional and genuine conversations about core attachment needs.

Multidimensional family therapy (MDFT; Liddle et al. 2001) has made many contributions to ABFT. First, it demonstrated how psychological science can be used to understand psychotherapy processes in family therapy. MDFT used research on theories from social learning theory and parenting, as well as child, and adolescent development to inform how therapists think about treatment. ABFT adopted a similar, empirically informed approach to model development. MDFT and ABFT conceptualize therapy as a series of *processes* that lead to *an* intended outcome. The five-task structure of ABFT evolved from the four-component model of MDFT (Diamond and Liddle 1999).

ABFT is often referred to as the emotionally focused therapy (EFT) for families because of the use of emotional processes as an active therapeutic process (Greenberg 2011; Johnson 2004). ABFT therapists use the emotional intensity in the room to motivate change. This intentional effort to increase intensity is often used to activate the attachment instinct of the adolescent and the parent. Furthermore, in both EFT and ABFT, emotion is targeted and viewed as a critical agent of change. Tracking emotion in the session helps the therapist identify core attachment themes and elicit new responses from family members.

Contextual family therapy introduced the concept of trust and fairness into family therapy (Böszörményi-Nagy and Spark 1973). In childhood, attachment is negotiated through behaviors (e.g., parent picks child up and comforts him or her). In adolescence, attachment is negotiated through conversation, and trust forms the foundation of conversation. Without trust and a mutual feeling of fairness, family members will not enter into meaningful conversations about interpersonal challenges. Consequently, forgiveness is an essential theme in ABFT. Apology and forgiveness are often directly or indirectly part of the conversation when attachment ruptures are being repaired (Pargament et al. 2000). The reestablishment of fairness, trust, and love helps family members start to view one another as humans that have strengths and good intentions (I-Thou) rather than as rivals or enemies (I-It) (Buber 1937).

Improving attachment security between the adolescent and his or her parents is the primary target of change in ABFT. The proposed mechanism of change occurs at several levels. On one level, this task aims to address or resolve the interpersonal injuries that have damaged trust between parents and adolescent. If they have a more trusting relationship, then the next time the adolescent feels suicidal, he or she might turn to his or her parents for help instead of hurting himself or herself. On another level, learning to work through these kinds of interpersonal conflicts requires mastering and practicing many new interpersonal skills, such as putting feelings into words, controlling impulses, regulating emotion, and resolving conflict. In this way, these conversations become in vivo, emotionally charged, therapeutic events. On a third level, these conversations also serve as corrective attachment experiences. The adolescent turns to his or her parents and feels free to express hurt, pain, fear, and other vulnerable emotions, while the parents remain emotionally receptive and available. These positive experiences of secure attachment revise the adolescent's internal working model of what to expect from parents in times of emotional need. These three proposed mechanisms of change lead to better management of emotions, better conflict resolution skills, and better relationships with parents who can help buffer against suicide-promoting stress.

Review of Empirical Evidence

ABFT research is conducted at the Center for Family Intervention Science at Drexel University and at partnering sites throughout the world (see full review in G. Diamond et al. 2016). ABFT research has focused primarily on reducing depression, suicidal ideation, and suicide attempts in adolescents, ages 12–18 years. To date, several studies have demonstrated that ABFT is more effective than wait-list control groups or treatment as usual in reducing depression and suicidal ideation (Diamond et al. 2002, 2010). In two of these studies (e.g., Diamond et al. 2002, 2010) and in a small pilot study (G. Diamond, S. Levy, T. Creed, "Feasibility, acceptability, and outcomes of attachment-based family therapy as an aftercare model for suicidal youth," manuscript in preparation, 2018), the ABFT treatment had more success in reducing suicide attempts than wait-list control or treatment as usual, but more research with a population who attempted suicide is needed to fully test this. ABFT has also been adapted for use with suicidal lesbian, gay, and bisexual adolescents (G.M. Diamond et al. 2012) and with young adults with unresolved anger toward a caregiver (G.M. Diamond et al. 2016). Secondary data analysis indicates that ABFT is effective for severely depressed adolescents and for those with a history of sexual trauma, both of which are predictors of poor response in treatment with combined medication and cognitive-behavioral therapy (Asarnow et al. 2009; Barbe et al. 2004; G. Diamond et al. 2012). Several process studies (e.g., G. Diamond et al. 2012; Ibrahim et al. 2018) have also explored the proposed mechanisms of change.

Several effectiveness research projects have been conducted or are currently underway. Israel and Diamond (2013) explored the feasibility of training therapists to conduct ABFT in a hospital setting in Norway. Similar implementation challenges are explored in three recent papers on implementing ABFT in Australia (G.S. Diamond et al. 2016), Belgium (Santens et al. 2016), and Sweden (Ringborg 2016). In the United States, we have recently partnered with a youth community health center (CHC) to conduct an implementation study of ABFT in a CHC working with a population of lesbian, gay, bisexual, transgender, and queer (LGBTQ) youth. ABFT also has a long history of success with low-income, minority youth who have been remarkably absent from many of the clinical trials testing interventions for depression and suicidality (Bernal et al. 2009).

ABFT has been evaluated with youth with mental health problems other than depression and suicidality and when depression and suicidality are comorbid with other mental health problems. There are published studies focused on anxiety (G. Diamond et al. 2012; Siqueland et al. 2005), unresolved anger (G.M. Diamond et al. 2016), and suicidal youth with anorexia nervosa (Wagner et al. 2016). In more recent years, ABFT has been expanded to include training and implementation in Belgium (Santens et al. 2016), Sweden (Ringborg 2016), and Norway (Israel and Diamond 2013). All of this empirical research had helped ABFT meet the criteria for a promising intervention (Chambless and Hollon 1998), and ABFT is currently listed on the National Registry of Evidence-Based Programs and Practices (NREPP) as a program with effective outcomes for depression, depressive symptoms, and suicidal thoughts and behaviors.

Treatment Components and Primary Intervention Strategies

In general, ABFT is recommended for clients 12 years of age and older and is not limited by treatment context. The model is used in outpatient, inpatient, home-based, hospital, and residential care settings. ABFT is also often done in conjunction with other individual psychotherapies (e.g., cognitive-behavioral therapy, dialectical behavioral therapy) and/or medication. Collaboration and coordination with these other providers are essential. ABFT is not recommended as a treatment approach for clients who have active psychosis, low-functioning autism spectrum disorders, borderline intellectual functioning, or severe externalizing behaviors. However, the guiding principles and tasks of ABFT can be applied when working with any family.

The treatment is conceptualized as five specific therapy tasks. A task is not a session; rather, a *task* represents a unique set of operations deemed important to the change process. Five tasks have been operationalized: relational reframe, adolescent alliance, parent alliance, attachment, and promoting autonomy. Each task has its own set of procedures, steps, and process and outcome goals. The reframe is typically one session, but the other tasks can require from one to four sessions. The tasks do not necessarily have to be completed in the order stipulated, but there is a certain elegant, logical flow to this sequence. On another level, each task represents a process that family therapists think about all the time: "Am I joined with the parents? Are we discussing the right content? Does the family still agree that relationship development is our goal?" Each task thus targets specific processes. If the therapist is in Task 4 (attachment task) but feeling stuck, he or she might think about what they did not accomplish in Task 3 (establishing parent alliance). Returning to a previous process, either in said session or in a separate session, might help to get the attachment task unstuck in the next attempt.

Task 1: Relational Reframing

The main goal for the first session is to shift the focus of the treatment from fixing the adolescent to strengthening family relationships, setting the foundation for the remainder of the therapy. The therapist begins the session by joining with all members of the family, coming to understand the severity of and past treatment for the suicidal thoughts and behaviors and exploring the impact of the youth's suicidality on other systems (e.g., family, school, health, other children, if relevant). Once this "intake" information is sufficiently complete, the therapist asks the adolescent, "When you are up in your room thinking of hurting yourself, what keeps you from going to your parents for support and help?" This question shifts the focus of the conversation from the adolescent's symptoms and problems to the quality of trust in the parent-child relationship. The ABFT model assumes that relational disappointments and conflict have damaged the attachment bond. Without this bond, adolescents do not use their parents as a resource, even when faced with life-threatening distress. The conversation sensitively, but intentionally, helps the family to identify these relational ruptures and their effects on the closeness of the parents and the adolescent. The therapist does not try to resolve the ruptures in this session but rather use them to activate family members' motivation to engage in the therapy. The therapist says to the parents, for example, "These ruptures have created distance between you and your child/children, which is getting in the way of them turning to you for help. Would you like to change that?" The session ends with an agreement to make relationship repair the first goal of therapy. Of course, some individuals in the family may be hesitant about this goal, but the therapist invites them back to discuss it more in the alliance-building sessions. The first session always ends with family-focused safety planning and an exploration of lethal means restrictions (if this has not already been completed as part of a separate intake).

Task 2: Establishing Adolescent Alliance

In the adolescent alliance task, the therapist meets alone with the adolescent (two to four sessions). The task has three phases: getting to know the adolescent better (bond), exploring the attachment narrative and obtaining the adolescent's agreement to discuss these ruptures directly with his or her parents (goal), and preparing the adolescent for the discussion with his or her parents (task). The therapist begins the task by explaining about confidentiality and its limits. In order to get to know the adolescent better, the therapist then asks about music, friends, hobbies, relationships, sex, substance use, sexual orientation, race, and life goals. When adolescents are involved in risky behaviors, therapists take a harm reduction approach. Throughout this joining process, the therapist tries to identify adolescent strengths, hopes, and dreams.

In the second phase of the task, the conversation shifts to depression and suicidal thoughts and behaviors. The therapist's goal here is not just to understand the symptoms and problems but also to see how well the adolescent understands some of the experiences and triggers that lead to his or her suicidal feelings and behaviors. Helping an adolescent to understand this depression/suicide narrative more coherently also helps him or her to see the link between these behaviors and some of the problems in his or her life (e.g., bullying, family conflict). The conversation then moves on to uncovering the attachment narrative. The therapist aims to help the adolescent to more honestly acknowledge the ways in which his or her parents have let him or her down, failed to protect him or her, or in some cases actually abused him or her and to understand the impact of these parental failures. Depressed adolescents generally have a conflict avoidant approach to interpersonal problems. They are easily angered, which can result in behavioral problems, but rarely feel comfortable or entitled to identify and talk about deeper interpersonal injuries that drive some of the anger, as well as their suicidal feelings. The therapist helps the adolescent to do so by linking these attachment narratives to the depression and suicidal feelings, which, in turn, helps motivate the adolescent to participate in the attachment task and address these ruptures more directly with his or her parents. In the third phase, the therapist prepares the adolescent for conversations with his or her parents about these relational ruptures.

Task 3: Establishing Parent Alliance

In the parent alliance task, the therapist meets alone with the parents for two to four sessions. Like the adolescent alliance task, this task has three phases: getting to know the parents better (bond), getting the parents to commit to wanting to support their adolescent in a different way (goal), and preparing the parents for the discussion with the adolescent (task). Generally, the therapist begins the task by trying to understand the current stressors that prevent the parents from being more available for their child. For example, many parents struggle with depression, marital conflicts, economic stress, or discrimination. Additionally, low-income parents often struggle with the impact of poverty, unsafe neighborhoods, bad schools, and lack of support. These conversations often lead to case management services or referrals to therapy for the parents. Simply by listening to these struggles, the therapist helps the parents to feel that the therapist understands the contextual challenges that affect them as adults (not just as parents), which, in turn, helps them to be more open to considering, and be insightful about, how the stressors in their lives impact their parenting and/or their adolescent directly.

The joining phase of Task 3 also focuses on the parents' own attachment history. Parents often fail to understand how their own histories of attachment relationships as children affect their ability to provide good parenting in the present. More importantly, the therapist helps parents to remember how a child feels when parents are not protective and available. As parents develop empathy for their own experiences as children, they become better able to sympathize with their adolescent's feelings. This reflective moment prepares the parents to be more attuned to the emotional needs of their child.

While parents are in this more reflective state, the therapist asks the parents if they would be interested in offering the support to their adolescent that they never received as a child. If the parents agree, the therapist begins to prepare the parents for the attachment task by helping them discuss and prepare for their fears about the conversation. The preparation work also involves some psychoeducational work with the parents, including emotion-coaching skills to help them remain available during Task 4.

Task 4: Attachment Task

The fourth task, repairing attachment, aims to produce a corrective attachment experience in which adolescents share their difficult and often painful stories while the parents provide support, understanding, and empathy. This task is typically broken down into one to four sessions. Initially, the adolescent opens up to his or her parents about the attachment ruptures and unmet attachment needs that he or she has experienced. The parents have been primed and coached to remain emotionally available in order to acknowledge the needs of the adolescent, and the adolescent has been primed and coached to speak about these difficult topics in a more mature, direct, and regulated manner. Sometimes, when appropriate, the parent apologizes for his or her contribution to the adolescent's feelings (e.g., divorce, alcoholism, marital conflict, unavailability). These kinds of conversations can go on for several sessions, depending on how many rupture themes or experiences the adolescent needs to discuss. This task is much more process and experience oriented than the others; there is no concrete ending point. The goal is for the parents and adolescent to tolerate the exploration of emotionally difficult material. For many adolescents, these conversations help to resolve their feelings of hurt and pain, whereas for others, they are merely a starting point and the adolescent needs to see how his or her parents will respond moving forward.

Task 5: Promoting Autonomy

After the existing relational ruptures have been addressed, trust begins to emerge. Even if there are still ruptures that have not been addressed or resolved, the mere permission to discuss them seems to lift a tension in the relationship. The goal of the attachment task is to revise the adolescent's expectation of his or her parents' availability, thus creating a more secure base relationship; in Task 5, this new expectation is put to the test. Treatment focuses on getting the adolescent back on his or her developmental track and promoting opportunities for competency and autonomy. Autonomy, however, does not come at the expense of attachment. Bowlby (1988) calls this phase a goal-corrected partnership: both parents and adolescent are equally responsible for maintaining the trustworthiness of the relationship. Both parents and adolescent must be willing to compromise to maintain the relationship.

These autonomy-promoting conversations usually happen at many levels. Potential topics include issues driving the depression or suicidality (e.g., being bullied or raped), cooperation around the home (e.g., doing chores or homework, following a curfew), or activities outside the home (e.g., getting back into school, restarting a hobby, managing other relationships, such as visiting one's father who had previously been abusive). These conversations might also focus on identity development: helping the family discuss racial or sexual marginalization or planning for the future (e.g., leaving home). Such conversations are new ones in that parents promote autonomy while the adolescent focuses on compromise. Because the process of developing and promoting autonomy is different for an 18-year-old preparing for college than for a 13-year-old struggling to adjust to middle school, therapists need to be careful to address the adolescent at a developmentally appropriate level. This task can last anywhere from a few sessions to many sessions, depending on the issues the family is facing. The therapist may also return to Tasks 2, 3, or 4 as needed.

Case Example

Alicia was a 17-year-old African American female living with her mother and younger sister. She was in the eleventh grade, was an A student, and played violin in the school orchestra. She had struggled with health problems (i.e., weak immune system) most of her life, but she had an optimistic attitude and a big, engaging personality. She had a small peer group of close friends, occasionally smoked marijuana, and had a history of fighting in school. She claimed that fighting "is just the way of life in the neighborhood where she lives." Her mother worked as an office staff member in a medical office, and her father was a computer repairman. The family had been a strong unit for many years, with both parents involved in their children's school life, Alicia's music performances, and the neighborhood community. The father, however, had been unhappy in the marriage for many years and had moved out 3 years before the family began treatment, after having an affair with another woman. When therapy began, he was still dating the other woman, although she remained married to her husband. Because of this complex situation, the children had no relationship with their father's new partner. The mother was very angry about the breakup and wanted the father to move back in with the family, although she struggled with whether or not she could forgive him. Alicia was referred for treatment after a fighting incident at school. During the evaluation by the school counselor, it was uncovered that Alicia had been severely depressed for a long time and had thoughts of hurting herself. She had also engaged in some nonsuicidal self-harm by marking her wrist with a knife. The parents were shocked that these problems were back; Alicia had been hospitalized for a suicide attempt 2 years prior to being referred for ABFT, but she had been doing well since the hospitalization. At the time of intake, Alicia's score on the Suicide Ideation Questionnaire (SIQ; Reynolds and Mazza 1999) was 45 (above 31 is clinical cutoff of risk for suicide), and her score on the Beck Depression Inventory-II (BDI-II; Beck et al. 1996) was 32 (29–63 represents severe depression).

Task 1: Relational Reframing

Only the father and Alicia attended the first session (Task 1). Initially, Alicia's father reported that the mother had to work, but during the session he disclosed that the mother felt burdened by raising the children alone, so she wanted him to bring Alicia to therapy. The therapist did not invite the younger sister because the first goal is to stabilize the suicidal patient and perform some initial attachment repair work with the parents. (We usually consider bringing siblings or other family members in during the second half of treatment.) Even though the mother did not attend, the first session still had a large impact.

After some initial bonding and history taking, the therapist spent some time trying to understand Alicia's suicidal impulses. Alicia said that she felt hopeless about life. She reported that some of her illnesses (particularly recent problems with her eyesight) made school more difficult. She had always been an A student, and now she was failing several classes, which exacerbated the fighting at school and increased her social isolation. The therapist listened carefully to these stories, looking for themes, challenges, and triggers. The conversation then moved on to the father-daughter relationship. When the therapist asked Alicia why she no longer turned to her father for support, she went silent. She shrugged her shoulders and turned away, almost in tears. The therapist asked the father why he thought his daughter was tearful. He could not answer. The father had previously been very attuned to Alicia's feelings, but he had started to drift apart from her when she started to push him away after the separation from her mother.

The therapist noted how unfortunate it was that they were now so distant when they had previously been so close. The father admitted that their relationship had been much more tense since he had moved out of the house, and Alicia agreed. The therapist explored this theme briefly but not too extensively. Instead, the therapist commented that it was tragic that these family events and other problems had created such distance between them. The therapist then said, "Without trying to sort out all these issues now, I do wonder if you miss your daughter [*activating his caregiving instinct*]? You have lost touch with her and that must sadden you…I wonder if you could turn to her now and tell her." With some hesitation from the father and coaching from the therapist, the father turned to his daughter and said he missed her. The daughter started to get defensive and accused the father of causing all the problems, but the therapist stopped her. The goal of a first session is not to go deeply into all these issues. In a first session, the family is not prepared to have a more productive conversation.

Instead, the therapist said, "Alicia, I know you are angry at your father. I think you have a right to feel that way. I would like to talk with you more about that when you and I meet alone next week. I wonder, though, if right now you could tell us if part of you misses your father? You know, when you are not feeling angry." Alicia again went silent. The therapist let this moment linger in the room before validating her anger, her sadness, and her hesitation to talk about any of this. The therapist then said to both of them, "Look, a lot has gone on in this family, a lot of challenging things, but it is clear to me that you two have lost a closeness that you once had—a closeness that I think could help you, Alicia, cope with some of the stress that leads to your thoughts about killing yourself." The therapist looked for verbal or nonverbal cues that the family members were at least interested in these ideas and then continued, "I wonder if we could spend the first part of this therapy focusing on finding out and working through as best we can the things that have gotten in the way of your dad being a resource to you, Alicia? Could we do that in here?" The father eagerly agreed, but Alicia only gave a shrug and a nonverbal "okay."

The session finished with the discussion of a safety plan and of bringing the mother in for treatment. A common safety plan worksheet was used to scaffold the strategies for Alicia to distract herself or seek help if suicidal feelings became too strong. She was hesitant to put her father down as one of the resources if she was feeling bad. She had some ambivalence about using her mother in this way as well, but she agreed that her mother was in closer proximity and that Alicia needed someone to turn to if things became difficult. Both Alicia and her father laughed when the therapist talked about bringing the mother into therapy. Alicia's father said she would not be in the same room with him. The therapist explained that might not be necessary; the therapist could work with each of them alone. Alicia and her father said that her mother was not the "therapy type" and might refuse to attend. This was the first moment of cooperation, if not tenderness, between them in the session. The family members were assured by the therapist that a sincere effort would be made to reach out to Alicia's mother.

Task 2: Establishing Adolescent Alliance

The therapist next met with Alicia alone to begin the Task 2 sessions. Alicia had much to talk about. She talked about her violin practice and concerts with great pride. Her friendship network was small, but long-standing. She aspired to be a veterinarian. She also talked about being an African American female and how much that was part of her identity. She was very proud of this identity and felt that her parents had instilled in her great values about her culture and the struggles African American females had been through. (The topic of identity usually gets discussed again in Task 5.)

The therapist then turned the conversation to Alicia's depression and suicidality. Her understanding of these was limited. She felt like she had struggled with depression most of her life but that things got worse when she turned 13. The nonsuicidal self-injury behaviors were her attempt to manage her pain. At times, she felt like she was too much of a burden to her parents, or she felt hopeless that things would ever get better. Both these feelings led her to want to kill herself. The therapist explored triggers for her prior suicide attempt, the value of the hospitalization, and what she felt kept her alive (reasons for living). Her primary motivation was her protectiveness of her sister.

In the next session, the discussion focused on Alicia's attachment rupture narrative. In this phase, the therapist tries to help the patient understand how disappointments related to family relationships might be contributing to suicidal thoughts. At first, Alicia, like many youth, denied that her parents contributed to the reasons why she had suicidal thoughts. The therapist started the attachment narrative by exploring Alicia's experience of her parents' divorce. The therapist elicited an episodic memory by asking Alicia how she learned about it, how she felt about it, and how it affected her life. Alicia described her family as a "happy family" before the divorce. The parents were very involved in the lives of the two kids and seemed to get along okay, so the divorce was a total shock to Alicia. Alicia started to talk about how it devastated her and her sister, as if her life had been ripped out from under her. They moved, they lost money, and the father was no longer there to protect her when her mother became enraged, as she often did. Alicia's mother, although a committed parent, had a difficult personality, was prone to anger, rigid in her expectations, and lacking in warmth and affection. Her father had served as a buffer against her mother's coldness, often comforting, if not protecting Alicia from her mother's frequent anger.

To shift the conversation from details to meaning, the therapist began to use more attachment language and more vulnerable emotions to frame and explore Alicia's story. The therapist empathically pointed out that the divorce resulted in not just a loss of the family but also a devastating loss of her father's closeness and protection. Although she loved her mother, she now had much more contact with her around management of daily tasks, a source of usual conflict. The daughter softened and said she had never thought about it that way. The therapist did not blame Alicia's parents for her suicidal feelings, although clearly the loss of her father and increased stress contributed to her feelings of despair and hopelessness. Instead, the therapist helped Alicia to articulate a more coherent narrative of how the loss and family conflict contributed to her suicidal feelings.

Developing her story was therapeutic in and of itself, but it also motivated Alicia to engage in the upcoming attachment task. Problems with her parents were contributing to her suicidal feelings. Therefore, if she could resolve some of these feelings, it might help her reduce some of the stress. Once Alicia accepted that strategy, the therapist prepared her for the upcoming conversation in the attachment task.

Task 3: Establishing Parent Alliance

Task 3 initially focused on the father and spanned three sessions. The therapist began the conversation by explaining how important it is for the therapist to better understand the parent's life when trying to help the parent heal his or her child. The father initially talked about his professional life. He had become a computer repairman, but he felt that he could have gone further in his education and made more money. He seemed a bit defeated by life, unhappy with this career, disappointed about his marriage, and worried about his kids. Still, he had a kind heart, a sensitive soul, and deep empathy for his daughter. He too tended to minimize the impact of the divorce on his kids, claiming that he came to the house at least once a week and continued to provide financial support to his wife and children. Over the course of these sessions, however, he came to understand how different a weekly visit was from putting the kids to bed every night, especially for Alicia. He found himself saying he was worried about how Alicia and her mother were getting along and how he used to mediate this relationship. An exploration of his early attachment history revealed a very punitive father and passive mother. The more he explored these memories, the more he began to see how his departure from his wife might have affected his daughters. He knew the feeling of being unprotected from an abusive parent figure. In the depth of that memory, he began to understand what his daughters were experiencing. This insight was used to motivate him to help his daughter talk more about these experiences directly and to begin to think about some behavioral changes he could make to better support his daughters.

Building a relationship with the mother in Task 3 took more effort. After a tense phone call during which she remained defensive, blaming the father for all the family's problems, and hesitant about the idea of therapy, the therapist offered to meet her for coffee near her place of work. The mother was surprised at this and welcomed the invitation. In ABFT, the parents are as much our patients as the adolescent. Reaching out and gaining trust are essential for alliance formation. In a small fast food restaurant, Alicia's mother told the therapist about the divorce, her anger at her husband, and her concerns about her daughter. By validating, empathizing, and showing genuine interest in her point of view, the therapist built up some trust with a woman that everyone said would never come to therapy. In a therapy session the next week, after exploring her own attachment history with the therapist, the mother also softened her view of her daughter's emotional needs. Admitting that she could be a bit harsh, she agreed to talk with her daughter during her first attachment session.

Task 4: Attachment Task

If parents are divorced, Task 4 may occur with each parent separately. (Given space limitations, we only summarize the attachment task with the father.) In the first Task 4 session, the father began by immediately apologizing for the divorce and its impact on his daughters. Although this was an admirable gesture, the therapist wanted to slow the conversation down. When apologies are appropriate, it is best when they come toward the end of the conversation, after the parent has given the adolescent an opportunity to put words to his or her inner, emotional turmoil. The therapist encouraged the father to ask more questions, which gave Alicia permission to talk about the divorce. She talked about how different things were after the divorce, how hard it was on everyone, and how she understood why he would want to leave, stating that "mom can be pretty difficult." The therapist blocked the conversation focused on empathizing with the father, asking instead if it was hard for Alicia to share her anger that was directed at her father. Alicia became uncomfortable. Her father assured her it was okay. Alicia said she was scared to show anger at her father for fear that he would come over even less than he did already. Her father was saddened to hear Alicia's dilemma and moved over on the couch and hugged her. Alicia melted in his arms, for the first time in a long time. This tender moment set the foundation for the rest of the conversation. The father encouraged Alicia to tell the truth about anything on her mind, and he remained attentive and close to her on the couch. Although such conversations do not necessarily resolve all issues, this one did help to revise the daughter's internal working model of her expectation of her father's availability.

Conversations with the mother were not as emotional. Alicia was less comfortable being honest with her mother. Instead, the therapist encouraged the mother to talk about herself. The mother was eager to apologize for her harsh ways. In a moment of surprising insight, the mother acknowledged the ways she was hard on Alicia. Some of it was well intended ("You are so talented, I just want to push you"), and some was just impatient and rigid. The shift in the conversation came when the mother talked about her own abusive childhood. Alicia knew some of these stories but had not heard them since becoming an adolescent. Gaining this perspective helped expand Alicia's view of her mother. The therapist helped the mother assure Alicia that this did not excuse the mother's behavior, but the therapist suggested that maybe they both had to change some. They left the session feeling a bit more compassionate for each other and a bit more like a team working to make a fatherless home a successful home.

Task 5: Promoting Autonomy

After a few more attachment tasks with each parent, the father become more engaged in his daughter's life. He could now distinguish between separating from his wife and abandoning his children. He became more committed to spending time at the house and getting a bigger apartment so the children could stay with him. He reinstituted his "Sunday with the girls" tradition and became reengaged with his daughter's health care and school life. His reengagement with the children helped reduce hostility between him and Alicia's mother. With hostility decreasing between them, they finally agreed to go through with the eye surgery for Alicia that had been postponed for a year.

Alicia's suicide scores continued to drop across the course of treatment ending far below clinical cutoffs (SIQ > 16; BDI > 12). Each week the session ended with a review of the safety plan. Each week the parents played an increasing role in the safety plan, whether it was reviewing feelings at night or being the primary contact when distraction did not work. Alicia and her mother decided to take an exercise class together so her mother could lose some weight and Alicia could burn off some tension from school. Alicia and her sister started to stay every other weekend at their father's new apartment. Unfortunately, the eye surgery was complicated, and Alicia missed a lot of school the second half of the year. Instead of repeating eleventh grade, the parents agreed to support Alicia's desire to go to Job Corp, a federally funded residential job-training program.

Recommendations for Clinicians Interested in Using This Treatment Approach

Adopting and Adapting the Treatment Across Various Practice Settings

The ABFT model lends itself to monitoring fidelity and adaptability across different practice settings. Several tools are used to monitor fidelity. First, because the model rests on the task structure and every session conducted falls within the goals and processes of at least one task, in preparing for a session or reviewing the work in supervision, the therapist can always ask himself or herself, "What task am I working on and what needs to be accomplished today to move it forward?" However, each task also represents a set of processes and goals. Sometimes when a task is not going well, the therapist can think back to those processes in past tasks to reduce the barrier to completing the current task. In this way, the task structure provides focus, directionality, and intentionality. Additionally, Table 8–1 presents a checklist that can help a therapist to prepare before they go into the session or to evaluate what happened after the session. Therapists are encouraged to use this measure, which includes the most essential elements of each of the five tasks, to "self-supervise" the work they are doing. Other versions of the "adherence" measure exist that have more detail; however, we included this version because it provides a good overview of the components of each task. We are experimenting with using this version of the adherence measure to reinforce or enhance learning when we disseminate ABFT in the community.

The task structure also helps make this treatment exportable to various settings. We are currently experimenting with acute or residential inpatient treatment programs. In the acute setting, families show high motivation to be involved in the treatment by either taking off work or coming every evening. This setup creates a unique opportunity for family intervention. In one acute inpatient facility, the clinical team requires the family to come to the hospital all day for 2 days. Families from out of town stay in a hotel across the street. Therapists conduct Task 1 in the morning and then start Task 2 and/or Task 3 over the next 2 days. Given the crisis nature of the work, many families may not get to Task 4; however, many can complete Task 4 back at home with their outpatient therapists. The crisis team is currently working to develop ABFT capacity in the hospital outpatient department to provide greater continuity of care in the transition from inpatient to outpatient treatment.

Clinical Implementation

Table 8–2 lists the treatment elements that can be implemented in everyday clinical practice.

TABLE 8-1. Tasks and phases of attachment-based family therapy

Task 1: Relational reframing

    Phase 1: Bond and understand the depression.

    Phase 2: Shift to attachment themes.

    Phase 3: Make improving the relationship the goal of treatment.

Task 2: Establishing adolescent alliance

    Phase 1: Bond and explore the depression.

    Phase 2: Develop an attachment narrative and connect it to depression.

    Phase 3: Choose, discuss, and practice content for Task 4.

Task 3: Establishing parent alliance

    Phase 1: Explore parents' current stressors and own attachment ruptures.

    Phase 2: Connect these themes to adolescent's experience.

    Phase 3: Prepare and practice emotion coaching/get permission to coach parents.

Task 4: Attachment task

    Phase 1: Adolescent discloses; parents listen.

    Phase 2: Parents disclose.

    Phase 3: Adolescent and parents engage in mutual explorative conversation.

Task 5: Promoting autonomy

    Discuss daily responsibility and mutual cooperation at home.

    Promote competency and autonomy outside the home.

    Engage in conversations that explore identity formation (sexual, racial, religious, etc.).

TABLE 8-2. Elements of the treatment that can be easily implemented in everyday practice

- Focus on improving the parent-adolescent relationship to increase the likelihood the adolescent will go to the parent for help in a suicidal crisis.
- Try to think, assess, and focus on the quality of the relationship rather than on behaviors.
- Try to identify ruptures in the relationships that have damaged trust in the relationships.
- Help families talk about these ruptures without getting defensive or argumentative.

Conclusion

In ABFT, the therapist helps adolescents explore avoided self-destructive attachment schemas and the vulnerable feelings that accompany them, providing a safe relational context where patients can develop a more coherent understanding of these attachment injuries and ruptures. In individual therapy, the therapist serves as the "good parent," helping the adolescent learn that relationships can be trustworthy again. In ABFT, the therapist functions as a transitional object. Sessions alone with the adolescent are therapeutic in and of themselves, but they also serve to prepare the adolescent for direct conversations with his or her parents. Before these conversations occur, however, the therapist has several sessions with the parents to help them understand their own attachment injuries in order activate their empathy for their child's longing for attachment security. The therapist then brings the family together for conversations specifically about past and current attachment rupture (e.g., "You abandoned me after the divorce!"). The adolescent expresses memories and feelings of vulnerability, and parents provide empathy and support. ABFT therapists assume that getting validation—often from the parent that neglected them—will have more "existential" impact than validation and empathy from a therapist. These "corrective attachment conversations" further help insecure attachment narratives become more coherent and help reestablish a more securely based family environment.

Although this clinical theory is compelling, much work remains to test these basis assumptions and theory application. Does the attachment task increase felt security and help reestablish the secure base of family life? Or does this occur in task 5, in which the adolescent really begins to trust that his or her parents can be different? Can these clinical processes be taught to therapists in real-world settings? What kinds of institutional changes would be needed to fully integrate and sustain this approach? Can the model be transported into other settings such as short-term inpatient units? Would the modular structure of ABFT lend itself to short-term intensive treating settings? These are some of the many questions we hope to address in the next decade.

Resource for Additional Training

Visit our website www.drexel.edu/abft.

Suggested Readings

Allen JP, Land D: Attachment in adolescence, in Handbook of Attachment Theory and Research and Clinical Applications. Edited by Cassidy J, Shaver PR. New York, Guilford, 1999, pp 319–335

Angus LE, Greenberg LS: Working With Narrative in Emotion-Focused Therapy: Changing Stories, Healing Lives. Washington, DC, American Psychological Association, 2011

Brent DA, Poling KD, Goldstein TR: Treating Adolescent Depression and Suicide: A Clinician's Guide. New York, Guilford, 2011

Diamond GS, Diamond GM, Levy SA: Attachment-Based Family Therapy for Depressed Adolescents. Washington, DC, American Psychological Association, 2014

Faber A, Mazlish E: How to Talk So Kids Will Listen and Listen So Kids Will Talk. New York, Simon & Schuster, 2012

Johnson S: Attachment Processes in Couple and Family Therapy. New York, Guilford, 2003

Joiner TE, Coyne JC: The Interactional Nature of Depression: Advances in Interpersonal Approaches. Washington, DC, American Psychological Association, 1999

Kobak R, Duemmler S: Attachment and conversation: toward a discourse analysis of adolescent and adult security, in Advances in Personal Relationships, Vol 5. Attachment Processes in Adulthood. Edited by Bartholomew K, Perlman D. London, Jessica Kingsley Publishers, 1994, pp 121–149

Garfinkel LF, Slaby AE: No One Saw My Pain: Why Teens Kill Themselves. New York, WW Norton, 1996

Gottman JM, Katz LF, Hooven C: Parental meta-emotion philosophy and the emotional life of families: theoretical models and preliminary data. Journal of Family Psychology 10(3):243–268, 1996

Gottman JM, DeClaire J: The Heart of Parenting: How to Raise an Emotionally Intelligent Child. New York, Simon & Schuster, 1997

References

Asarnow JR, Miranda J: Improving care for depression and suicide risk in adolescents: innovative strategies for bringing treatments to community settings. Annu Rev Clin Psychol 10:275–303, 2014 24437432

Asarnow JR, Jaycox LH, Tang L, et al: Long-term benefits of short-term quality improvement interventions for depressed youths in primary care. Am J Psychiatry 166(9):1002–1010, 2009 19651711

Barbe RP, Bridge JA, Birmaher B, et al: Lifetime history of sexual abuse, clinical presentation, and outcome in a clinical trial for adolescent depression. J Clin Psychiatry 65(1):77–83, 2004 14744173

Beautrais AL, Joyce PR, Mulder RT, et al: Prevalence and comorbidity of mental disorders in persons making serious suicide attempts: a case-control study. Am J Psychiatry 153(8):1009–1014, 1996 8678168

Beck AT, Steer RA, Ball R, Ranieri W: Comparison of Beck Depression Inventories -IA and -II in psychiatric outpatients. J Pers Assess 67(3):588–597, 1996 8991972

Bernal G, Jimenez-Chafey MI, Rodriguez MM: Cultural adaptation of treatments: a resource for considering culture in evidence-based practice. Professional Psychology: Research and Practice 40(4):361–368, 2009

Böszörményi-Nagy I, Spark GM: Invisible Loyalties: Reciprocity in Intergenerational Family Therapy. Hagerstown, MD, Routledge, 1973

Bowlby J: A Secure Base: Parent-Child Attachment and Healthy Human Development. London, Basic Books, 1988

Brent DA, McMakin DL, Kennard BD, et al: Protecting adolescents from self-harm: a critical review of intervention studies. J Am Acad Child and Adolesc Psychiatry 52(12):1260–1271, 2013 24290459

Buber M: I and Thou. Translated by Smith RG. Edinburgh, Scotland, Clark, 1937

Chambless DL, Hollon SD: Defining empirically supported therapies. J Consult Clin Psychol 66(1):7–18, 1998 9489259

Diamond G, Creed T, Gillham J, et al: Sexual trauma history does not moderate treatment outcome in Attachment-Based Family Therapy (ABFT) for adolescents with suicide ideation. J Fam Psychol 26(4):595–605, 2012 22709259

Diamond G, Russon J, Levy S: Attachment-based family therapy: A review of the empirical support. Fam Process 55(3):595–610, 2016 27541199

Diamond GM, Diamond GS, Levy S, et al: Attachment-based family therapy for suicidal lesbian, gay, and bisexual adolescents: a treatment development study and open trial with preliminary findings. Psychotherapy (Chic) 49(1):62–71, 2012 22181026

Diamond GM, Shahar B, Sabo D, et al: Attachment-based family therapy and emotion-focused therapy for unresolved anger: the role of productive emotional processing. Psychotherapy (Chic) 53(1):34–44, 2016 26828910

Diamond GS, Liddle HA: Transforming negative parent-adolescent interactions: from impasse to dialogue. Fam Process 38(1):5–26, 1999 10207708

Diamond GS, Reis BF, Diamond GM, et al: Attachment-based family therapy for depressed adolescents: a treatment development study. J Am Acad Child Adolesc Psychiatry 41(10):1190–1196, 2002 12364840

Diamond GS, Wintersteen MB, Brown GK, et al: Attachment-based family therapy for adolescents with suicidal ideation: a randomized controlled trial. J Am Acad Child Adolesc Psychiatry 49(2):122–131, 2010 20215934

Diamond GS, Diamond GM, Levy SA: Attachment-Based Family Therapy for Depressed Adolescents. Washington, DC, American Psychological Association Press, 2014

Diamond GS, Wagner I, Levy SA: Attachment-based family therapy in Australia: introduction to a special issue. Australian and New Zealand Journal of Family Therapy 37:143–153, 2016

Frey LM, Hunt QA: Treatment for suicidal thoughts and behavior: a review of family-based interventions. J Marital Fam Ther 44(1):107–124, 2018 28394014

Greenberg LS: Theories of Psychotherapy: Emotion-Focused Therapy. Washington, DC, American Psychological Association, 2011

Ibrahim M, Jin B, Russon J, et al: Predicting alliance for depressed and suicidal adolescents: the role of perceived attachment to mothers. Evid Based Pract Child Adolesc Ment Health 3(1):42–56, 2018

Israel P, Diamond GS: Feasibility of attachment based family therapy for depressed clinic-referred Norwegian adolescents. Clin Child Psychol Psychiatry 18(3):334–350, 2013 22930777

Johnson SM: The Practice of Emotionally Focused Marital Therapy: Creating Connection, 2nd Edition. New York, Brunner/Routledge, 2004

Kobak R, Cassidy J, Lyons-Ruth K, et al: Attachment, stress, and psychopathology: a developmental pathways model, in Developmental Psychopathology: Vol 1. Theory and Method, 2nd Edition. Edited by Cicchetti D, Cohen DJ. Hoboken, NJ, Wiley, 2006, pp 333–369

Liddle HA, Dakof GA, Parker K, et al: Multidimensional family therapy for adolescent drug abuse: results of a randomized clinical trial. Am J Drug Alcohol Abuse 27(4):651–688, 2001 11727882

McKeown RE, Garrison CZ, Cuffe SP, et al: Incidence and predictors of suicidal behaviors in a longitudinal sample of young adolescents. J Am Acad Child Adolesc Psychiatry 37(6):612–619, 1998 9628081

Minuchin S: Families and Family Therapy. Cambridge, MA, Harvard University Press, 1974

Pargament KI, McCullough ME, Thoresen CE: The frontier of forgiveness: seven directions for psychological study and practice, in Forgiveness: Theory, Research, and Practice. Edited by McCullough ME, Paragment KI, Thoresen CE. New York, Guilford, 2000, pp 299–319

Restifo K, Bögels S: Family processes in the development of youth depression: translating the evidence to treatment. Clin Psychol Rev 29(4):294–316, 2009 19356833

Reynolds WM, Mazza JJ: Assessment of suicidal ideation in inner-city children and young adolescents: reliability and validity of the Suicidal Ideation Questionnaire-JR. School Psychology Review 28(1):17–30, 1999

Ringborg M: Dissemination of attachment-based family therapy in Sweden. Australian and New Zealand Journal of Family Therapy 37:228–239, 2016

Rubenstein JL, Halton A, Kasten L, et al: Suicidal behavior in adolescents: stress and protection in different family contexts. Am J Orthopsychiatry 68(2):274–284, 1998 9589765

Rushton JL, Forcier M, Schectman RM: Epidemiology of depressive symptoms in the national longitudinal study of adolescent health. J Am Acad Child Adolesc Psychiatry 41(2):199–205, 2002 11837410

Santens T, Devacht I, Dewulk S, et al: Attachment-based family therapy between Magritte and Poirot: dissemination dreams, challenges and solutions in Belgium. Australian and New Zealand Journal of Family Therapy 37:240–250, 2016

Sheeber L, Hops H, Davis B: Family processes in adolescent depression. Clin Child Fam Psychol Rev 4(1):19–35, 2001 11388562

Sheftall AH, Mathias CW, Furr RM, et al: Adolescent attachment security, family functioning, and suicide attempts. Attach Hum Dev 15(4):368–383, 2013 23560608

Siqueland L, Rynn M, Diamond GS: Cognitive behavioral and attachment based family therapy for anxious adolescents: Phase I and II studies. J Anxiety Disord 19(4):361–381, 2005 15721570

Summerville MB, Kaslow NJ, Doepke KJ: Psychopathology and cognitive and family functioning in suicidal African-American adolescents. Curr Dir Psychol Sci 5:7–11, 1996

Wagner B, Silverman MAC, Martin CE: Family factors in youth suicidal behaviors. Am Behav Sci 46:1171–1191, 2003

Wagner I, Diamond GS, Levy S, et al: Attachment-based family therapy as an adjunct to family-based treatment for adolescent anorexia nervosa. Australian and New Zealand Journal of Family Therapy 37:207–227, 2016

The SAFETY Program

A Youth and Family-Centered
Cognitive-Behavioral Intervention Informed by
Dialectical Behavior Therapy

Jennifer L. Hughes, Ph.D., M.P.H.
Kalina Babeva, Ph.D.
Joan R. Asarnow, Ph.D.

Introduction

Adolescent suicide is a major public health problem; innovative strategies and interventions are needed to address youth safety and well-being when an increase in suicidal thinking or behavior occurs. Unfortunately, adolescent suicidal behavior is common; it is the second leading cause of death for ages 15–24 years and the fourth for ages 5–14 years (Centers for Disease Control and Prevention [CDC] 2014). Additionally, for every one adolescent death by suicide in the United States, there are an estimated 100–200 nonlethal suicide attempts made by adolescents (Moskos et al. 2004). Adolescent suicidality, more broadly defined as suicidal ideation and behavior, is common: 17.7% of high school students reported that they had seriously considered attempting suicide over the course of the year, 8.6% reported attempting suicide one or more times, and 2.8% reported making a suicide attempt that required medical attention (Kann et

255

al. 2016). Developing, testing, and disseminating effective prevention and treatment strategies for suicidal behavior in youth is critical, given the high costs of suicide to individuals, families, communities, and society.

Brief Overview of the Safe Alternatives for Teens and Youths (SAFETY) Intervention

The Safe Alternatives for Teens and Youths (SAFETY) program is a family-based, cognitive-behavioral therapy (CBT) intervention designed to provide treatment over a 12-week period in the aftermath of a suicide attempt or self-harm behavior (Asarnow et al. 2015, 2017). Although the SAFETY program is informed by dialectical behavior therapy (DBT), SAFETY offers a less intensive and more family- and community-centered approach that is tailored to meet the needs of the diverse group of youth presenting with suicidal and self-harm behavior. The SAFETY intervention is brief (3 months), individually tailored, and directly focused on preventing suicidal behavior. Treatment for the youth and family is principle guided, is based on a social-ecological and cognitive-behavioral model of behavior change, and targets risk and protective factors in the environment. These include targets such as building protective support within family, peer, and community systems; restricting access to dangerous and potentially lethal methods of self-harm; enhancing safe and adaptive thoughts, actions, behaviors, coping, and stress reactions; and addressing the individual through environment interactions that can enhance safety and reduce suicide attempt risk (e.g., developing cope-ahead plans for responding safely in situations associated with increased risk of suicidal urges and behavior). The treatment plan is based on a case conceptualization for each youth/family developed through a "cognitive-behavioral fit analysis" that identifies proximal risk factors associated with increased suicide attempt risk as well as protective processes for each youth. This cognitive-behavioral fit analysis considers emotional and cognitive-behavioral processes within the youth, family, and broader social systems affecting the youth (e.g., peers, school, community).

Theoretical Model of SAFETY and Proposed Mechanism of Change

The SAFETY program was originally designed to be incorporated within the emergency response to suicide attempts, and it expands on the Family

Intervention for Suicide Prevention (FISP; Asarnow et al. 2008, 2009a), a second-generation adaptation of the Specialized Emergency Room Intervention (Rotheram-Borus et al. 2000). FISP is an enhanced mental health intervention for youth presenting to emergency departments (EDs) with suicidal episodes and aims to provide a therapeutic "behavioral assessment" of risk, with the primary goal of increasing the likelihood that youth will link to appropriate follow-up treatment. This is in line with Objective 8.4 of the National Strategy for Suicide Prevention, which emphasizes the need to "promote continuity of care and the safety and well-being of all patients treated for suicide risk in emergency departments or hospital inpatient units" (U.S. Department of Health and Human Services (HHS) Office of the Surgeon General and National Action Alliance for Suicide Prevention 2012, p. 54). As such, FISP presents the youth and family with a series of behavioral challenges designed to "drag out" skills and behaviors that are incompatible with suicidal behavior and thus support increased safety. Additionally, FISP aims to enhance motivation for follow-up treatment through providing a therapeutic experience that is supportive, while addressing and reducing barriers to treatment using motivational enhancement strategies in a population known to have low rates of follow-up care. The intervention components provided in FISP are also designed to enhance safety and reduce suicide attempt risk. Importantly, FISP is the initial session of SAFETY with subsequent sessions addressing proximal risk and protective factors for suicidal behavior within the context of the youth's and family's social-ecological niche.

By targeting the period following a suicide attempt, the SAFETY program focuses on a time of elevated risk for suicide attempts and deaths—the immediate aftermath of a suicidal episode as youth are transitioning to outpatient care from the ED or hospital (Brent et al. 2009, 2013; Bridge et al. 2014). Developed through a unique "incubator model," the SAFETY treatment development process was rooted in partnerships with community care settings, clinicians, families, and youth. The treatment development process included extensive needs assessments, with community partners, therapists, parents, and youth providing information to guide treatment development. The intervention was pretested in collaboration with community partners under routine care conditions, while controlled trials were conducted in the laboratory (Asarnow et al. 2015, 2017). This incubator model created a "two-way street" in which information on the needs of consumers and community settings informed the treatment development process throughout development and testing. These partnerships and pretesting under routine practice conditions aimed to improve upon the long gap (often cited as 17 years) between the demonstration of efficacy in laboratory-based trials and treatment availability in community practice (Institute of Medicine 2001).

The SAFETY program is rooted in a family-based social-ecological cognitive-behavioral model of behavior change (Henggeler et al. 2002; see Table 9–1). This model views individual, family, social-ecological, and interactional processes as critical change targets (Asarnow and Miranda 2014). The SAFETY approach thus aims to address the multiple determinants of suicidal behavior with consideration of the multiple systems in which a youth is involved, including the family, peers, school, and community. This individualized approach is designed to address the heterogeneity among the diverse youth with suicidal and self-harm behavior and risk.

Many risk factors have been implicated in suicidality (Bridge et al. 2006; Cha et al. 2018). The SAFETY approach recognizes that there is considerable heterogeneity among youth who attempt suicide, thus requiring that the treatment be guided by a case formulation/cognitive-behavioral fit analysis that identifies proximal risk and protective processes associated with suicide attempt risk for each individual youth, as well as the youth's social-ecological context. This is consistent with recent analyses that have indicated that individual risk and protective factors viewed in isolation have relatively weak power for predicting suicide attempts and deaths; that it is likely that there are many paths to nonfatal and fatal suicide attempts (equifinality); and that intervention and prediction models will likely need to consider many risk and protective factors in combination as well as time-varying patterns (Franklin et al. 2017). For instance, risk for suicide death is likely to be substantially higher in an impulsive, depressed, aggressive male faced with what he perceives to be an unresolvable problem who has ready access to a firearm compared with a male with the same characteristics and no access to a firearm. The cognitive-behavioral fit analysis–driven treatment plan is designed to allow consideration of complex interactions across a range of individual and environmental characteristics that impact suicide and suicide attempt risk.

SAFETY specifically targets individuals with prior suicide attempts and self-harm, including nonsuicidal self-injury characteristics that have been

TABLE 9-1. SAFETY program principles

1. The primary purpose of assessment is to understand the "fit" between suicide attempts, their broader systemic context, and cognitive-behavioral processes.

2. The primary purpose of the intervention is to enhance safety and reduce suicide attempt risk; sessions focus on factors/processes identified in the cognitive-behavioral fit analysis as contributing to or reducing suicide attempt risk and targeted in the intervention plan.

3. Interventions should be designed to promote SAFE vs. UNSAFE actions/ behavior, activities, thoughts, coping, stress reactions and promote contact and relationships with SAFE people in SAFE settings/environments. (See SAFETY pyramid.)

4. Assessment is continuous and linked with intervention; information on the youth and their systemic context emerges throughout the intervention period and is used to refine the cognitive-behavioral fit analysis and intervention plan.

5. Intervention contacts should build on strengths as levers of change and emphasize positives.

6. Interventions should be present focused, action oriented, and require consistent (daily or weekly) effort by the youth and family members to promote youth safety and reduce suicide attempt risk.

7. Interventions should target sequences of behaviors within and between multiple systems that maintain or reduce suicide attempt risk.

8. Interventions should be developmentally appropriate and culturally sensitive, fitting the developmental needs of the youth and cultural context of the youth and family.

9. Intervention outcomes are evaluated continuously from multiple perspectives (e.g., youth, family, clinician); therapists assume accountability for overcoming barriers to successful outcomes.

10. Attention is directed to promoting intervention generalization and persistence from the start; the role of caregivers in nurturing, protecting, and addressing family members' needs across multiple systemic contexts is emphasized.

Note. SAFETY = Safe Alternatives for Teens and Youths.
Source. Adapted from multisystemic therapy (Henggeler et al. 2002). © Joan R. Asarnow.

shown to be among the most reliable predictors of future suicide attempts and death, including premature death from alcohol or drug poisoning and other unnatural causes of death (Asarnow et al. 2011b; Joiner et al. 2005; Morgan et al. 2017; Shaffer et al. 1996; Taliaferro and Muehlenkamp, 2014; Wilkinson et al. 2011). Although there are many and varied risk factors for an individual youth, risk factors that have frequently been noted include the presence of a psychiatric disorder, with over 90% of youth who die by suicide estimated to have suffered from a mental health disorder such as depression, bipolar disorder, or substance abuse (Cha et al. 2018; O'Connor and Nock 2014). Hopelessness has also been related to attempted suicide and death by suicide (Goldston et al. 2001; Lewinsohn et al. 1994; Shaffer et al. 1996), and impulsivity and impulsive aggression are associated with adolescent suicidal behavior and suicidal ideation (Beautrais et al. 1999; Brent et al. 1999; Bridge et al. 2006; Brodsky et al. 2008; Conner et al. 2004). Other psychological variables associated with risk for suicidality include low self-esteem, high levels of neuroticism, and gender and sexual minority status (Bridge et al. 2006). Although female gender is associated with increased risk of suicide attempts, suicide deaths are more common in males (Centers for Disease Control and Prevention 2014).

The strong family-centered approach in SAFETY is based on recognition that the family and other social systems can serve a major protective role, and family factors as well as environmental stresses and strengths can affect the risk of suicidality. Again, each youth's social-ecological niche is likely to have particular combinations of risk and protective factors that can be targeted in treatment. For instance, a family history of suicidal behavior is associated with risk for suicidal behavior, and parents and other family members of suicidal youth may also be at heightened risk for suicide and suicide attempts (Brent et al. 2015; Qin and Mortensen 2003). Bidirectional patterns are often observed where suicidal and self-harm behavior, mental health problems, and stress in children contribute to increasing mental health problems and stress in parents, leading to elevated risk across the family (Asarnow et al. 2008; Bridge et al. 2006; Hammen 2006; Pfeffer et al. 1998). Stressful life events and traumatic stress, such as being the victim of bullying, abuse, getting pregnant/getting someone else pregnant, or loss of a loved one, can also increase suicide attempt risk (Asarnow et al. 2008; Brent et al. 2009; Bridge et al. 2006; Brodsky et al. 2008; Gabrielli et al. 2015; Goldston et al. 2016; Gould and Kramer 2001; Stein et al. 2017; Steinhausen et al. 2006).

In addition to focusing on reducing risk factors, SAFETY aims to enhance protective factors and processes that can reduce suicide attempt risk in each youth. Some of these factors are family variables, such as parent-child connectedness, support, and protective monitoring and supervision; school variables, such as strong positive ties to the school; and cultural variables, such as religious or cultural beliefs opposed to suicide (Borowsky et al. 2001; Bridge et al. 2006; Resnick et al. 1997).

Given the many risk and protective factors associated with youth suicide, and the uniqueness of each youth presenting for treatment after a suicide attempt, the SAFETY approach uses the cognitive-behavioral fit analysis to create a case conceptualization and treatment plan that is individualized to the risk and protective factors for the youth and family. Drawing on the cognitive-behavioral fit analysis, therapists select specific evidence-based therapy modules designed to promote protective processes and decrease risk factors. The fit analysis, case conceptualization, and treatment plan are designed around a "SAFETY pyramid" (see Figure 9–1), which emphasizes five elements. At the base of the pyramid, treatment aims to build *safe settings* (e.g., restricting access to dangerous suicide attempt methods and addressing both risk and protective processes in the home, at school, among peers, in the community). Second, treatment promotes interactions with *safe people* and actively works to strengthen family interactions that would lead to increased safety (e.g., helping youth and parents develop validating and supportive listening and communication styles that enhance the likelihood that youth will turn to parents for protection and support rather than harming themselves when feeling suicidal or depressed). Third, treatment encourages *safe activities and actions* that will promote reasons for living rather than activities and behaviors associated with increased risk (e.g., nonsuicidal self-injury, drug use). Fourth, treatment emphasizes *safe thoughts* that support safe and adaptive behaviors—as opposed to unsafe thoughts that can contribute to suicidal risk—and encourage self-validation and recognition that there are multiple ways to view any situation (e.g., dialectical thinking). Finally, at the top pyramid level, treatment emphasizes *safe stress reactions* and coping strategies that can de-escalate unsafe suicidal and self-harm tendencies and help the youth to cope safely and effectively with stressors. These include emotion regulation and distress tolerance strategies as well as turning to others, safe people, for support and protection when emotional reactions reach a point where the youth may have difficulties responding safely without the support of others.

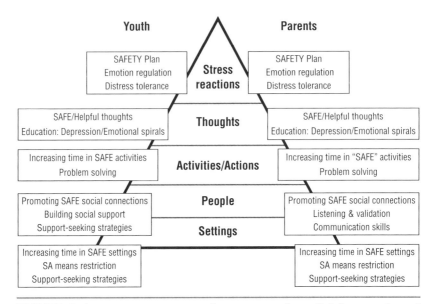

FIGURE 9-1.   SAFETY pyramid: conceptual model for youth and parent intervention.

SA = suicide attempt; SAFETY = Safe Alternatives for Teens and Youths. © Joan R. Asarnow.

Throughout the intervention, the SAFETY program is designed to emphasize enhancing protective supports within the social systems in which the youth is embedded (e.g., family, peers, community) to decrease subsequent suicidal behavior (Asarnow et al. 2015; King et al. 2010). With this focus, SAFETY aims to decrease the youth's feelings of burdensomeness and disconnectedness, two increasingly important constructs found to be related to Joiner's Interpersonal Psychological Theory of Suicide (IPTS; Joiner 2005; Joiner and Van Orden 2008), through the promotion of safe social supports and connection to one's social network. The IPTS has increasingly been shown to be applicable to adolescent suicide risk (Czyz et al. 2012; Horton et al. 2016; King et al. 2017; Stewart et al. 2015).

Given the focus on tailoring the SAFETY treatment plan to the cognitive-behavioral fit analysis for each youth, as in multisystemic therapy (MST; Henggeler et al. 2009), core principles guide the assessment and intervention process. Through these principles, the intervention model is specified and is also responsive to the unique presentations and needs of each youth and family and their environmental context. The SAFETY manual includes general guidelines; therapists select modules and emphasis based on the youth's cognitive-behavioral fit analysis.

Empirical Evidence Supporting Efficacy of SAFETY Program

The SAFETY intervention was developed and tested using a series of treatment development trials. In the initial treatment development trial, 35 suicide-attempting youth, ages 11–18 years, were enrolled in a 12-week open trial of the SAFETY Program. At the 3-month posttreatment assessment, there were statistically significant improvements on measures of suicidal behavior (medium effect size), nonsuicidal self-injury (medium effect size), hopelessness (large effect size), youth depression (large effect size), youth social adjustment (large effect size), and parent depression (medium effect size). Treatment satisfaction was high (Asarnow et al. 2015). There was one reported suicide attempt by 3 months and another by 6 months, yielding cumulative attempt rates of 3% and 6% at 3 and 6 months, respectively (Asarnow et al. 2015).

In the preliminary randomized controlled trial, 42 adolescents, ages 12–18 years with suicide attempts or other self-harm behavior in the past 3 months were randomly assigned to the SAFETY intervention or treatment as usual enhanced by parent education and support accessing community treatment (E-TAU). Survival analyses indicated a significantly higher probability of survival without a suicide attempt by the 3-month follow-up point in those youth who received the SAFETY intervention compared with youth receiving E-TAU (Asarnow et al. 2017). At the 3-month follow-up, four individuals in the E-TAU intervention group reported one or more suicide attempts, resulting in a total of six suicide attempts, with survival analyses yielding a survival analysis risk estimate of 0.33, standard error (SE) 0.13 at 3 months, compared with 0 in the SAFETY condition group. Two additional individuals engaged in preparatory behavior but did not initiate suicide attempts; one was in the E-TAU intervention group, and one was in the SAFETY intervention group. At approximately 5 months post baseline, one youth in the SAFETY intervention group, who had reported preparatory behavior at 3 months, reported a suicide attempt, yielding a survival analysis risk estimate of 0.08, SE 0.07, by 6 months

(Asarnow et al. 2017). The SAFETY intervention was also associated with a significantly lower risk of ED visits and hospitalizations, compared with E-TAU during the 3-month treatment period.

The results of these two studies are promising given the suicide attempt rate in a similar sample of 181 youth presenting to an ED with suicidal episodes—9% and 14% of youth had attempted suicide at roughly 2 and 7 months, respectively (Asarnow et al. 2011a). Moreover, youth suicide attempt rates in control conditions in the literature range from about 11% to 35% (Ougrin et al. 2015).

Treatment Components and Primary Intervention Strategies

SAFETY uses a two-therapist model, with sessions including three components: 1) individual treatment time with the youth; 2) individual treatment time with the parent(s) (provided at the same time as youth individual treatment); and 3) family treatment with youth and parent(s) together. One therapist has a primary youth focus and the other a primary parent/caregiver focus, allowing individual work with the youth and parent(s) to occur simultaneously (see Table 9–2). This format allows for focused individual time to address issues/concerns and enhance skills with the youth and parent(s) separately, plus time with the family together to practice newly learned skills with the aim of addressing risk and enhancing protective factors identified in the cognitive-behavioral fit analysis.

Interestingly, a two-therapist model has been used in the two cognitive-behavioral treatments that have been shown to be effective in reducing suicide attempts in suicidal youth (SAFETY and integrated CBT for suicidal substance-abusing youth, Esposito-Smythers et al. 2011). A second therapist is also used in DBT in the multifamily group, with the group therapist or cotherapist (specifically, a therapist other than the youth's individual therapist) providing parent coaching as needed (McCauley et al. 2016; Mehlum et al. 2014). In this context, it is important to note that in addition to providing critical protection and support for their children, parents whose children have attempted suicide are often experiencing trauma, anxiety, or depressive symptoms after their child's suicide attempt or self-harm behavior. Although much work has been done to understand the unique risk of suicide bereavement in those close to the one who died by suicide

TABLE 9-2.   SAFETY program "basics"

	Youth session	Parent session	Family session
Clinician	Youth therapist	Parent therapist	Youth and parent therapists
Session time	Concurrent 45–60 minutes	Concurrent 45–60 minutes	Joint 20–30 minutes
Session agenda	1. Agenda setting	1. Agenda setting	1. Thanks notes
	2. Bridging to prior session	2. Bridging to prior session	2. Capsule summaries
	3. Safety check	3. Safety check	3. In-session practice/skill application
	4. Practice/homework review	4. Practice/homework review	4. Practice assignment
	5. Work on a session-specific skill or topic	5. Work on a session-specific skill or topic	
	6. Address issues identified by youth/parent	6. Address issues identified by youth/parent	
	7. Review/update SAFETY plan	7. Review/update SAFETY plan	
	8. Practice assignments	8. Practice assignments	

Note.   SAFETY = Safe Alternatives for Teens and Youths. © Joan R. Asarnow.

(Pitman et al. 2014), less is known about the psychological and health consequences of caring for a youth who has made a suicide attempt. The parent therapist is able to provide support to the parent(s) during this distressing time and can focus on the unique questions and needs of the parent(s) related to the youth's treatment. The SAFETY two-therapist family-centered model also facilitates treatment adherence, a known challenge for suicidal youth, by increasing motivation of the parent(s) to attend and bring their children to sessions. As in DBT and MST, SAFETY therapists are available for phone coaching 24 hours a day, every day. Home visits are used as needed, with the first session usually held in the home to support the family in restricting access to dangerous self-harm methods and to assess and understand the youth's family and social-ecological context. For instance, this provides an opportunity to see the youth's room and neighborhood and to meet the family pet; this can strengthen the therapeutic relationship and ability of the therapist to structure treatment to build on strengths in the environment and address potential dangers.

Another benefit of the two-therapist model is the support that therapists are able to provide to one another while working with a high-risk youth and family and in developing the cognitive-behavioral fit analysis and treatment plan. Therapists have a brief scheduled check-in (2–3 minutes) following individual youth and parent sessions/immediately prior to the family session. Therapists can also contact each other rapidly during individual sessions (e.g., page, message) to convey information regarding between-session suicidal behavior, imminent risk, or issues that need to be immediately addressed and/or would require restructuring the session plan. This allows for an integration of treatment goals and for coping skills to be taught in the "same therapeutic language," making it easier for parents to support youth in using skills and for true application work to be done in the family session.

The standard agenda for "family sessions" includes 1) a round of "thanks notes" (described in greater detail in subsection "Phase 1 of SAFETY program"); 2) capsule summaries where youth and parents share and teach what they learned in the individual sessions to help consolidate skills and strengthen the "family team" approach; 3) work on specific problem areas or skills; and 4) "assigning" a family "practice," which always includes giving each other thanks notes during the week and optional other practices, such as "active listening."

Sessions are typically held weekly (or more frequently if needed). The SAFETY intervention uses a standard structure with three phases; sessions include both required and individually tailored treatment components (see Table 9–3). In Phase 1, the focus is on establishing safety, developing the cognitive-behavioral fit analysis, treatment planning, and goal setting. Initial sessions focus on 1) identifying the chain of triggering events, vulnerabilities, thoughts, actions, emotions, and environmental processes leading to suicide attempt or self-harm behavior and the consequences of this behavior; 2) protective processes that could prevent suicide attempts in the future; and 3) a consideration of the youth's suicidal behavior within broader social systems, such as their peer, school, or neighborhood environments. This information is integrated into the cognitive-behavioral fit analysis, and the treatment plan is developed to target skills, behaviors, and supports that would enhance protective processes. In Phase 2, the focus is on implementing this treatment plan by selecting specific modules targeting the risk and protective processes identified through the cognitive-behavioral fit analysis and working on skills training, problem solving, and promoting strengths and reasons for living during the individual and family sessions. Skills are prioritized and ordered based on the cognitive-behavioral fit analysis. Aims of Phase 3 include continued skills practice, with a focus on consolidation of treatment gains, addressing relapse prevention through the development and guided practice of a relapse prevention plan, and addressing emotions and reactions to treatment and termination. A care linkage plan is developed to connect youth and families to continued services if desired and recommended.

Phase 1 of SAFETY Program

Phase 1 is typically three sessions. Unless the family refuses, the first session is conducted in the home. This home treatment option was included in SAFETY because suicidal youth and their families typically struggle to follow-up with treatment; past studies have found low rates of treatment attendance and engagement (Asarnow and Miranda 2014; Asarnow et al. 2011a; National Prevention Council 2011; Ougrin et al. 2012; Rotheram-Borus et al. 2000). An added benefit of in-home sessions is that the youth and parent therapists see the home and neighborhood, which allows for a more productive discussion of safety and opportunities to restrict access to dangerous suicide attempt methods. For example, one youth reported hav-

TABLE 9-3.   SAFETY treatment phases and objectives

Session/week	Major objectives and focus
Session 1	Initial cognitive-behavioral fit analysis of suicidal behavior, build protective support and monitoring in the home, restrict access to potentially lethal methods of self-harm, develop initial SAFETY plan (Principles 1, 2, 4, 5, and 6).
Sessions 2–3	Expand cognitive-behavioral fit analysis to explain how suicidal behavior "fits" within multiple systems (families, peers, school, community), conduct chain analysis of index suicidal behavior from both youth and parent perspectives, and identify risk and protective factors to be targeted through intervention plan. Review and update SAFETY plan (Principles 3, 4, 5, 6, 7, and 8).
Session 4	Collaborate with youth and family to develop the initial intervention plan and targets, considering all levels of the SAFETY pyramid: 1) settings/environment, 2) people and relationships, 3) activities, actions, behavior, 4) thoughts, 5) stress reactions and coping. (Acronym = SAFE SPATS to facilitate recall and adherence, Principles 1, 2, 3, 7). The intervention plan specifies the targets/modules and module components used and their sequence in order to reduce suicide attempt risk. Modules developed to date include Building Hope and Safe Coping—The Hope Box; Cognitive Module; Communication and Problem-Solving; Building Family Support–Family Album; Building Social Support; Emotion Regulation and Distress Tolerance. Modules may also be selected from other manuals (e.g., Youth Partners in Care Depression Module, Dialectical Behavior Therapy, Cognitive–Behavior Therapy for Anxiety). Needs for non-study services are evaluated, and youth and family are supported in linking to other needed services as appropriate (see Principle 10).

TABLE 9-3. SAFETY treatment phases and objectives *(continued)*

Session/week	Major objectives and focus
Session 5–Week 9	Implement intervention plan, refine as new information is acquired and the cognitive-behavioral fit analysis is refined. Monitor youth and family response and revise intervention plan as appropriate (see Principles 4 and 9). Ensure that need for non-study services, follow-up care, factors contributing to intervention generalization and persistence are addressed throughout intervention period.
Weeks 10–12	Consolidate gains, relapse prevention, link to follow-up care as indicated. Final session is standard across participants, emphasizes relapse prevention and linkage to follow-up care and other needed services.

Note. As in MST, the frequency and timing of sessions is adjusted to meet youth and family needs. Each session follows a standard structure: 1) set agenda, 2) review practice/homework and SAFETY plan since last contact, 3) session-specific skill/topic based on treatment plan and cognitive-behavioral fit analysis, 4) address youth and family issues as needed, 5) review and update of SAFETY plan, 6) assign practices and prepare for following week. Fit analysis and treatment plan evolve over time as new information is acquired. Other treatment and community resources are accessed as needed. MST=multisystemic therapy; SAFETY= Safe Alternatives for Teens and Youths. © Joan R. Asarnow.

ing recurrent thoughts to jump from high places as a means to die; the home visit gave the parent therapist a chance to discuss how to secure access to balconies and open stairwell rails to increase the youth's safety at home.

This first session is modeled after FISP (Asarnow et al. 2008, 2009a). Goals of the first session include highlighting the seriousness of suicidal behavior and the importance of committing to treatment and maximizing safety through protective monitoring and lethal means restriction; fostering protective family support and effective communication; developing a "feelings thermometer" to illustrate a hierarchy of suicide-eliciting situations and related feelings, thoughts, physiological sensations, and urges; developing a safety plan that youth can use to reduce their "emotional temperature" and, thus, risk for suicidality; and developing a "safety plan card" to use when the adolescent is feeling suicidal, with youth and parents practicing use of the safety plan in session. Therapists work with both the adolescent and parents to commit to using the SAFETY plan rather than engaging in suicidal behavior if intense distress and/or a state of risk emerges; thus, a commitment to safe behavior is made. In addition, therapists bring a locked box to the home and work with parents and youth to lock up or remove potentially lethal means. The SAFETY plan is supplemented with a hope box filled with cues for safe coping and reasons for living (Asarnow et al. 2009a); this is typically the first practice assignment developed with the youth at the end of the in-home session.

The remaining Phase 1 sessions focus on conducting a *chain analysis* (a detailed examination of events, vulnerabilities, emotions, thoughts, and actions leading up to the suicidal event)—similar to that used in DBT and other CBT approaches—with the youth and parent(s) to understand the most recent suicidal or self-harm event, as well as on further evaluation of risk and protective factors to complete the cognitive-behavior fit analysis. This evaluation is completed using the SAFETY pyramid as a guide. Throughout Phase 1, the youth therapist works to instill hope and build upon the youth's existing reasons for living. Safety and suicidal thoughts and behavior are reviewed each session, and the DBT hierarchy for structuring sessions is used, with the agenda focusing on any life-threatening (suicidal or self-harm) behavior first, followed by therapy-threatening and quality of life behaviors. If there has been any suicidal or self-harm behavior or urges, a chain analysis of the incident is conducted, the safety plan is reviewed, and a commitment to treatment and using the safety plan revisited. As new skills are introduced, the safety plan is also revised to incorporate skills that the youth finds helpful. In Phase 1 parent sessions, the focus is on understanding the parents' perspective of the suicide risk, as well as understanding their current thoughts and feelings related to the youth's suicidality and other needs and strengths within the family. If needed, a parent safety plan is developed to aid the parent in effective coping during a youth's suicidal crisis. Initial family sessions focus on teaching about and completing thanks notes and addressing factors related to imminent safety, such as increasing active listening and validation, minimizing conflict around "hot topics," and developing supportive strategies for protective safety monitoring. The thanks notes intervention is introduced and conducted in the first session in conjunction with a focus on family strengths. In session, the youth, parent(s), and therapists complete a *round of thanks notes*, in which each individual writes one thing she or he is thankful for or appreciates about the other people in the room. These are written on post-it notes and given to the recipient. The youth, parent(s), and therapists each choose one to share with the group. This intervention aims to increase the youth's sense of support and belonging and shift the focus in the family to positive strengths versus negative behaviors; additionally, thanks notes can be used to reinforce any effective behavior. Thereafter, the thanks notes action is completed at the beginning of each family session, and the family is encouraged to complete these as an ongoing at-home practice assignment beginning in Phase 1. Families often adapt the thanks notes task to their individual styles, for instance developing thanks texts or including a thanks note in a child's lunch bag.

Phase 2 of SAFETY Program

Phase 2 focuses on continued use of the safety plan and learning new coping skills. For the youth, these skills include a range of techniques derived from CBT and DBT, including use of the feelings thermometer to self-monitor mood and suicidal urges, emotion regulation, use of distress tolerance skills, understanding depression and emotional spirals, problem solving, behavioral activation, sleep interventions, and social support interventions, as warranted (Asarnow et al. 2009b; Miller et al. 2007). For the parent, the focus is on using his or her parent safety plan, active listening and validation, communication and problem solving, education about depression and emotional spirals, and wellness strategies for taking care of themselves (Asarnow et al. 2005; Miller et al. 2007). Common family session skills include active listening and validation, problem solving, and behavioral activation through safe family activities.

Phase 3 of SAFETY Program

In Phase 3, youth and parent(s) consolidate learned skills through continued practice assignments and application of the safety plan. The therapists work with the youth and parent(s) to address relapse prevention planning. This generally begins with a relapse prevention task in which the youth is guided through a situation associated with suicidal urges (often the situation leading to the index suicide attempt); this is a technique modeled after one used in CBT for adult suicide attempters and adapted for adolescents (Berk et al. 2004; Brown et al. 2002; Stanley et al. 2009). The youth's ability to independently generate and use/practice the skills on the safety plan is assessed, with guided skills training and practice used as needed until the youth can demonstrate an ability to use the safety plan without therapist prompting. Ongoing and potential future treatment needs are also assessed, and the youth and family are linked to other needed services (e.g., mental health, school) as well as longer-term services that can provide regular monitoring (e.g., primary care). A common intervention in Phase 3 is the development of the family album, which can create a treatment-ending ritual conveying the love and support of the family. For instance, one parent created a photo album including pictures of the child and family, letters the child had sent from camp, a medal that the parent had earned, and a note sharing how much the child meant to the parent. This intervention is initially discussed and developed through parent sessions, and then the family album is presented to the youth by the parents in the family session component (Rotheram-Borus et al. 1994).

Case Example

Marissa, a 14-year-old girl, presented to the SAFETY program after being seen at a local ED for a suicide attempt by overdose. She had taken eight Tylenol tablets and then had fallen asleep. When her aunt tried to wake her up to get her to finish her homework, Marissa told her aunt about the intentional ingestions, stating, "I'd rather be dead than feel like this." Her aunt and mother took her to the ED, where she received medical intervention and was then seen by a consult psychiatrist. Given her denial of current suicidal thinking during the ED assessment, her willingness to talk to her mother if suicidal thoughts or self-harm urges returned, and her mother's agreement to monitor her and take her to outpatient treatment, she was discharged home under the care of her mother.

Background and Initial Presentation

Marissa lives with her mother and aunt; she has never had a relationship with her father. Mother reported that Marissa's aunt has lived with them since Marissa was in early grade school and that she "feels like her second parent." Marissa is in ninth grade at an arts magnet high school, having previously attended the neighborhood middle school. She was accepted into the arts magnet program this year; however, both she and her mother report this transition has been difficult, as she does not have many friends at her new school.

Marissa and her mother reported that she had been "fine" until age 13, when she began eighth grade. At that time, she experienced bullying by a group of girls at school; after she had refused to let one of the girls take credit for more work than she had done on a group project, the group of girls began calling her names and putting negative posts on her social media accounts. Although Marissa had moved to a different school for ninth grade, she continued to experience frequent sadness and irritability, as well as trouble falling asleep, feeling "bored" often, and not enjoying her art and piano lessons as much as she had before. She also reported that her grades had dropped over the course of eighth grade and that she continued to have "lower than usual" grades (Bs and Cs) at her new school, stating, "I just can't focus like I used to; but I also think my new school is harder." Per her mother, she had gained 15 pounds in the past year, which had a negative impact on her view of herself. Additionally, Marissa reported having suicidal thoughts multiple times each week, frequently late at night when she couldn't sleep or was looking at pictures on social media, thinking, "I just can't be happy like other people; no one really cares about me." Marissa denied any prior suicide attempts, reporting she had thought about the pills that afternoon when she saw the bottle on the counter in the kitchen.

Phase 1

The SAFETY parent therapist called Marissa's mother to introduce herself and schedule the first SAFETY session. Mother was hesitant to schedule a session at her home, stating, "Oh, it's fine; we can just come to you!" The parent therapist then explained the purpose of the home visit: to make it easy to begin treatment, for the treatment team to see the family's home to get to know them better, and for the parent therapist to be able to assist the parent in addressing safety concerns at the home. After hearing this rationale, Mother quickly agreed and asked whether her sister, Marissa's aunt, could be there as well. The parent therapist and Mother discussed Marissa's relationship with her aunt and decided that it would be good for her to attend, given that she lives in the home and is involved in Marissa's daily life. The parent therapist let the youth therapist know about this decision, and they planned to discuss early in the home session whether Marissa would like her aunt involved in all parts of the initial session or just those that involved Mother and the parent therapist.

The in-home session was set for after school on a Thursday. The youth and parent therapist arrived and found the family awaiting the visit. The family dog greeted the therapists at the door. The therapists, Marissa, Mom, and Aunt sat at the kitchen table for the session. The youth and parent therapists introduced themselves, with the youth therapist taking the lead in setting the agenda for the first session. She stated, "Thank you again for having us in your home. We are glad that you have agreed to be part of the SAFETY program, and we are glad to see that your family is here, ready to support Marissa in moving forward through this difficult time." The joint session agenda is as follows: introductions, a review of the SAFETY program expectations and limits of confidentiality, the individual and family strengths activity, and development of the feelings thermometer. After that, the youth therapist and Marissa would "tour" her room, and the parent therapist, Mom, and Aunt would discuss safety in the home.

Following review of the SAFETY program expectations and confidentiality limits, the parent therapist introduced the individual and family strengths activity. Marissa was easily able to state the following positive attributes: "I like that I'm creative, I'm a good friend, and I guess I'm smart sometimes." Mother and Aunt quickly chimed in with similar statements about Marissa, including that they love her and that she is very helpful around the home. The parent therapist went on to describe the thanks notes practice assignment, in which Marissa and her family will be asked to write notes to one another with a statement of specific or general appreciation each day. The therapists and family did a quick practice round of thanks notes, and each person shared one that she had received.

The youth therapist then introduced the feelings thermometer concept. Marissa worked with the therapist to identify feelings, thoughts, physiological sensations (body feelings), and actions associated with different levels, 1–10, on the thermometer, with 10 being "most distressed." Marissa briefly described the day of the suicide attempt, stating that was her 10. Mother and Aunt listened attentively throughout this activity, occasionally asking clarifying questions with the support of the parent therapist. The youth therapist thanked Marissa for her willingness to share about these feelings, particularly with Mother and Aunt present, while underscoring the importance of their presence in better understanding Marissa's perspective and how they can notice when she is distressed using this feelings thermometer language. For example, if Mother noted that Marissa appeared upset when she was picking her up from school, she could ask, "What's your number on the feelings thermometer?" The youth therapist explained that over time, the parent therapist would work with Mother and Aunt to teach them skills to support Marissa at the higher levels on the feelings thermometer, just as she would be learning skills to help herself at those times, and that family sessions in SAFETY would be used to make sure all of these skills were indeed helpful in keeping Marissa safe.

Marissa and the youth therapist then went to her room. Marissa gave the youth therapist a "tour" of her room; the youth therapist asked specific questions about where Marissa spends time in the house (she noted she spends a lot of time in her room, as the house "feels crowded sometimes") and where she goes in her room to calm herself down (Marissa pointed to a beanbag chair in the corner with a record player and her vinyl collection). The youth therapist and Marissa worked to complete the remainder of the feelings thermometer details, as Marissa told the therapist additional information that she had not wanted to say in front of her Mother and Aunt about a difficult conversation with a guy she liked on the day of the suicide attempt. Marissa and the youth therapist then began to create a written safety plan, using Marissa's existing distress tolerance skills. She stated that listening to her records, walking and petting her dog, and looking at art websites helped distract her and bring her temperature down when she is upset. She reported she also liked painting with her Aunt, watching cooking shows with her Mother, and going to record stores with her best friend. Marissa agreed that if she were to have suicidal thoughts prior to the next session, she would be willing to talk to her Aunt, her art teacher, or the school counselor. She noted that she "doesn't like to bother Mom with problems because she already has enough to deal with, between working two jobs and going to school, and she usually just freaks out anyway." The youth therapist validated Marissa's concern and worked to instill hope that through SAFETY, the parent therapist would help Mother learn more skills to effectively support Marissa during crises. The youth therapist also gave Marissa her emergency contact information and discussed phone coaching as an option. After obtaining a verbal commitment from Marissa to use the safety plan or call for coaching if she were to become distressed or suicidal, the youth therapist had Marissa take a picture of the safety plan with her cell phone so she'd have it at all times. They wrapped up their time together and returned to the kitchen.

While Marissa and the youth therapist were meeting, the parent therapist, Mother, and Aunt walked through the home with the lockbox that the SAFETY team had brought to the session. They collected all medications in the home, and Mother put the kitchen knife set in the box as well. Aunt mentioned that she has certain medications that must be refrigerated; the parent therapist helped Aunt make a plan for getting a lockbox specific to those medications to keep in the refrigerator. Given Marissa's past suicidal behavior involving pills, all agreed that this would be an important step in supporting immediate safety. The parent therapist discussed a safety plan with Mother and Aunt, which included monitoring Marissa when she reported being at an "8 or higher" on the feelings thermometer (as the therapist had requested during the family session) and calling the parent therapist for coaching if they wanted support. The parent therapist worked to instill hope that Mother and Aunt would be able to learn ways to support Marissa during her times of distress. They wrapped up their time together and returned to the kitchen, where Marissa described her safety plan to Mother and Aunt. Mother was able to share with Marissa that she wanted to be there for Marissa if she was upset or feeling unsafe. Marissa shared with Mother what she wanted Mother to do if approached for support, and Marissa and Mother practiced sequences where Marissa approached Mother because of unsafe feelings and Mother responded in ways that increased the likelihood that Marissa would feel comfortable approaching Mother in the future. The parent and youth therapists reminded the family about the thanks notes practice assignment and set the next session appointment.

Session two, held early the following week, began with the youth therapist meeting with Marissa while the parent therapist met with Mother and Aunt. In both sessions, the therapist focused on conducting a chain analysis to better understand the events on the day of suicide attempt and to inform the cognitive-behavioral fit analysis. Marissa described that she had been feeling depressed for several months and had not slept well the night before the attempt. She also noted that she and Mother had been fighting about her grades that week and that she was "really just over it" when she woke up that day. Marissa went on to describe that she had found herself thinking a lot about the events of the past year and had seen a post on social media from one of the girls that had been bullying her. The post was not directed at Marissa, but she stated she started to think about how unfair it was that this girl seemed so happy after she had "ruined my life." Marissa revealed that she had an awkward moment with a guy she likes after school and that she found herself ruminating about this moment as she walked home from school. She stated she felt ashamed about it, thinking, "I'm a complete failure as a person." Marissa reported she walked into the house, saw the medicine bottle on the kitchen counter, and thought, "I'm done." She got a glass of water, poured out the contents of the bottle, and took the eight pills. Marissa then went to sleep on the couch. The next thing she remembered is Aunt shaking her to wake up and feeling groggy. She told Aunt what she had done, and Aunt called Mother, who was pulling into the driveway. They immediately put her in the car and drove to the hospital ED. Marissa said that she felt bad about the whole thing and felt embarrassed by what had happened.

The youth therapist validated that it had to be tough to think back through that day and thanked Marissa for sharing her story. They then continued to work on her safety plan and discussed Marissa developing a hope box as a physical reminder of her safety plan and reasons for living (see also Chapter 3, "Safety Planning and Risk Management," for a detailed discussion of using a hope box for safety planning). They started working on the hope box in session, printing off some pictures of Marissa's favorite art and writing lyrics from her favorite songs on coping cards. They decided the hope box would be her practice assignment for the week and discussed what they might say about the session in the joint family session (i.e., the youth session capsule summary).

In the session with the parent therapist, Mother described a similar conflict-filled week prior to the suicide attempt. She expressed frustration at Marissa's grades and "constant complaining" about her piano lessons. The parent therapist provided psychoeducation about depression and tied these concerns to symptoms. Mother and Aunt recounted the events after the suicide attempt, both describing feeling fearful and frustrated by what had happened. The parent therapist provided validation and focused on how both women's quick action had been a safe response. The parent therapist checked back about home safety. Mother stated that all medication remained locked up and that Aunt had secured her medications, too. The parent therapist presented the SAFETY pyramid and began discussing how this approach would aid the caregivers in helping Marissa. The group decided that Mother and Aunt would review youth depression handouts provided by the parent therapist for a practice assignment for the week and discussed what they might say about the session in the joint family session (i.e., the parent session capsule summary).

After the youth and parent sessions, therapists met briefly to check in and plan for the family session. The therapists, Marissa, and her caregivers then all met together. A round of thanks notes was completed and each participant shared one with the group. Mother reported they had forgotten to do thanks notes after the second day; all agreed to do them in the coming week. In sharing capsule summaries, Marissa told Mother and Aunt about her hope box and how she thought it would help to put it in her room, next to her beanbag chair, "for those tough moments." The parent therapist, Mother, and Aunt shared about their discussion of what had happened that day and how all are looking forward to supporting Marissa. The youth and parent therapists then provided some psychoeducation on depression, using the emotional spirals handout (Asarnow et al. 2005). The session wrapped up after setting the next appointment.

The remainder of Phase 1 treatment focused on the youth and parent therapists collaborating to develop a cognitive-behavioral fit analysis (see Figure 9–2) for Marissa, a case conceptualization, and treatment plan. In session three, this was presented separately to Marissa and to her Mother (Aunt could not attend the session), and treatment goals were agreed upon. Goals included addressing depressive symptoms through psychoeducation and behavioral activation, active listening/validation skills to decrease family conflict, cognitive skills to address Marissa's depressive

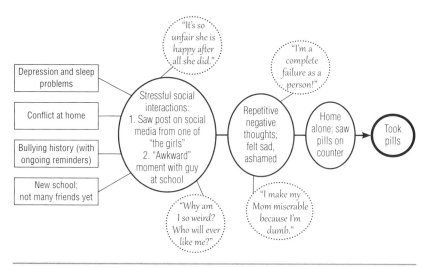

FIGURE 9-2. Cognitive-behavioral fit analysis.

© Joan R. Asarnow.

thinking (particularly related to social stressors and social comparisons), and problem-solving skills for the family.

Phase 2

Sessions continued weekly (see Figure 9–3), with skills being taught and added to the safety plan. In the youth sessions, Marissa completed her hope box and learned about behavioral activation. She worked with Mother and Aunt to plan some activities with her best friend and some family activities. Additionally, Marissa learned cognitive skills to notice and identify helpful and unhelpful (e.g., "I'm a complete failure as a person") thoughts and strategies for generating helpful thoughts (e.g., In response to the thought "I am always messing up, I am really stupid," a more helpful thought might be "Yes, I did mess up, and I'm human, I mess up. Everyone makes mistakes, I will have other days when things go better, just hang in there and keep trying"). She shared these strategies with Mother and Aunt in the family sessions. Marissa developed a sleep health plan to address her habit of late night social media scrolling, committing to plugging in her phone in the hallway. All strategies were added to her safety plan, as applicable. During Phase 2, Marissa had a difficult week (session 8) after seeing one of "the girls" at her school. The therapist

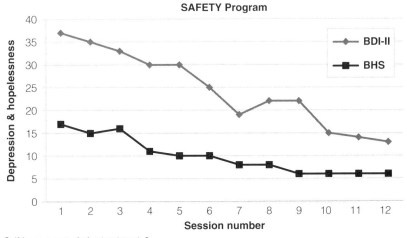

SAFETY Program Dashboard

Patient name: Marissa   Gender: Female   Age: 14

Diagnosis: major depressive disorder

Treatment targets (based on cognitive-behavioral fit analysis): vulnerabilities (depression, sleep, family environment), behavioral activation, thoughts (especially related to social stressors/social comparisons), problem solving

Self-harm events during treatment: 0

Suicidal behavior during treatment: 0

FIGURE 9-3.   SAFETY program dashboard.

BDI-II=Beck Depression Inventory–II; BHS=Beck Hopelessness Scale; SAFETY=Safe Alternatives for Teens and Youths. © Joan R. Asarnow.

worked with her to make a coping card specific to this situation that included distress tolerance skills and thoughts related to that specific risk situation (see Figure 9–4). Depressive symptoms and suicidal thinking were assessed at each session, both by self-report on questionnaires and in discussion. The youth therapist reviewed the safety plan and commitment to safety in each session.

The parent therapist continued working through the SAFETY pyramid with Mother and Aunt. They worked to develop contingency management plans to support Marissa in keeping up with behavioral activation activities and schoolwork. They also focused on learning and practicing active listening and validation, with Mother additionally identifying some distress tolerance skills to help her de-escalate her emotional response during conflict at home.

Treatment Components

Session	1	2	3	4	5	6	7	8	9	10	11	12
Youth interventions												
Safety plan	X	X	X	X	X	X	X	X	X	X	X	X
Feelings thermometer	X	X	X	X	X	X	X	X	X	X	X	X
Chain analysis		X										
Hope box		X	X		X							
Psychoeducation: depression			X	X								
Emotion regulation	X	X						X				
Behavioral activation			X	X	X							
Sleep hygiene			X	X								
Cognitive skills					X	X	X	X	X	X		
Social support					X	X	X					
Problem solving									X	X	X	
Relapse prevention											X	X
Parent interventions												
Parent safety plan	X	X	X	X								
Safe settings	X	X	X	X			X					
Chain analysis		X	X									
Psychoeducation: depression		X	X	X								
Contingency management				X	X	X						
Problem solving									X	X	X	
Relapse prevention											X	X
Family interventions												
Family positives	X											
Thanks notes	X	X	X	X	X	X	X	X	X	X	X	X
Active listening/validation			X	X	X							
Safe activities			X	X								
Family album											X	X
Relapse prevention											X	X

FIGURE 9-3. SAFETY program dashboard (*continued*).

The family sessions consisted of thanks notes, review of capsule summaries, and in-session practice related to the skills Marissa and her family were learning. In particular, the family sessions included repeated practice of active listening, validation, and problem solving with a focus on strengthening Marissa's relationship with Mother and Aunt such that she would feel more comfortable going to them for help, rather than think she was bothering them. All agreed that this part of the SAFETY program was particularly useful, as the family was spending more time together at home and "actually talking about things that matter" (quote from Marissa on a thanks note in session 9).

Situation	Plan
See one of "the girls" at school	• Tell myself: "It feels hard now AND it will get better." • Tell myself: "Not everyone at this schools knows about what they did. I'm sure people are focused on other things now." • Take deep breaths (focus on belly rising/falling; notice temperature difference). • Focus intensely on school work. • Find new friends for distraction or support. • Talk to Mrs. P (English teacher) or Ms. C (counselor). • Use SAFETY plan or hope box. • Call Mom. • Call SAFETY therapist for coaching.

FIGURE 9-4.   SAFETY coping card.

SAFETY= Safe Alternatives for Teens and Youths. © Joan R. Asarnow.

Phase 3

The youth therapist prepared Marissa for the relapse prevention session in the last session of Phase 2, providing the rationale for reviewing the suicide attempt in detail again so that she and Marissa would be able to assess Marissa's ability to tolerate going through the story, particularly with the use of her new skills! Marissa initially expressed hesitation, noting she had come so far and doesn't think about that anymore. With additional support, she agreed to go through the relapse prevention task. In session 9, the youth therapist led Marissa through a guided imagery exercise, reviewing the prior suicide attempt (similar to the chain analysis exercise) and then reviewing with Marissa what she would do differently now. She noted she would have made sure to use her coping card if she were to see a post like that from one of "the girls" and that she easily would have called her Mother or Aunt to pick her up that day and take her to do a family behavioral activation activity, rather than going home to an empty house. Marissa also named several helpful thoughts she would use to counter the negative thinking related to "the girls" and the "awkward situation" with the guy. Last, she named specific distress tolerance skills from her SAFETY plan and mentioned using her hope box, as part of her new SAFETY strategies. The youth therapist then guided Marissa through the task again, and this time Marissa produced and practiced using the skills she had described. The therapist praised Marissa for her hard work throughout the sessions. The remainder of Phase 3 in youth therapy was spent continuing to practice skills, planning for Marissa's next steps in treatment (i.e., referral to a therapist in her neighborhood, who often works with her pediatrician), anticipating and planning ahead for likely stresses in the near future, and planning for termination of treatment with the SAFETY team through reflecting on the strong collaboration and Marissa's increased sense of hope now that she knows therapy can work for her.

The parent therapist went through a similar relapse prevention exercise with Mother and Aunt. They focused on how they would now monitor Marissa's depression more closely, in collaboration with the new therapist and her pediatrician, and they would continue to use the active listening, validation, and problem-solving skills to support safety. Mother also described her own safety plan to use distress tolerance skills when she is upset with Marissa, so she is able to calm down and better use her listening skills. The parent therapist introduced the family album activity, in which Mother and Aunt were encouraged to create an album that represented their family, focusing on their sense of belonging together, their family strengths, and hope. Mother expressed excitement about this activity and decided to take the lead; Aunt agreed to contribute one section related to her relationship with Marissa. The caregivers worked on the family album as a practice assignment, with a plan to present this to Marissa at session 11. The parent therapist also worked with Mother to plan for Marissa's ongoing treatment, as all agreed she would benefit from continued CBT to treat remaining depression symptoms and to help her to strengthen her social relationships and network. Marissa was seeing her pediatrician for medication management, and all agreed that this was effective.

Phase 3 family sessions focused on continued practice of skills and planning for termination. In session 11, Mother brought in the family album. Marissa initially appeared embarrassed when it was presented but then began laughing and smiling as Mother described the different pictures and quotes. Marissa, Mother, and Aunt took turns describing each page to the therapists and clearly enjoyed sharing about their family. In the final family session, the therapists worked to instill hope about the next treatment stage and praised the family for their commitment, follow-through, and hard work in the SAFETY program. The session concluded with a final round of thanks notes, with the therapists having written personalized cards to each family member.

Recommendations for Clinicians Interested in Using This Treatment Approach

Adopting and Adapting the Treatment Across Various Practice Settings

In our previous work, we have found that treatments are more likely to be adopted and sustained when there is some adaptation for the specific needs of each practice setting (Asarnow et al. 2005, 2009a, 2009b). This generally involves use of a leadership team and/or "champions" who consider and adapt the treatment program for the needs of each setting. With respect to SAFETY specifically, we have found that in some settings there have been difficulties implementing the two-therapist model. The use of two separate therapists, one who focuses mostly on the youth and the other whose focus is on the parent(s), generally does not involve additional therapist time because additional therapy time is often needed to address the needs of both the youth and family, and there are clear clinical advantages of the two-therapist model (e.g., greater motivation to attend, increased therapeutic intervention in fixed-time interval, ability to address parent/family issues that parent(s) may not be able to share with the youth without losing therapy time with the youth). Nevertheless, scheduling two therapists at the same treatment hour can be challenging, and billing rules may limit reimbursement. It is important to note that the evaluation of the SAFETY treatment's efficacy has been conducted with the two-therapist model. Furthermore, in youth presenting with suicide attempts (like many youth), confidentiality concerns may limit openness if a single therapist works with the youth and parent(s). Finally, existing evidence on treatments for suicide-attempting youth suggests greater benefits for treatments with strong family components (Ougrin et al. 2015). Therefore, we encourage clinicians in various practice settings to develop strategies for using the two-therapist model, although we recognize that this may be challenging and need some adaptation (e.g., fewer sessions with the second therapist, phone contacts, etc.).

Clinical Implementation

Table 9–4 lists treatment elements that can be implemented in everyday clinical practice.

TABLE 9-4. Elements of the treatment that can be easily implemented in everyday practice

- Include family/caregivers in treatment and build support within the youth's multiple social-ecological contexts.
- Address both youth and family needs.
- In the aftermath of a suicide attempt, retain a strong focus on safety and factors related to safety rather than any other concerns parent(s) may bring up (e.g., academic performance, poor chore completion).
- All families should receive counseling on the importance of lethal means restriction and supportive protective monitoring.
- Given heterogeneity in the presentation of youth with suicidality, carefully assess (using a cognitive-behavioral fit analysis) each youth's unique pattern of risk and protective factors, considering the multiple systems within which the youth interacts (e.g., family, school, peers, community), and develop the treatment plan to address each youth's unique risk and protective processes.
- Increase youth's and family's understanding of the situations that tend to lead to unsafe behavior and develop skills and plans for reducing suicide attempt risk.
- Obtain a clear commitment from youth in each session to use safe coping rather than engaging in suicidal/self-harm behavior.
- Be aware of parent's own needs and possible difficulties, including stresses, physical and mental health and functioning problems, traumatic stress, and emotion regulation difficulties.
- Recognize and support strengths in parents/caregivers and families and support them in creating safe coping plans to be used when feeling overwhelmed and/or in need of support.
- Remain strengths focused throughout treatment, emphasizing youth and family courage, perseverance, and skillfulness as frequently as possible.
- Build strengths in the youth, family, and other environments that support reasons for living and adaptive coping and functioning.
- Strengthen supportive communication (e.g., active listening, validation, thanks notes) and protections and the ability of youth to reach out to responsible adults and/or peers at times when they are feeling unsafe.
- Choose specific intervention components strategically and *collaboratively* with each youth and family, based on their own unique risk and protective factors and processes.
- Collaboratively set clear treatment goals and articulate rationale to youth and family.

TABLE 9-4.   Elements of the treatment that can be easily implemented in everyday practice *(continued)*

- Enhance cognitive-behavioral, emotion regulation, distress tolerance, and interpersonal skills that allow the youth to cope effectively and build reasons for living.
- Teach skills to parents/caregivers and youth in the "same therapeutic language" to improve parents/caregivers' ability to support youth in using skills.
- Practice skills in session as much as possible (rather than just explaining/talking about skills) and assign relevant practices between sessions.
- Risk persists after acute treatment; consider and plan for future stresses, assess relapse prevention skills, develop and practice a relapse prevention plan, and link to treatment and other services as needed (e.g., primary care, school, mental health care, community supports).

Conclusion

In conclusion, the SAFETY intervention is a promising DBT-informed family- and youth-centered cognitive-behavioral approach for reducing suicide attempt risk. Future research is needed to further evaluate efficacy, effectiveness in real-world settings, and cost-effectiveness of SAFETY. Given that risk often extends beyond the 12-week acute treatment period used in SAFETY, future work is needed to explore continuation and maintenance treatment strategies, as well as optimal strategies for transitioning youth to routine care services. Although risk is particularly elevated in the period shortly after a suicide attempt, risk can become elevated again in response to stressors. This underscores the importance of continued monitoring and support to increase the likelihood that youth will seek help should suicidal and/or self-harm urges recur. Strategies will also be needed to adapt this approach across the diverse settings represented in routine care, including those where the two-therapist model is challenging to implement.

Resources for Additional Training

Center for Trauma-Informed Adolescent Suicide, Self-Harm, and Substance Abuse Treatment and Prevention, Semel Institute for Neuroscience and Human Behavior, https://www.semel.ucla.edu/youth-stress/research/asap-center-trauma-informed-adolescent-suicide-self-harm-and-substance-abuse

Treatment and Services Adaptation Center, https://www.asapnctsn.org/

National Child Traumatic Stress Network, https://www.nctsn.org/resources/training

National Registry of Evidence-based Programs and Practices (NREPP), Substance Abuse and Mental Health Services Administration, https://nrepp.samhsa.gov/Legacy/ViewIntervention.aspx?id=377

Suggested Readings

SAFETY Program

Asarnow JR, Berk MS, Hughes JL, et al: The SAFETY Program: a treatment development trial of a cognitive-behavioral family treatment for adolescent suicide attempters. J Clin Child Adolesc Psychol 44(1):194–203, 2015

Asarnow JR, Hughes JL, Babeva KN, et al: Cognitive-behavioral family treatment for suicide attempt prevention: a randomized controlled trial. J Am Acad Child Adolesc Psychiatry 56(6):506–514, 2017

Family Intervention for Suicide Prevention: SAFETY Session 1

Asarnow JR, Berk MS, Baraff LJ: Family Intervention for Suicide Prevention: a specialized emergency department intervention for suicidal youth. Prof Psychol Res Pr 40(2):118–125, 2009

Asarnow JR, Baraff LJ, Berk M, et al: Effects of an emergency department mental health intervention for linking pediatric suicidal patients to follow-up mental health treatment: a randomized controlled trial. Psychiatr Serv 62(11):1303–1309, 2011

Hughes JL, Asarnow JR: Enhanced mental health interventions in the emergency department: suicide and suicide attempt prevention in the ED. Clin Pediatr Emerg Med 14(1):28–34, 2013

References

Asarnow JR, Miranda J: Improving care for depression and suicide risk in adolescents: innovative strategies for bringing treatments to community settings. Annu Rev Clin Psychol 10:275–303, 2014 24437432

Asarnow JR, Jaycox LH, Duan N, et al: Effectiveness of a quality improvement intervention for adolescent depression in primary care clinics: a randomized controlled trial. JAMA 293(3):311–319, 2005 15657324

Asarnow JR, Baraff LJ, Berk M, et al: Pediatric emergency department suicidal patients: two-site evaluation of suicide ideators, single attempters, and repeat attempters. J Am Acad Child Adolesc Psychiatry 47(8):958–966, 2008 18596552

Asarnow JR, Berk MS, Baraff LJ: Family Intervention for Suicide Prevention: A specialized emergency department intervention for suicidal youth. Prof Psychol Res Pr 40:118–125, 2009a

Asarnow JR, McKowen J, Jaycox LH: Improving care for depression: integrating evidence-based depression treatment within primary care services, in Treatment of Adolescent Depression. Edited by Essau CA. London, Oxford University Press, 2009b, pp 159–174

Asarnow JR, Baraff L, Berk M, et al: An emergency department intervention for linking pediatric suicidal patients to follow-up mental health treatment. Psychiatr Serv 62(11):1303–1309, 2011a 22211209

Asarnow JR, Porta G, Spirito A, et al: Suicide attempts and nonsuicidal self-injury in the treatment of resistant depression in adolescents: findings from the TORDIA study. J Am Acad Child Adolesc Psychiatry 50(8):772–781, 2011b 21784297

Asarnow JR, Berk MS, Hughes JL, et al: The SAFETY Program: a cognitive-behavioral family treatment for youths after a suicide attempt. J Consult Clin Psychol 44(1):194–203, 2015

Asarnow JR, Hughes JL, Babeva KN, et al: Cognitive-behavioral family treatment for suicide attempt prevention: a randomized controlled trial. J Am Acad Child Adolesc Psychiatry 56(6):506–514, 2017 28545756

Beautrais AL, Joyce PR, Mulder RT: Personality traits and cognitive styles as risk factors for serious suicide attempts among young people. Suicide Life Threat Behav 29(1):37–47, 1999 10322619

Berk MS, Henriques GR, Warman DM, et al: A cognitive therapy for suicide attempters: An overview of the treatment and case examples. Cognit Behav Pract 11(3):265–277, 2004

Borowsky IW, Ireland M, Resnick MD: Adolescent suicide attempts: risks and protectors. Pediatrics 107(3):485–493, 2001 11230587

Brent DA, Baugher M, Bridge J, et al: Age- and sex-related risk factors for adolescent suicide. J Am Acad Child Adolesc Psychiatry 38(12):1497–1505, 1999 10596249

Brent D, Greenhill L, Compton S, et al: The Treatment of Adolescent Suicide Attempters study (TASA): predictors of suicidal events in an open treatment trial. J Am Acad Child Adolesc Psychiatry 48:987–996, 2009 19730274

Brent DA, McMakin DL, Kennard BD, et al: Protecting adolescents from self-harm: a critical review of intervention studies. J Am Acad Child Adolesc Psychiatry 52(12):1260–1271, 2013 24290459

Brent DA, Melhem NM, Oquendo M, et al: Familial pathways to early onset suicide attempt: a 5.6-year prospective study. JAMA Psychiatry 72(2):160–168, 2015 25548996

Bridge JA, Goldstein TR, Brent DA: Adolescent suicide and suicidal behavior. J Child Psychol Psychiatry 47(3–4):372–394, 2006 16492264

Bridge JA, Horowitz LM, Fontanella CA, et al: Prioritizing research to reduce youth suicide and suicidal behavior. Am J Prev Med 47(3) (suppl 2):S229–S234, 2014 25145744

Brodsky BS, Mann JJ, Stanley B, et al: Familial transmission of suicidal behavior: factors mediating the relationship between childhood abuse and offspring suicide attempts. J Clin Psychiatry 69(4):584–596, 2008 18373384

Brown GK, Henriques G, Ratto C, Beck AT: A Cognitive Therapy Intervention for Suicide Attempters. Philadelphia, PA, University of Pennsylvania, 2002

Centers for Disease Control and Prevention: Suicide prevention: youth suicide. 2014. Available at: http://www.cdc.gov/violenceprevention/pub/youth_suicide.html. Accessed July 2, 2018.

Cha CB, Franz PJ, M Guzmán E, et al: Annual Research Review: suicide among youth—epidemiology, (potential) etiology, and treatment. J Child Psychol Psychiatry 59(4):460–482, 2018 29090457

Conner KR, Meldrum S, Wieczorek WF, et al: The association of irritability and impulsivity with suicidal ideation among 15- to 20-year-old males. Suicide Life Threat Behav 34(4):363–373, 2004 15585458

Czyz EK, Liu Z, King CA: Social connectedness and one-year trajectories among suicidal adolescents following psychiatric hospitalization. J Clin Child Adolesc Psychol 41(2):214–226, 2012 22417194

Esposito-Smythers C, Spirito A, Kahler CW, et al: Treatment of co-occurring substance abuse and suicidality among adolescents: a randomized trial. J Consult Clin Psychol 79(6):728–739, 2011 22004303

Franklin JC, Ribeiro JD, Fox KR, et al: Risk factors for suicidal thoughts and behaviors: a meta-analysis of 50 years of research. Psychol Bull 143(2):187–232, 2017 27841450

Gabrielli J, Hambrick EP, Tunno AM, et al: Longitudinal assessment of self-harm statements of youth in foster care: rates, reporters, and related factors. Child Psychiatry Hum Dev 46(6):893–902, 2015 25534966

Goldston DB, Daniel SS, Reboussin BA, et al: Cognitive risk factors and suicide attempts among formerly hospitalized adolescents: a prospective naturalistic study. J Am Acad Child Adolesc Psychiatry 40(1):91–99, 2001 11195570

Goldston DB, Erkanli A, Daniel SS, et al: Developmental trajectories of suicidal thoughts and behaviors from adolescence through adulthood. J Am Acad Child Adolesc Psychiatry 55(5):400–407.e1, 2016 27126854

Gould MS, Kramer RA: Youth suicide prevention. Suicide Life Threat Behav 31(suppl):6–31, 2001 11326760

Hammen C: Stress generation in depression: reflections on origins, research, and future directions. J Clin Psychol 62(9):1065–1082, 2006 16810666

Henggeler S, Schoenwald SK, Rowland MD, et al: Serious Emotional Disturbance in Children and Adolescents: Multisystemic Therapy. New York, Guilford, 2002

Henggeler SW, Schoenwald SK, Borduin CM, et al: Multisystemic Therapy for Antisocial Behavior in Children and Adolescents, 2nd Edition. New York, Guilford, 2009

Horton SE, Hughes JL, King JD, et al: Preliminary examination of the interpersonal psychological theory of suicide in an adolescent clinical sample. J Abnorm Child Psychol 44(6):1133–1144, 2016 26667025

Institute of Medicine: Crossing the quality chasm: a new health system for the 21st century. March 2001. Available at: https://www.ncbi.nlm.nih.gov/pubmed/25057539. Accessed July 2, 2018.

Joiner TE: Why People Die by Suicide. Cambridge, MA, Harvard University Press, 2005

Joiner TE Jr, Conwell Y, Fitzpatrick KK, et al: Four studies on how past and current suicidality relate even when "everything but the kitchen sink" is covaried. J Abnorm Psychol 114(2):291–303, 2005 15869359

Joiner TE, Van Orden KA: The interpersonal–psychological theory of suicidal behavior indicates specific and crucial psychotherapeutic targets. Int J Cogn 1(1):80–89, 2008

Kann L, McManus T, Harris WA, et al: Youth Risk Behavior Surveillance—United States, 2015. MMWR Surveill Summ 65(6)(No. SS-6):1–174, 2016 27280474

King CA, Kerr DCR, Passarelli MN, et al: One-year follow-up of suicidal adolescents: parental history of mental health problems and time to post-hospitalization attempt. J Youth Adolesc 39(3):219–232, 2010 19967398

King JD, Horton SE, Hughes JL, et al: The interpersonal-psychological theory of suicide in adolescents: a preliminary report of changes following treatment. Suicide Life Threat Behav 31:1–11, 2017 28370278

Lewinsohn PM, Rohde P, Seeley JR: Psychosocial risk factors for future adolescent suicide attempts. J Consult Clin Psychol 62(2):297–305, 1994 8201067

McCauley E, Berk MS, Asarnow JR, et al: Collaborative adolescent research on emotions and suicide (CARES): a randomized controlled trial of DBT with highly suicidal adolescents, in New Outcome Data on Treatments for Suicidal Adolescents. Berk MS, Adrian M (Chairs). Symposium conducted at the meeting of the 50th Annual Convention of the Association for Behavioral and Cognitive Therapies (ABCT), New York, October 27–30, 2016

Mehlum L, Tørmoen AJ, Ramberg M, et al: Dialectical behavior therapy for adolescents with repeated suicidal and self-harming behavior: a randomized trial. J Am Acad Child Adolesc Psychiatry 53(10):1082–1091, 2014 25245352

Miller A, Rathus J, Linehan M: Dialectical Behavior Therapy with Suicidal Adolescents. New York, Guilford, 2007

Morgan C, Webb RT, Carr MJ, et al: Incidence, clinical management, and mortality risk following self harm among children and adolescents: cohort study in primary care. BMJ 359:j4351, 2017 29046278

Moskos MA, Achilles J, Gray D: Adolescent suicide myths in the United States. Crisis 25(4):176–182, 2004 15580853

National Prevention Council. National prevention strategy. June 26, 2011. Available at: https://www.surgeongeneral.gov/priorities/prevention/strategy/index.html. Accessed July 2, 2018.

O'Connor RC, Nock MK: The psychology of suicidal behaviour. Lancet Psychiatry 1(1):73–85, 2014 26360404

Ougrin D, Tranah T, Leigh E, et al: Practitioner review: Self-harm in adolescents. J Child Psychol Psychiatry 53(4):337–350, 2012 22329807

Ougrin D, Tranah T, Stahl D, et al: Therapeutic interventions for suicide attempts and self-harm in adolescents: systematic review and meta-analysis. J Am Acad Child Adolesc Psychiatry 54(2):97.e2–107.e2, 2015 25617250

Pfeffer CR, Normandin L, Kakuma T: Suicidal children grow up: relations between family psychopathology and adolescents' lifetime suicidal behavior. J Nerv Ment Dis 186(5):269–275, 1998 9612443

Pitman A, Osborn D, King M, et al: Effects of suicide bereavement on mental health and suicide risk. Lancet Psychiatry 1(1):86–94, 2014 26360405

Qin P, Mortensen PB: The impact of parental status on the risk of completed suicide. Arch Gen Psychiatry 60(8):797–802, 2003 12912763

Resnick MD, Bearman PS, Blum RW, et al; Findings from the National Longitudinal Study on Adolescent Health: Protecting adolescents from harm. JAMA 278(10):823–832, 1997 9293990

Rotheram-Borus MJ, Piacentini J, Miller S, et al: Brief cognitive-behavioral treatment for adolescent suicide attempters and their families. J Am Acad Child Adolesc Psychiatry 33(4):508–517, 1994 8005904

Rotheram-Borus MJ, Piacentini J, Cantwell C, et al: The 18-month impact of an emergency room intervention for adolescent female suicide attempters. J Consult Clin Psychol 68(6):1081–1093, 2000 11142542

Shaffer D, Gould MS, Fisher P, et al: Psychiatric diagnosis in child and adolescent suicide. Arch Gen Psychiatry 53(4):339–348, 1996 8634012

Stanley B, Brown G, Brent DA, et al: Cognitive-behavioral therapy for suicide prevention (CBT-SP): treatment model, feasibility, and acceptability. J Am Acad Child Adolesc Psychiatry 48(10):1005–1013, 2009 19730273

Stein MB, Campbell-Sills L, Ursano RJ, et al: Childhood maltreatment and lifetime suicidal behaviors among new soldiers in the US Army: results from the Army Study to Assess Risk and Resilience in Servicemembers (Army STARRS). J Clin Psychiatry 79(2):pii: 16m10900, 2017 28541647

Steinhausen HC, Bösiger R, Metzke CW: Stability, correlates, and outcome of adolescent suicidal risk. J Child Psychol Psychiatry 47(7):713–722, 2006 16790006

Stewart S, Eaddy M, Ezzell S, et al: The validity of the interpersonal theory of suicide in adolescence: a review. J Clin Child Adolesc Psychol 11:1–13, 2015 25864500

Taliaferro LA, Muehlenkamp JJ: Risk and protective factors that distinguish adolescents who attempt suicide from those who only consider suicide in the past year. Suicide Life Threat Behav 44(1):6–22, 2014 23855367

U.S. Department of Health and Human Services (HHS) Office of the Surgeon General and National Action Alliance for Suicide Prevention: 2012 National Strategy for Suicide Prevention: Goals and Objectives for Action. Washington, DC, U.S. Department of Health and Human Services, 2012

Wilkinson P, Kelvin R, Roberts C, et al: Clinical and psychosocial predictors of suicide attempts and nonsuicidal self-injury in the Adolescent Depression Antidepressants and Psychotherapy Trial (ADAPT). Am J Psychiatry 168(5):495–501, 2011 21285141

10

Pharmacological Approaches for Treating Suicidality in Adolescents

Isheeta Zalpuri, M.D.
Manpreet K. Singh, M.D., M.S.

Introduction

Suicide is a complex and multidetermined behavior that has been recognized as an urgent public health concern, and it is a leading cause of death among youth in the United States (Centers for Disease Control and Prevention 2017). The estimated lifetime prevalence of suicidal ideation, plans, and attempts in adolescents ages 13–18 years is 12.1%, 4.0%, and 4.1%, respectively (Nock et al. 2013). Around one-third of youth with suicidal ideation go on to develop a suicide plan during adolescence, and approximately 60% of those with a plan will attempt suicide (Nock et al. 2013). The focus of this chapter is on pharmacological approaches to the treatment of suicidal behavior among adolescents. We will address both the transdiagnostic nature of suicidal behavior, as well as its association with particular psychiatric diagnoses.

In this chapter, we provide a review of the psychiatric medications commonly prescribed to youth, the research data supporting the use of each medication with suicidal youth, and the consequences of overdose with each medication. Following this general review, we will address four assumptions that frequently complicate the pharmacological management of suicidal behavior. First, pharmacological treatments may increase suicide risk in some patients because of the risk of overdose with these medications. Second, there is a lack of a strong evidence base for pharmacological approaches to treating suicidal behavior. No pharmacological intervention has been found to conclusively decrease self-harm behaviors in a randomized controlled trial (RCT) in children and adolescents (Hawton et al. 2015), and the RCTs in the extant literature have specific selection criteria that may not apply to all patients (Weisberg et al. 2009). Third, clinicians must weigh the risks of increased suicidality from exposure to certain pharmacological agents, such as selective serotonin reuptake inhibitors (SSRIs), which include a black box warning, against the risks of increased suicidality when suicidal symptoms are untreated. Although it is important to be careful with medication dosing, at times medications need to be started as first-line treatment and titrated accordingly to address the severity of symptoms. This decision is frequently made in urgent settings such as inpatient psychiatric hospitalizations or other settings that permit close clinical follow-up and reassessment of suicide risk and monitoring of medication safety and tolerability. Fourth, given that suicidal behavior is transdiagnostic, there are advantages and pitfalls to treating suicidal behavior as a symptom rather than as part of various psychiatric disorders. Moderators and neurobiological factors that personalize treatment responses are largely untested but may inform successful targeted outcomes. The goal of this chapter is to provide a framework for successfully addressing these assumptions in clinical practice, using continual assessment and reassessment, patient education, and timely modification of treatment to minimize risk and optimize treatment response.

Review of Published Data on Potential Pharmacological Agents Typically Used With Suicidal Youth

To date, there is no medication approved by the U.S. Food and Drug Administration (FDA) for the treatment of suicide-related symptoms or self-harm behaviors in youth. Antidepressants may or may not play a direct therapeutic role in the acute management of suicidal ideation or suicide attempts in adolescents. However, they are considered first-line pharmacological agents for treatment of depression and anxiety in youth, which are commonly comorbid with suicidality. In most studies reviewed, suicide-related symptoms were considered in post hoc analyses of depression treatment trials, providing inferential efficacy for the treatment of suicidal thoughts and behaviors. Thus, explicit data linking antidepressants to reduction in suicidal thoughts and behaviors is lacking because most studies primarily focus on the treatment of affective or anxiety disorders and usually do not examine suicide as a primary end point. We now review current available pharmacological options according to drug class and medication for the treatment of suicidal ideation and behavior in adolescents.

Antidepressants

Depression is common in adolescents presenting with suicide-related behaviors and is an important predictor of future episodes of self-harm (Hawton et al. 1999) and suicide (Kovacs 1996). Although not all suicidal youth are depressed, if youth present with depressive symptoms, it is essential to target these symptoms and reduce the severity of the current episode, while preventing future episodes with appropriate treatment. Indeed, if depressive symptoms are decreased, research shows that nonsuicidal self-injury drops in frequency (Wilkinson et al. 2011). Thus, on the basis of this principle, clinicians will target treatment of depression with medication to reduce suicide-related behaviors. Figure 10–1 provides a flow chart of possible decision trees clinicians may use for the pharmacological treatment of a depressed youth with suicide-related symptoms.

The FDA has approved two antidepressants for the treatment of depression in children and adolescents. Fluoxetine was approved in 2002 (for ages 7–17 years), and escitalopram was approved in 2009 (for ages 12–19 years). There is evidence that youth treated with an antidepressant had lower depression severity scores and higher rates of response and remission than those taking placebo, which may reduce suicidal symptoms and behaviors (Hetrick et al. 2012). Although it may be reasonable to treat mild-moderate depression with therapy first, if the depression is severe or impacting functioning or is associated with poor sleep and other neurovegetative symptoms, increased irritability, or agitation, it may be reasonable to start a medication as these symptoms can increase the risk of suicide.

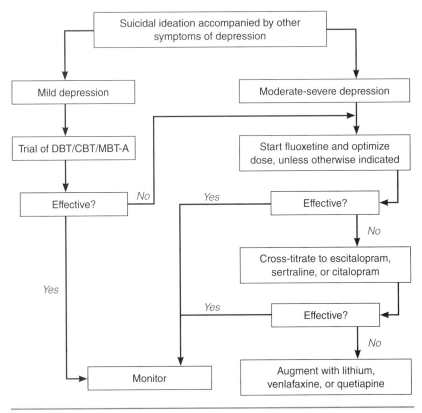

FIGURE 10-1.   A possible approach to pharmacological treatment of a depressed suicidal adolescent.

CBT = cognitive-behavioral therapy; DBT = dialectical behavior therapy; MBT-A = mentalization-based treatment for adolescents.

The Treatment of Adolescent Depression Study (TADS) found that a combination of fluoxetine and cognitive-behavioral therapy (CBT) was the best treatment approach for adolescents with depression compared with either of these interventions alone. This study included 439 adolescents ages 12–17 years with a diagnosis of major depressive disorder (MDD) divided into four treatment groups: fluoxetine alone, CBT alone, combination of fluoxetine and CBT, and placebo. After 12 weeks, 71% of the participants responded to combination treatment, 61% responded to fluoxetine-only treatment, 43% responded to CBT-only treatment, and 35% responded to placebo-only treatment. At the beginning of the trial, 29% of the participants had clinically significant suicidal thoughts. Importantly, rates of suicidal thinking were reduced among all treatment groups, but the combination treatment showed the greatest reduction in suicidal thinking. Suicide-related events were twice as common among those participants who were treated with fluoxetine alone, and only the fluoxetine treatment arm was associated with more suicide-related events than placebo (15% vs. 8% for combination and 6% for CBT alone). However, a causal relationship between fluoxetine and suicidal events was not established.

Prior to initiating antidepressant treatment in children and adolescents, it is prudent to screen for a personal or family history of mania or hypomania because of the potential risk of activation-related increased suicidality. Here, *activation-related suicidal ideation* is defined as the presentation of suicidal ideation or behavior in the context of a pharmacological exposure or dose increase (Delavenne et al. 2013; Goldsmith and Moncrieff 2011). It is also essential to establish a safety plan, ascertain a schedule for close follow-up, and communicate and review with patients and families short- and long-term side effects of medications and warning signs that require immediate attention. A patient's response to the pace of dose titration may delineate natural illness course (e.g., symptom worsening) from treatment-emergent agitation or activation-related suicidal symptoms. For example, an abrupt increase in frequency or intensity of suicidal symptoms that coincides with a medication dose increase might lead a clinician to suspect that the antidepressant is worsening rather than ameliorating suicidal symptoms, and thus the clinician may reduce or taper off the antidepressant. Alternatively, if a patient is experiencing a psychosocially triggered increase in suicidal ideation in the context of a stable antidepressant dose, a clinician might consider titrating the medication to address the symptom worsening. Collaboration with a child's parent(s) and teachers can aid in determining whether to taper or titrate, as well as facilitate an accurate understanding of treatment adherence and prevent hoarding of antidepressants in suicidal youth. Hence, unless otherwise indicated, parents should oversee administering medications to suicidal adolescents. Factors that contribute to treatment failure must be carefully considered, including misdiagnosis, unrecognized or untreated comorbid psychiatric or medical disorders (e.g., anxiety, eating, substance use, and personality disorders, hypothyroidism), undetected bipolar disorder, inappropriate pharmacotherapy or psychotherapy, inadequate length of treatment or dose, lack of adherence to treatment, medication side effects, exposure to chronic or severe life events (e.g., sexual abuse, ongoing family conflicts), and cultural, religious, or ethnic factors.

Although there is evidence that fluoxetine leads to faster and greater improvement in depressive symptoms when compared with placebo or psychotherapy, treatment with an antidepressant is most commonly initiated in adolescents after carefully assessing an initial psychotherapeutic response. Thus, antidepressants should be used for those with moderate-severe depression after psychosocial interventions have been determined to be ineffective or not feasible (Vitiello and Ordóñez 2016). Indeed, antidepressants may reduce risk of relapse and recurrence of depression in the maintenance phase of treatment. Data are mixed about whether combination (antidepressants and psychotherapy) treatments are superior to antidepressant monotherapy (Vitiello and Ordóñez 2016).

Fluoxetine, escitalopram, citalopram, and sertraline are the only SSRIs that have been found to be consistently efficacious in reducing depression in RCTs when compared with placebo. Among other classes of antidepressants, including selective norepinephrine reuptake inhibitors (SNRIs), tricyclic antidepressants (TCAs), and other agents commonly used for depression, only extended-release venlafaxine has been found to be effective in the treatment of depression in adolescents by randomized controlled design (Brent et al. 2008). In the subsections below, we review specific antidepressant classes and medications.

Selective Serotonin Reuptake Inhibitors

SSRIs can treat depression, anxiety, and irritability, which may reduce the risk of suicidality. In general, SSRIs are the preferred first-line medication choice for pharmacologically treating adolescents with depression. A post hoc analysis of the Treatment of SSRI-Resistant Depression in Adolescents (TORDIA) study demonstrated similar results (Brent et al. 2008). In this study, authors identified predictors for self-harm adverse events (suicidal and nonsuicidal self-injury) in adolescents with treatment-resistant depression. Adolescents who did not respond to a prior trial of an SSRI were randomly assigned to an alternative SSRI (either fluoxetine, citalopram, or paroxetine) or venlafaxine in TORDIA. The four treatment arms were an alternative SSRI, venlafaxine, SSRI with CBT, and venlafaxine with CBT. Although there were no completed suicides, there were 58 suicidal adverse events in 48 participants and 50 nonsuicidal adverse events in 31 participants (11 of these participants also had a suicidal adverse event). There was a significant reduction in suicidal ideation, but no differences were found between the different treatment arms for suicidality or self-harm. However, a secondary analysis found that venlafaxine was associated with an increased risk of self-harm events when compared with SSRIs. In addition, those who received an antianxiety medication were more likely to engage in both suicidal and nonsuicidal self-injurious behaviors. Unlike TADS, there was no decrease in suicide-related events from the addition of CBT. This could be related to increased severity of symptoms found in the TORDIA sample.

Fluoxetine

Randomized controlled trials (Almeida-Montes and Friederichsen 2005; Emslie et al. 1997, 2002; March et al. 2004) and systematic reviews suggest that fluoxetine is an effective treatment for adolescent depression. A meta-analysis from four RCTs, which included intervention for 708 youth with major depression, which lasted 6 weeks and compared fluoxetine and venlafaxine with placebo, found that the response rate was greater for those treated with fluoxetine than placebo (30% vs. 6%) (Gibbons et al. 2012b). Similar results have been found in other meta-analyses as well, and fluoxetine is considered to be the best available agent for treatment of moderate-severe depression (Cipriani et al. 2016). Indeed, fluoxetine has the most evidence to support efficacy compared with placebo and is often used as a first-line antidepressant choice. Factors that may make fluoxetine a less favorable choice include family history of response to another antidepressant or preference for an alternative treatment, a history of previous side effects, drug-drug interaction, or response to a different antidepressant during a previous episode.

Fluoxetine is also efficacious for the maintenance phase of treatment in pediatric depression (Emslie et al. 2008). The Adolescent Depression Antidepressant and Psychotherapy Trial (ADAPT) (Goodyer et al. 2007), a publicly funded clinical trial for adolescent depression in the United Kingdom, assessed whether combination therapy with fluoxetine and CBT was superior to fluoxetine monotherapy in 208 adolescents, ages 11–17 years, with moderate to severe major depression. Compared with the TORDIA sample, ADAPT participants had much higher risks of both suicidal (30% vs. 5%) and nonsuicidal (37% vs. 9%) self-harm acts. On average, there was a decrease in suicidal thoughts and self-harm in all treatment arms of ADAPT, but there was no evidence of added benefit of CBT on suicidal thinking or action. Specifically, the study found no benefit of adding CBT to medication and no decrease in suicidality risk with combined medication and CBT treatment. In fact, there were more participant suicide attempts and nonsuicidal self-injury over the study period (28 weeks) than in the month before baseline. Relative to baseline, more suicide-related behavior during the study period may have been related to participants being assessed and followed with greater frequency than they were prior to study participation and compared with other trials. This methodological confound makes it challenging to delineate true risk from an ascertainment bias. Nevertheless, a meta-analysis of RCTs of newer-generation antidepressants and CBT in adolescent depression showed that addition of CBT to medication management provided minimal benefit to depressive symptomatology and suicidality (Dubicka et al. 2010). However, variation in sampling, methodological differences among studies, and few trials examining suicide as a primary outcome limit the generalizability of these results.

The Treatment of Adolescent Suicide Attempters (TASA) study was an open treatment trial in which Brent and colleagues (2009) studied predictors of suicide attempts and events in adolescents who were diagnosed with depression. Adolescents, ages 12–18 years, with recent suicide attempt and unipolar depression, were given a choice of either psychotherapy specific for suicide (TASA CBT, $n=17$), medication management alone ($n=14$), or combination psychotherapy and fluoxetine treatment ($n=93$). Twenty-four participants in this study experienced a suicidal event during a 6-month enrollment period, and 10 events occurred within the first 4 weeks. The rate of suicidal events was highest in the combination group compared with the other two groups (23.7% [22 participants with suicidal events, 93 total number of participants in the combined group] vs. 6.5% [2 participants with suicidal events in both medication and psychotherapy groups, 31 total number of participants in the two groups]; Fisher, $P<0.04$). However, post hoc analyses suggested that participants in the combination group were at higher risk for suicide because of higher self-rated depression scores and hopelessness, lower levels of functioning, higher levels of suicidal ideation, and higher number of prior suicide attempts compared with the other groups. After controlling for these baseline differences, there was no significant difference in the type of treatment on suicidal outcomes (Brent et al. 2009). This study highlights the importance of early therapeutic contact in the course of treatment and careful safety planning and that key participant characteristics prior to an intervention may determine clinical response.

Fluoxetine has a long half-life, and in the event of an overdose, most of the fluoxetine ingesters remain asymptomatic. Most frequently reported symptoms after an overdose include nausea, vomiting, somnolence, tremor, agitation, and tachycardia.

Importantly, about 30% of the depressive episodes do not remit with fluoxetine (Gibbons et al. 2012b). For those cases, a suggested next step would be to try an alternative SSRI such as escitalopram, sertraline, or citalopram. For partial responders to an SSRI, an augmentation agent, such as mirtazapine or bupropion, may be considered as a reasonable next step. However, for nonresponders to SSRIs and after two failed trials, switching to an alternate antidepressant such as bupropion, venlafaxine, mirtazapine, or duloxetine may be considered. However, these recommendations have largely been based on data derived from adults (Hughes et al. 2007).

Escitalopram

Escitalopram is FDA approved for pediatric depression to as young as age 12. Escitalopram has shown positive effects compared with placebo (Emslie et al. 2009; Hetrick et al. 2012), but these effects have reflected modest (5%–10%) improvements in standardized depression severity scores in adolescents with at least moderate symptoms of major depression (Findling et al. 2013). Escitalopram is rarely associated with a prolonged QTc interval, which has been observed in case reports of escitalopram overdose (Schreffler et al. 2013). Indeed, the cardiotoxic effects of escitalopram may contribute to its lethality during an overdose. Electrocardiogram monitoring for widening QRS complex or prolonged QT interval is currently only recommended in the context of an overdose. A risk to benefit ratio of escitalopram should be carefully considered for patients with personal or family histories of cardiac abnormalities.

Sertraline

Sertraline has been found to be effective in depression (Wagner et al. 2003), and a favorable benefit to suicide risk ratio has been demonstrated for sertraline for the treatment of MDD in adolescents and obsessive-compulsive disorder in children and adolescents (March et al. 2006). Case reports on sertraline overdose warn of serotonin syndrome and asynchrony between psychiatric and organic symptoms (Pitzianti et al. 2016).

Citalopram

When compared with placebo, citalopram has been found to be effective in treating depression in adolescents in one randomized controlled trial (Wagner et al. 2004). Similar to escitalopram, however, citalopram has a high risk of lethality in overdose due to its cardiotoxic potential.

Paroxetine

Although paroxetine has been found to have some beneficial antidepressant effect on secondary clinical outcome measures, improvements in depression severity in pediatric populations have not been demonstrated to date. In July 2003, the FDA issued a warning against the use of paroxetine in those younger than 18 years because of increased suicidal impulses. The potential of self-harm and suicidal behavior has been found to be 1.5–3.2 times higher in those taking this medication compared with placebo. Indeed, in both young adults (Carpenter et al. 2011) and youth (Apter et al. 2006), paroxetine use has been associated with higher risk of suicide-related events compared with placebo. Importantly, in the pediatric trials, such treatment arm differences were not derived from analyses of suicide-related items in rating scales, suggesting that suicide-related events may be conceptually different when reported as an adverse event versus as a symptom of a broader syndrome. Although paroxetine has the highest rate of discontinuation symptoms among SSRIs, it is relatively safe in overdose; symptoms include vomiting, drowsiness, tremors, dizziness, and sinus tachycardia.

Fluvoxamine

Fluvoxamine is often used as one of the first-line pharmacological agents for the treatment of obsessive-compulsive disorder in adolescents. Overdose is generally considered safe with mild to moderate ingestion and can include symptoms of drowsiness, tremor, diarrhea, vomiting, abdominal pain, dizziness, mydriasis, and sinus tachycardia; although at higher doses, seizures have been reported.

Bupropion

Although not applicable to depressed youth, in adult depressed patients with greater baseline suicidal ideation, treatment with paroxetine compared with bupropion resulted in greater acute improvement in suicidal ideation, after adjusting for global depression (Grunebaum et al. 2012). Risk of fatal or nonfatal self-harm has not been demonstrated when bupropion was used for smoking cessation in adults (Thomas et al. 2013). In a small open-label trial, sustained-release bupropion has shown some efficacy in the treatment of major depression in adolescents (Glod et al. 2003). In an overdose, bupropion causes cardiovascular events such as tachycardia and hypertension. It has also been reported to lower seizure thresholds in adolescents (Storrow 1994).

Venlafaxine and Other Selective Norepinephrine Reuptake Inhibitors

In the TORDIA study, venlafaxine was equally as efficacious as SSRIs (Brent et al. 2008); however, it manifested with more side effects than SSRIs. Also, those with high suicidal ideation had a higher rate of self-harm events when treated with venlafaxine compared with those treated with an SSRI. Moreover, the data for venlafaxine in pediatric depression are mixed, with some placebo-controlled trials not demonstrating a significant difference from placebo (Emslie et al. 2007). On the basis of the extant data in adults, several clinical guidelines for pediatric depression (Hughes et al. 2007) suggest that if a patient has experienced two failed trials of SSRIs, venlafaxine may be a reasonable next option with close monitoring for suicide risk. Although venlafaxine and the broader class of SNRIs may not be consistently more effective than placebo for treatment response, they have been found to be effective in adolescents to achieve remission. Importantly, there is no significant statistical difference in suicide-related risk outcomes between SNRIs and placebo (five trials: risk ratio $[RR] = 1.09$; 95% confidence interval $[CI] = 0.60–1.99$; $P = 0.78$; Xu et al. 2016). In an overdose, venlafaxine can cause cardiovascular events including ventricular arrhythmia and cardiac arrest.

Tricyclic Antidepressants

Tricyclic agents have not been found to be superior to placebo (Hazell and Mirzaie 2013), and they are frequently associated with significant adverse events in the pediatric population, including cardiotoxicity and lethality in overdose. Thus, there is little justification for the use of this medication class for the treatment of depression in children and adolescents.

Mood Stabilizers

A systematic literature review of all studies until August 2012 to assess the incidence and prevalence of suicidal ideation and suicide attempts in children and adolescents with bipolar spectrum disorders found that both ideation and attempts were common in the past and at the time the study was conducted (Hauser et al. 2013). As many as at least one out of two youth had either a current or a past history of suicidal ideation, and one out of four or five youth had either a current or a past history of suicide attempt. Most patients with suicidal ideation were white, and suicide attempts were significantly associated with female sex and older age. The past-year suicidal ideation prevalence rates in youth with bipolar disorder were higher than in those with depression (72.2% vs. 52.4%). Although suicide attempts were less frequent than suicidal ideation, the weighted past and current suicidal ideation was 57.4% and 21.3%, whereas current and past suicide attempt was 50.4% and 25.5%. In adults, long-term lithium treatment has been known to reduce both attempted and completed suicides in unipolar major depression and in bipolar patients (Baldessarini et al. 2006). Although less robust than lithium, divalproex and carbamazapine have also been known to have antisuicidal effects (Goodwin et al. 2003; Patorno et al. 2010).

Lithium

Lithium was the first drug approved by the FDA for the treatment of mania in children 12 years and older. In a multicenter randomized, double-blind placebo-controlled study of children and adolescents (ages 7–17 years) with a diagnosis of bipolar disorder I, Findling et al. (2015) found better response (32% vs. 21%) and remission (26% vs. 14%) rates in symptoms with lithium than placebo. Although suicidal ideation was an adverse event, it was not related to and did not increase with lithium treatment.

In a controlled, randomized, no-patient-choice, 8-week protocol, participants, ages 6–15 years, with a DSM-IV (American Psychiatric Association 1994) diagnosis of bipolar I disorder (manic or mixed phase) were randomly assigned to risperidone, lithium, or divalproex sodium; suicidality significantly decreased for all medication groups when compared from baseline to 8 weeks posttreatment (risperidone: 48.7% vs. 6.4%; lithium: 29% vs. 11.3%; divalproex sodium: 36.8% vs. 7.9%) (Geller et al. 2012).

Apart from nausea, vomiting, and diarrhea, acute lithium toxicity can cause electrocardiogram changes; neurotoxicity, including sluggishness, ataxia, confusion, agitation; and in severe cases, encephalopathy and seizures.

Lamotrigine

Lamotrigine has not been found to be more effective than placebo in reducing suicide risk in adults with bipolar I disorder during a depressive episode (Calabrese et al. 2003). There are no data available to ascertain the role of lamotrigine in suicidality in the pediatric population. In an overdose, lamotrigine can cause seizures, movement disorders, altered consciousness, hypersensitivity reactions, and electrocardiogram changes.

Topiramate

A retrospective chart review suggested that topiramate might be beneficial as an adjunctive treatment for mania in children and adolescents with bipolar disorder (Barzman et al. 2005). Topiramate overdose can be associated with somnolence and at times vertigo, mydriasis, and agitation. Both lamotrigine and topiramate have been found to have efficacy in treatment of impulsivity (a risk factor for suicidality and self-harm) in adults with borderline personality disorder: however, this has not been studied in pediatric populations (Lieb et al. 2010).

Atypical Antipsychotics

A small open trial of 9- to 17-year-old youth found that quetiapine (average dose of 390 mg/day) added as an adjunct to SSRIs resulted in a significant reduction in aggression, irritability, affect instability, suicidality, and depressive symptoms (Podobnik et al. 2012). This small open trial merits replication and consideration of rational drug combinations, particularly in youth with treatment-refractory or treatment-resistant depression. Combination treatments are considered after initial, sequential monotherapy trials have failed.

Children and adolescents with first-episode psychosis are far more likely to attempt suicide than those without a history of psychosis (Falcone et al. 2010). Adolescents diagnosed with depressive and psychotic symptoms are at a much higher risk of more severe suicidal behavior (e.g., suicide plans, suicide acts) compared with adolescents with depressive symptoms only (Kelleher et al. 2012). One possible explanation for this is the presence of command type auditory hallucinations, directing individuals to harm themselves. Alternatively, this may be related to an indirect cognitive mechanism and a sense of disintegration and fragmentation of the self, resulting from intrusive thoughts and voices in psychosis (Kelleher et al. 2012). A meta-analysis that assessed factors associated with suicide attempts or deliberate self-harm before and after treatment found that the strongest predictors of deliberate self-harm in early psychosis were depressed mood and prior deliberate self-harm. Although positive symptoms of psychosis were unrelated to self-harm before or after treatment, negative symptoms had an association with self-harm after treatment (Challis et al. 2013).

Several multisite clinical trials of atypical antipsychotics have found that olanzapine, risperidone, and aripiprazole are efficacious in the acute treatment of adolescents with psychosis when compared with placebo.

Risperidone and olanzapine have been associated with a lower risk of suicidality when compared with first-generation antipsychotics in adults with schizophrenia. Moreover, clozapine has been known to have a clinically relevant advantage over other antipsychotics in reducing suicidality in adults (Aguilar and Siris 2007). There are, however, no trials assessing the efficacy of antipsychotic medications in suicidal adolescents. Aripiprazole has been found to be efficacious as an adjunctive therapy in major depressive disorder in adults, but there are no RCTs with adolescents (Marcus et al. 2008).

Owing to their relatively favorable receptor profile (when compared with typical antipsychotics), atypical antipsychotics cause mild to moderate toxicity syndromes in most patients, although children are more sensitive to these effects. An overdose has been related to central nervous system depression, appetite stimulation, hypotension (H_1 receptor antagonism), dizziness, orthostatic hypotension, reflex tachycardia, miosis, nasal congestion (α_1 receptor antagonism), dry skin, urinary retention, blurry vision, tachycardia, constipation, agitation, and hallucinations (M_1 receptor antagonism).

Anxiolytic Agents

Anxiety and subthreshold anxiety symptoms are associated with an increased suicide risk. Severe ruminative anxiety, panic attacks, and agitation are particularly important to assess as these can lead to depressive symptoms and manifest as risk factors for suicide. In addition to SSRIs and SNRIs described above, benzodiazepines have been used for treatment of anxiety in adults who are acutely suicidal. For example, lorazepam has been used in an acute situation where there is a risk of suicidality or self-harm due to agitation (Neale and Smith 2007). However, benzodiazepines have a limited role in the longer-term treatment for adolescent anxiety and agitation, with their use typically restricted to severe and treatment-refractory anxiety that is impacting day-to-day functioning. Moreover, this class has been associated with paradoxical agitation, irritability, and oppositional behavior in adolescents, mitigating their use on a regular basis.

Stimulants

A small pilot study assessing the relationship between attention-deficit/ hyperactivity disorder (ADHD) and suicidality in adolescents ($n=23$; ages 12–18 years) as an independent phenotype found that the majority of the patients (65%) who attempted suicide met criteria for ADHD, predominantly inattentive type (Manor et al. 2010). In a retrospective population-based study of individuals ages 6–25 years who were treated with methylphenidate (Man et al. 2017), the incidence of suicide attempts prior to and immediately following initiation of methylphenidate increased but returned to baseline levels during ongoing treatment. Methylphenidate has also been shown to improve the severity of co-occurring ADHD and borderline personality disorder as well as aggressive behavior among female adolescents ages 14–19 years in a 12-week open-label study (Golubchik et al. 2008). However, these limited and uncontrolled results cannot be used to infer that stimulants have an effect on lowering suicidality.

Adolescents with depressive symptoms tend to self-medicate more frequently with stimulants (Zullig et al. 2015). When compared with population-based surveys, the California Poison Control System records revealed a significantly higher rate of suicidal ideation and suicide attempts in adolescents abusing methylphenidate. It was also noted that there is an increased incidence of suicidality in adolescent females abusing methamphetamine. Hence, this group is considered at high risk for suicidality (Auten et al. 2012), which could be due to increased severity of depression in this group or an exacerbation of depressive symptoms in those abusing stimulants. When compared with stimulants, atomoxetine has not been significantly associated with an increased risk of suicidal events in adolescents (Linden et al. 2016).

Analgesics

Psychological pain is a core feature of suicidality (Ducasse et al. 2017). Preceding the advent of antidepressants, opioids were widely used and considered effective for the treatment of the psychic pain associated with depression, suicidality, and related syndromes. Because of their addictive potential and lethality in overdose, they were replaced with contemporary antidepressants. Although the role of opioids has not yet been studied in the treatment of adolescent suicidality, very low dosages of the partial μ agonist and potent κ antagonist buprenorphine have been reported as a treatment option for severely suicidal adults. Results of a 4-week double-blind placebo-controlled trial suggest that in severely suicidal patients without substance use disorders, this time-limited, short-term use of very low sublingual doses of buprenorphine decreased suicidal ideation compared with placebo (Yovell et al. 2016). Interventions of this kind may play some role for youth with borderline personality traits, after first ruling out substance use disorders, given the frequent risk for use of and dependence on prescription opioids associated with the impulsivity features of borderline personality disorder (Tragesser et al. 2013).

Challenges in the Pharmacological Management of Suicidal Youth

Increased Overdose Risk With Pharmacological Treatments

The pharmacological management of suicidal ideation and behaviors among youth represents a double-edged sword. On the one hand, if used appropriately, medications may substantially improve suicidal symptoms and course among youth (Olfson et al. 2003). On the other hand, medications may also provide a mechanism by which youth may overdose to end their lives. Given that some studies have shown that antidepressants are associated with an increased risk of suicide attempts or completed suicides (Olfson et al. 2006), any time a medication is started with youth, prescribing clinicians must carefully review the risks and benefits of treatment and must develop a safety plan, including monitoring access to medication, because the medication can be used as a method to attempt suicide. After informed consent is obtained and treatment is initiated, clinicians must counsel youth and their families about lethal means of self-harm and develop strategies that prevent hoarding of medications for potential future use in a suicide attempt (Runyan et al. 2016). The ability of parents to effectively prevent access to lethal means of self-harm and to support teens during a suicidal crisis is important in addition to weighing the risks and benefits of pharmacological treatment options (Czyz et al. 2017). With regard to the risk of overdose with SSRIs, to date, there are no data to support preference for one SSRI over another. The decision is based on clinical judgment, family's preference, and any prior patient history or family history of antidepressant-related suicide attempt or completed suicide.

Morbidity (or serious disease-related outcomes) and mortality (fatal outcomes) risks due to medication overdose vary across medication classes, and differences in risk are important to consider when selecting treatments for youth at increased risk for suicide. For example, older-generation antidepressants such as tricyclic antidepressants and monoamine oxidase inhibitors are less favored for use in pediatric populations because of their high risk for morbidity or mortality in the context of an overdose. However, a recent study suggested that with the decrease in tricyclic antidepressant prescriptions and the increase in bupropion prescriptions, youth today are more likely to overdose on bupropion than on tricyclic antidepressants, and they experience significantly higher incidence of morbidity than youth who overdosed on a tricyclic antidepressant (Sheridan et al. 2018). In a recent review of the National Poison Data System for single-drug exposures in individuals age 12 and older, other contemporary psychotropic medications are similarly problematic (Nelson and Spyker 2017). Specifically, lithium, quetiapine, olanzapine, bupropion, and carbamazepine were associated with high *morbidity* indices (number of serious outcomes per 1,000 exposures), and lithium, venlafaxine, bupropion, quetiapine, olanzapine, ziprasidone, valproic acid, carbamazepine, and citalopram were associated with higher *mortality* indices (number of fatal outcomes per 10,000 exposures). Together, these data caution balancing consideration of the risk of suicide attempt by medication overdose with benefits of treatment.

Weighing the Risks of Treating Suicidality Versus Not Treating Suicidality in Adolescents With Antidepressant Medications

The association of antidepressant use with an increased risk for suicidality in adolescents is complicated by conflicting findings from multiple cohorts of youth. Clinicians must frequently and urgently weigh the risks of increased suicidality from exposure to certain pharmacological agents, such as antidepressants, against the risks of increased suicidality from leaving suicidal symptoms untreated (Rihmer and Akiskal 2006). Concerns about the use of antidepressants in children and adolescents were first raised in the United Kingdom in 2003 and the United States in 2004, followed by the FDA issuing a black box warning regarding increased risk of suicide with use of antidepressants. While reexamining analyses of published and unpublished data regarding suicidal thoughts and behaviors and their association with antidepressants in children and adolescents, the FDA advisory panel found that there is a small increased risk of suicidal thoughts or behavior in children taking antidepressants compared with placebo (RR =2.0, 95% CI=1.3–3.0) (Hammad et al. 2006). Following this warning, the rates of antidepressant prescriptions declined (Nemeroff et al. 2007) with a commensurate increase in suicide rates worldwide (Libby et al. 2009; Lu et al. 2014).

Multiple studies worldwide have unequivocally demonstrated the potential liabilities associated with undertreating suicidal behaviors, including the potential for increases in suicidal behaviors or completed suicides (Richmond and Rosen 2005). Although a reduction in risk of suicide-related events from antidepressants should not be overestimated, certain patient characteristics such as female sex, psychotic features, borderline personality disorder, and previous suicide-related events from antidepressant exposure may predict outcome and may be clinically informative (Kuba et al. 2011). If the relative benefits outweigh the risks, pharmacological management should be a part of an informed clinician's tool kit. Please refer to Table 10–1 for a summary of antidepressant efficacy and risk in overdose.

Data From Randomized Controlled Trials

Many adolescent depression trials have excluded participants at high risk of suicidal ideation or behavior or did not have adequate power to detect rare events such as suicide (Rappaport et al. 2005). In the context of a clin-

TABLE 10–1. Summary of efficacy and risk in overdose of currently available antidepressants for adolescents

Antidepressant	Efficacy in randomized controlled trials	Risk in overdose
Fluoxetine	+ Emslie et al. 1997, + Emslie et al. 2002, + March et al. 2004, + Almeida-Montes and Friederichsen 2005 – Simeon et al. 1990	Nausea, vomiting, somnolence, tremor, agitation, and tachycardia
Escitalopram	+ Emslie et al. 2009 – Wagner et al. 2006	Cardiac toxicity, vomiting, somnolence, tremor
Sertraline	+ Wagner et al. 2003	More common: nausea, tremor, and lethargy; less common: agitation, vomiting, tachycardia, and bradycardia
Citalopram	+ Wagner et al. 2004 – von Knorring et al. 2006	Cardiac toxicity, nausea, dizziness, tachycardia, tremor, and somnolence; rare, but in large doses: neurotoxicity
Paroxetine	– Keller et al. 2001, – Berard et al. 2006, – Emslie et al. 2006, – Apter et al. 2006	Vomiting, drowsiness, tremors, dizziness, and sinus tachycardia; rare and brief: self-limited seizures
Fluvoxamine	No RCTs in depression	Drowsiness, tremor, diarrhea, vomiting, abdominal pain, dizziness, mydriasis, and sinus tachycardia, although at higher doses, seizures have been reported
Venlafaxine	+ Brent et al. 2008 – Emslie et al. 2007	QT prolongation, QRS prolongation, tachycardia, cardiac arrest, seizures, and serotonin toxicity

TABLE 10–1. Summary of efficacy and risk in overdose of currently available antidepressants for adolescents *(continued)*

Antidepressant	Efficacy in randomized controlled trials	Risk in overdose
Bupropion	No RCTs	Lower seizure threshold, tachycardia, hypertension; malignant dysrhythmias are rare
Mirtazapine	– Dubitsky 2004	Sedation, some may experience sinus tachycardia, and mild hypertension
Duloxetine	– Emslie et al. 2015	Gastrointestinal or neurological, including central nervous system depression

Note. RCT = randomized controlled trials; SSRI = selective serotonin reuptake inhibitor. Most SSRI overdose can result in serotonin syndrome, although these are rarely serious.

+ Indicates studies where the antidepressant was found to be more efficacious than placebo in the treatment of depression.

– Indicates studies where the antidepressant was not significantly more efficacious than placebo.

ical trial, suicide-related behaviors have been recorded as adverse events and not events that were assessed as a primary outcome in the study (Mann et al. 2006).

As already discussed above, to assess the relation between antidepressants and suicidality in pediatric patients participating in randomized, placebo-controlled trials, Hammad et al. (2006) conducted a meta-analysis of 24 trials that were submitted to the FDA. Sixteen trials investigated participants with MDD; 4 trials, those with obsessive-compulsive disorder; 2 trials, those with generalized anxiety disorder; 1 trial, individuals with social anxiety disorder; and 1 trial, those with ADHD. There were no completed suicides in any of the trials. However, TADS showed a significant association of suicidality in the group treated with antidepressants compared with placebo. Specifically, in TADS, 10 suicidal events occurred in the fluoxetine-alone treatment arm (8 ideation, 2 attempts) versus 6 events in the combined treatment arm (2 attempts, 3 ideation, 1 self-harm), but this difference was not statistically significant at 12 weeks. However, TADS reported significantly more suicidal events in the fluoxetine-alone treatment arm at 36 weeks. Separate analyses for suicidal ideation and behavior for all the trials indicated that the RR for suicidal ideation was 1.74 (95% CI=1.06–2.86) and the RR for suicidal behavior was 1.90 (95% CI=1.00–3.63). The overall RR for suicidality for SSRIs (fluoxetine, sertraline, paroxetine, fluvoxamine, and citalopram) in depression trials was 1.66 (95% CI=1.02–2.68). Patients taking antidepressants had an increased risk of suicidality during the first few months of treatment compared with those taking placebo (4% vs. 2%). Importantly, most studies found that antidepressants neither worsened preexisting suicidal ideation prior to medication initiation nor induced suicidal ideation after participants were enrolled in these trials.

In a comprehensive review of pediatric trials conducted between 1998 and 2006, Bridge et al. (2007) noted that the benefits (number needed to treat=10) of antidepressants outweigh their risks of suicidal ideation/suicide attempt (number needed to harm=112) in children and adolescents who have major depression and anxiety disorders. It was also concluded that fluoxetine was the only agent that was more beneficial than placebo in children less than age 12. It is difficult to assess the risk of suicidality secondary to antidepressant use because depression in itself can lead to suicidal tendencies (in fact, suicidal ideation is a symptom in the diagnostic criteria for major depression).

To determine the efficacy and adverse outcomes associated with newer antidepressants, a review (Bridge et al. 2007) of published and unpublished RCTs, cross-over trials, and cluster trials compared newer-generation antidepressants with placebo in children and adolescents ages 6–18 years who were diagnosed with depression. A total of 19 trials with 3,335 participants were included. The drug classes included SSRIs (citalopram, escitalopram, fluoxetine, fluvoxamine, paroxetine, and sertraline), selective norepinephrine reuptake inhibitors (desvenlafaxine, duloxetine, milnacipran, and venlafaxine), norepinephrine reuptake inhibitors (reboxetine), norepinephrine dopamine reuptake inhibitors (bupropion), norepinephrine dopamine disinhibitors (agomelatine), and tetracyclic antidepressants (mirtazapine). On the basis of 17 trials (3,229 participants), suicidal ideation or behavior occurred more frequently in those who received antidepressants (RR=1.58, 95% CI=1.02–2.45).

To determine the short-term safety of antidepressants, a different meta-analysis of 4 randomized trials (708 children and adolescents with major depression) found that the risk of suicidal thoughts and behavior was comparable for fluoxetine and placebo. Moreover, antidepressants did not provide a protective effect against suicidality in youth (Gibbons et al. 2012a). As can be noted from these results, this meta-analysis has been inconclusive: there is an absence of reliable data on suicidality for many antidepressants, and many antidepressants have not been compared directly. In contrast, in a recent meta-analysis of double-blind RCTs comparing any antidepressant with placebo or another antidepressant as oral monotherapy in the acute treatment of MDD in children and adolescents ages 9–18 years, Cipriani et al. (2016) found robust evidence to suggest that the risk of suicidal ideation or behavior was greater with venlafaxine when compared with placebo (odds ratio 0.13, 95% CI=0.00–0.55) and five other antidepressants (duloxetine, escitalopram, fluoxetine, imipramine, and paroxetine).

Data From Observational Studies

Several observational studies provide additional context about the risk for suicide with antidepressant use. A review of observational studies in children ages 9–18 years with a diagnosis of depression has shown that during the first year of antidepressant use, 266 participants attempted and 3 completed suicide, which yielded an event rate of 27.04 suicidal acts per 1,000 person-years (95% CI=23.9–30.5 suicidal acts per 1,000 person-years). The risk was similar across SSRIs and SNRIs (Schneeweiss et al. 2010). In a retrospective cohort study that included 36,842 children ages 6–18 years enrolled in Tennessee Medicaid between 1995 and 2006, who were new users (defined as filling no prescriptions for antidepressants in the preceding 365 days) of one of the antidepressant medications (fluoxetine, citalopram, escitalopram, paroxetine, sertraline, or venlafaxine), the rate of suicide attempts for those on fluoxetine was relative to the rate for each of the other antidepressants (Cooper et al. 2014). However, because this study focused on suicide attempts resulting in death or medical treatment, it is likely that the less serious attempts or suicidal ideation were missed. The participants also included those in the Medicaid program, who may be exposed to different life stressors, compared with the general population. The study also found an increased risk of suicidal behavior for participants who used multiple, overlapping antidepressants, which likely reflects mental illness severity rather than true medication effect.

The ongoing discussion about the risks versus benefits of antidepressants in children and adolescents has a significant impact. It is likely that cognition and energy improve with pharmacotherapy more rapidly than mood; thus, patients may be at increased risk to act on suicidal ideation during the first few weeks of treatment. Hence, although there appears to be a slight increased risk in suicidal thoughts and behaviors after starting an antidepressant (when compared with placebo), the potential consequences of untreated depressive symptoms may be worse.

Advantages and Pitfalls for Treating Suicidal Behavior as a Symptom Rather Than as a Diagnostic Target

Suicidal behavior is transdiagnostic and frequently co-occurs with other psychiatric symptoms that are transdiagnostic such as insomnia, anhedonia, hopelessness, and irritability. In the literature on psychotherapy approaches for treating suicidal youth, there is the growing consensus that suicide attempts must be directly targeted in treatment versus indirectly in the context of treating of the underlying psychiatric disorder (Linehan 2008). In some cases, youth may present with traits similar to borderline personality disorder in adults. In the development of DSM-5 (American Psychiatric Association 2013) criteria for borderline personality disorder and other psychiatric disorders, provisions for dimensional traits were added and compared with categorical personality disorders (Calvo et al. 2016). DSM-5 cautions reserve in the diagnosis of personality disorders in children and adolescents unless there are unusually pervasive and persistent traits that are unlikely to be limited to a particular developmental stage or another mental disorder. Moreover, there are no psychotropic medications licensed for use in borderline personality disorder, either in adults or youth.

For the maladaptive personality traits or core traits associated with borderline personality disorder, various classes of medications have been deemed effective (Vita et al. 2011), but polypharmacy is common (Starcevic and Janca 2018). For example, in a large European database, 80% of patients with borderline personality disorder received two or more psychotropic medications concomitantly (Bridler et al. 2015). Prescribing trends also suggest that antidepressants are increasingly being replaced with mood stabilizers and atypical antipsychotics (Feurino and Silk 2011), which have their own complex adverse side-effect profiles, including weight gain and sedation. Few interventions have been evaluated for efficacy in youth with borderline personality disorder. Those interventions that have been evaluated are limited by small sample sizes, uncontrolled designs, or post hoc testing, or testing for the efficacy of an intervention to reduce suicide-related behaviors in adolescents as a primary outcome has not been done (Amminger et al. 2013; Golubchik et al. 2008; Kutcher et al. 1995; Sharp et al. 2013; Wöckel et al. 2010).

Given the limited evidence demonstrating efficacy for medications for borderline personality disorder, clinicians either completely avoid pharmacotherapy for patients with borderline personality disorder or use specific medications to target specific core symptoms, creating confusion and variable prescribing practices. Clinical guidelines consistently suggest use of medications with caution, for a short term, for mainly symptom relief, with frequent reevaluation of need for ongoing pharmacotherapy, and the avoidance of polypharmacy (Starcevic and Janca 2018). The weight of these guidelines is particularly salient for the developing brain, which may be at high risk when subject to many years of polypharmacy and variable prescribing practices that start in childhood. Whereas it is reasonable to use medications targeted at a certain diagnosis and for symptom relief, one must be careful to avoid polypharmacy.

Predicting Medication Response Based on Moderators of Suicide-Related Outcomes

Because suicidal behavior is transdiagnostic with inter-individual variability and remission rates after pharmacological treatment are low, recent efforts have been made to take a personalized medicine approach for its treatment, taking special care to understand sociodemographic, cultural, psychological, and neurobiological moderators of suicide-related outcomes that may contribute to improved treatment outcomes.

Sociodemographic and Cultural Predictors of Treatment Response

Suicide attempts are strong predictors of suicide, and suicide attempts are highly familial, such that parental history of suicide attempts conveys nearly a 5-fold increase of the odds of suicide attempt in offspring at risk for a mood disorder (Brent et al. 2015). Impulsive aggression and mood disorders are clear antecedents of early-onset suicidal behavior in genetically at-risk youth (Melhem et al. 2007) and may be important targets for pharmacological treatment in the prevention of suicidal behavior. Clinicians should consider antidepressants that are currently FDA approved for depressive symptoms, such as escitalopram or fluoxetine, and take into consideration family history of response to antidepressants, drug-drug interactions, and patient preference. Interestingly, in psychiatrically hospitalized youth, although family conflict is positively associated with suicidal ideation, it does not moderate the relation between anxiety and suicidal ideation (Machell et al. 2016). Nevertheless, family support may be an important intervention target to decrease suicide risk among anxious youth by integrating positive parenting techniques (e.g., providing praise, emotion coaching, attending to positive behaviors) and improved parent-child communication into treatment.

Hart and colleagues (2017) identified subtypes of suicide attempters using a latent profile analysis relating clinical symptoms manifesting in childhood (depression, anxiety, and aggression measured in second and fourth to seventh grades) to suicide attempts between the ages of 13–30 years. They found that the group with high depression, anxiety, and aggression was primarily composed of African American males with histories of substance use and violent, drug-related criminal convictions. This group had multiple and potentially medically lethal suicide attempts starting at a young age. Indeed, aggressive behavior is associated with earlier onset of MDD, younger age of completed suicide, and impulsive suicide attempts (Zouk et al. 2006). Combined with symptoms of anxiety and depression, aggression can increase impulsivity and reactivity, leading to lethal suicide attempts. Hence, treatment of suicidality should aim not only to target symptoms of depression and anxiety, which are commonly associated with suicidal thoughts and behaviors, but also target aggression and impulsivity.

It is also important to note age and sex differences in suicidal behavior. Older adolescents present with more severe acts of self-harm, yet receive the lowest intensity of assessment and aftercare, and 18- to 25-year-old young adults were more likely than younger adolescents to self-poison with prescription medicines, mixed overdoses, alcohol, or recreational drugs (Diggins et al. 2017). Another study found that suicidal ideation or suicide attempt during childhood and adolescence predicted a suicide attempt during young adulthood for female, but not male, adolescents (Lewinsohn et al. 2001). Indeed, female adolescents and youth (ages 13–22 years) have been seen to have a higher rate of suicide attempts before suicide completion when compared with their male counterparts. Female suicide victims also have higher rates of depression and tend to attempt suicide by overdosing more frequently (Marttunen et al. 1995). Together, these studies suggest important individual patient characteristics that may be of importance in the selection of pharmacological treatment for suicidal behavior in youth. Subtype and personalized approaches may permit enhanced precision of predictions for various markers of outcome.

Neurobiological Predictors of Treatment Response

Understanding neurobiological predictors of suicide may provide exciting new insights about underlying mechanisms of the origins of suicidal symptoms and thus inform treatment selection (Niculescu et al. 2017). Serotonergic dysfunction has frequently been implicated as a biological marker of suicide in adults; however, this has not been consistently replicated in adolescents, and a common genetic variant associated with suicidal behavior has not yet been identified (Picouto et al. 2015).

Psychological constructs of loss and hopelessness as well as impulsivity and aggression may be relevant in understanding characteristics that place youth at high risk for suicide-related behavior. For example, in a study of adolescents with a history of suicide attempt compared with a never-suicidal group, Bridge et al. (2015) found no overall difference between the two groups in delay discounting or impulsive aggression. Impulsive aggression was related to suicide attempts only in the absence of psychotropic drug use. It is known that antidepressants, specifically SSRIs may help reduce impulsivity and aggression, which can reduce the risk of suicide.

Other biological variables may also be in play. Recent evidence suggests that nocturnal wakefulness may be a previously unrecognized risk factor for suicide. These results are particularly salient for youth, who may be at high risk for sleep dysfunction during adolescence (Perlis et al. 2016). In a different study examining the pathophysiology of teen suicide, teen suicide victims were found, in postmortem studies, to have significantly low protein levels of mean protein, mRNA levels of β-catenin, and pGSK-3β-ser[9] in the prefrontal cortex and hippocampus, as well as reduced GSK-3β mRNA levels in the prefrontal cortex but not in the hippocampus, compared with healthy control subjects (Ren et al. 2013). Given that treatment with lithium and antipsychotic drugs causes changes in GSK-3β, their role in teen suicide should be assessed further. Another study found that the mRNA and protein expression levels of IL-1β, IL-6, and TNF-α were significantly increased in the Brodmann area 10 (BA-10) of suicide victims compared with nonsuicidal control subjects. These results suggest an important role for IL-1β, IL-6, and TNF-α in the pathophysiology of suicidal behavior, implying that proinflammatory cytokines may be an appropriate target for developing therapeutic agents (Pandey et al. 2012).

Future studies on the neurobiology of suicide in adolescence should consider the specific developmental and biological processes that may uniquely contribute to increasing risk. Prospective studies that are designed to integrate psychological and biological domains together may advance our understanding of how suicidal ideation progresses to an attempt or a completed suicide.

Future Directions

There are a number of areas for growth in developing improved approaches to the pharmacological treatment and prevention of suicidal behavior and self-injury in adolescents. First, studies that directly assess the efficacy and effectiveness of pharmacological treatments in reducing suicide-related symptoms and severity are needed to build an evidence base for treating self-harm and preventing adolescent suicide. Second, improving our ability to predict self-harm and suicide-related events in the context of pharmacological exposures would aid clinicians in selection and dosing strategies. Third, although there are several therapeutic intervention approaches that have demonstrated an ability to decrease risk and rates of suicide-related events among youth, most studies require replication for establishing an evidence base. Fourth, psychotropic medications appear to have differential safety profiles in the context of an overdose. Comparative effectiveness and safety assessments as well as personalized medicine approaches to understanding individualized responses to treatment may aid in improved treatment selection methods. Pharmacogenomics has recently emerged as one potential but yet to be tested approach to treatment selection (Niculescu et al. 2017), although polygenic score analyses for suicide attempts have not shown predictive ability for suicidal ideation (Mullins et al. 2014). Fifth, future randomized controlled trials should be designed in a fashion that enables investigation of potential mechanisms and moderators of change. Finally, longer-term observational and outcome data are needed to determine whether pharmacological treatments have indeed reduced or prevented suicide-related outcomes.

Recommendations and Conclusion

Given that there is still a dearth in the literature on the pharmacological treatment of suicidal behavior in adolescents, the decision to use pharmacotherapy for the treatment of depression should be made on a case-by-case basis, after discussion with the patient and family and after weighing possible risks, benefits, and alternatives. There is strong evidence that antidepressants can improve adolescent depressive symptoms, including suicidal ideation and behaviors, significantly better than placebo, even though the magnitude of the effects is, at best, modest. The evidence establishing an association between the improvement of depressive symptoms and treatment with antidepressants is still inconclusive to date. Most studies so far have not shown any completed suicides in this group following initiation of an antidepressant, and often the risk is higher prior to treatment. Hence, it is important to weigh the risks versus the benefits of prescribing medications and to ensure close and regular follow-up, again, particularly at the beginning of the treatment. A concern for increased suicide risk alone should not deter providers from prescribing antidepressants, especially when there is enough evidence of the benefits of antidepressants in depressed adolescents. It is also important to start children and adolescents on a low dose to avoid potential adverse outcomes, because for this group, therapy initiated at high therapeutic doses seems to be associated with heightened risk of deliberate self-harm (Miller et al. 2014). However, one must not deter from titrating dose on an as-needed basis for symptom relief, especially for those with severe symptoms or treatment-resistant depression.

Experience in clinical practice suggests the following actions to minimize risk and optimize treatment response: 1) continually assess and reassess suicidality in at-risk youth being treated with medication, 2) provide education to patients and families on the beneficial and harmful effects of medications, and 3) make timely adjustments to treatments if initial strategies are unsuccessful. We underscore that providing psychoeducation to families and regular follow-up is of utmost importance in developing a treatment partnership with adolescents at high risk for suicidal behavior or self-harm. Suicide-related behaviors are transdiagnostic and can be representative of a variety of psychiatric phenomenology. If suicidal behavior is treated as a symptom rather than as part of a diagnosis, clinicians should guard against polypharmacy. Thoughtful consideration of individual patient characteristics, risk factors, and neurobiological predictors of treatment response may improve treatment outcomes, but this needs to be tested. We need more research to help us intervene effectively to decrease suicidal and nonsuicidal self-harm and to help youth achieve favorable developmental outcomes.

References

Aguilar EJ, Siris SG: Do antipsychotic drugs influence suicidal behavior in schizophrenia? Psychopharmacol Bull 40(3):128–142, 2007 18007574

Almeida-Montes LG, Friederichsen A: Treatment of major depressive disorder with fluoxetine in children and adolescents. A double-blind, placebo-controlled study. Psiq Biol 12:198–205, 2005

American Psychiatric Association: Diagnostic and Statistical Manual of Mental Disorders, 4th Edition. Washington, DC, American Psychiatric Association, 1994

American Psychiatric Association: Diagnostic and Statistical Manual of Mental Disorders, 5th Edition. Arlington, VA, American Psychiatric Association, 2013

Amminger GP, Chanen AM, Ohmann S, et al: Omega-3 fatty acid supplementation in adolescents with borderline personality disorder and ultra-high risk criteria for psychosis: a post hoc subgroup analysis of a double-blind, randomized controlled trial. Can J Psychiatry 58(7):402–408, 2013 23870722

Apter A, Lipschitz A, Fong R, et al: Evaluation of suicidal thoughts and behaviors in children and adolescents taking paroxetine. J Child Adolesc Psychopharmacol 16(1–2):77–90, 2006 16553530

Auten JD, Matteucci MJ, Gaspary MJ, et al: Psychiatric implications of adolescent methamphetamine exposures. Pediatr Emerg Care 28(1):26–29, 2012 22193694

Baldessarini RJ, Tondo L, Davis P, et al: Decreased risk of suicides and attempts during long-term lithium treatment: a meta-analytic review. Bipolar Disord 8(5 Pt 2):625–639, 2006 17042835

Barzman DH, DelBello MP, Kowatch RA, et al: Adjunctive topiramate in hospitalized children and adolescents with bipolar disorders. J Child Adolesc Psychopharmacol 15(6):931–937, 2005 16379513

Berard R, Fong R, Carpenter DJ, et al: An international, multicenter, placebo-controlled trial of paroxetine in adolescents with major depressive disorder. J Child Adolesc Psychopharmacol 16(1-2):59-75, 2006 16553529

Brent D, Emslie G, Clarke G, et al: Switching to another SSRI or to venlafaxine with or without cognitive behavioral therapy for adolescents with SSRI-resistant depression: the TORDIA randomized controlled trial. JAMA 299(8):901–913, 2008 18314433

Brent DA, Greenhill LL, Compton S, et al: The Treatment of Adolescent Suicide Attempters study (TASA): predictors of suicidal events in an open treatment trial. J Am Acad Child Adolesc Psychiatry 48(10):987–996, 2009 19730274

Brent DA, Melhem NM, Oquendo M, et al: Familial pathways to early onset suicide attempt: a 5.6-year prospective study. JAMA Psychiatry 72(2):160–168, 2015 25548996

Bridge JA, Iyengar S, Salary CB, et al: Clinical response and risk for reported suicidal ideation and suicide attempts in pediatric antidepressant treatment: a meta-analysis of randomized controlled trials. JAMA 297(15):1683–1696, 2007 17440145

Bridge JA, Reynolds B, McBee-Strayer SM, et al: Impulsive aggression, delay discounting, and adolescent suicide attempts: effects of current psychotropic medication use and family history of suicidal behavior. J Child Adolesc Psychopharmacol 25(2):114–123, 2015 25745870

Bridler R, Häberle A, Müller ST, et al: Psychopharmacological treatment of 2195 inpatients with borderline personality disorder: a comparison with other psychiatric disorders. Eur Neuropsychopharmacol 25(6):763–772, 2015 25907249

Calabrese JR, Bowden CL, Sachs G, et al; Lamictal 605 Study Group: A placebo-controlled 18-month trial of lamotrigine and lithium maintenance treatment in recently depressed patients with bipolar I disorder. J Clin Psychiatry 64(9):1013–1024, 2003 14628976

Calvo N, Valero S, Sáez-Francàs N, et al: Borderline Personality Disorder and Personality Inventory for DSM-5 (PID-5): dimensional personality assessment with DSM-5. Compr Psychiatry 70:105–111, 2016 27624429

Carpenter DJ, Fong R, Kraus JE, et al: Meta-analysis of efficacy and treatment-emergent suicidality in adults by psychiatric indication and age subgroup following initiation of paroxetine therapy: a complete set of randomized placebo-controlled trials. J Clin Psychiatry 72(11):1503–1514, 2011 21367354

Challis S, Nielssen O, Harris A, et al: Systematic meta-analysis of the risk factors for deliberate self-harm before and after treatment for first-episode psychosis. Acta Psychiatr Scand 127(6):442–454, 2013 23298325

Centers for Disease Control and Prevention: QuickStats: suicide rates for teens aged 15–19 years, by sex—United States, 1975–2015. MMWR Morb Mortal Wkly Rep 66(30):816, 2017 28771461. Available at https://www.cdc.gov/mmwr/volumes/66/wr/mm6630a6.htm. Accessed December 6, 2018.

Cipriani A, Zhou X, Del Giovane C, et al: Comparative efficacy and tolerability of antidepressants for major depressive disorder in children and adolescents: a network meta-analysis. Lancet 388(10047):881–890, 2016 27289172

Cooper WO, Callahan ST, Shintani A, et al: Antidepressants and suicide attempts in children. Pediatrics 133(2):204–210, 2014 24394688

Czyz EK, Horwitz AG, Yeguez CE, et al: Parental self-efficacy to support teens during a suicidal crisis and future adolescent emergency department visits and suicide attempts. J Clin Child Adolesc Psychol 53(July):1–13, 2017 28715239

Delavenne H, Garcia FD, Thibaut F: Do antidepressant treatments influence self-harm and aggressive behaviors? [in French]. Presse Med 42(6 Pt 1):968–976, 2013 22959339

Diggins E, Kelley R, Cottrell D, et al: Age-related differences in self-harm presentations and subsequent management of adolescents and young adults at the emergency department. J Affect Disord 208:399–405, 2017 27810724

Dubicka B, Elvins R, Roberts C, et al: Combined treatment with cognitive-behavioural therapy in adolescent depression: meta-analysis. Br J Psychiatry 197(6):433–440, 2010 21119148

Dubitsky GM: Review and Evaluation of Clinical Data: Placebo-Controlled Antidepressant Studies in Pediatric Patients. Washington, DC, U.S. Food and Drug Administration, August 6, 2004

Ducasse D, Holden RR, Boyer L, et al: Psychological pain in suicidality: a meta-analysis. J Clin Psychiatry August 29, 2017 [Epub ahead of print], 28872267

Emslie GJ, Rush AJ, Weinberg WA, et al: A double-blind, randomized, placebo-controlled trial of fluoxetine in children and adolescents with depression. Arch Gen Psychiatry 54(11):1031–1037 1997 9366660

Emslie GJ, Heiligenstein JH, Wagner KD, et al: Fluoxetine for acute treatment of depression in children and adolescents: a placebo-controlled, randomized clinical trial. J Am Acad Child Adolesc Psychiatry 41(10):1205–1215, 2002 12364842

Emslie GJ, Wagner KD, Kutcher S, et al: Paroxetine treatment in children and adolescents with major depressive disorder: a randomized, multicenter, double-blind, placebo-controlled trial. J Am Acad Child Adolesc Psychiatry 45(6):709–719, 2006 16721321

Emslie GJ, Findling RL, Yeung PP, et al: Venlafaxine ER for the treatment of pediatric subjects with depression: results of two placebo-controlled trials. J Am Acad Child Adolesc Psychiatry 46(4):479–488, 2007 17420682

Emslie GJ, Kennard BD, Mayes TL, et al: Fluoxetine versus placebo in preventing relapse of major depression in children and adolescents. Am J Psychiatry 165(4):459–467, 2008 18281410

Emslie GJ, Ventura D, Korotzer A, Tourkodimitris S: Escitalopram in the treatment of adolescent depression: a randomized placebo-controlled multisite trial. J Am Acad Child Adolesc Psychiatry 48(7):721–729, 2009 19465881

Emslie GJ, Wells TG, Prakash A, et al: Acute and longer-term safety results from a pooled analysis of duloxetine studies for the treatment of children and adolescents with major depressive disorder. J Child Adolesc Psychopharmacol 25(4):293–305, 2015 25978741

Falcone T, Mishra L, Carlton E, et al: Suicidal behavior in adolescents with first-episode psychosis. Clin Schizophr Relat Psychoses 4(1):34–40, 2010 20643627

Feurino L 3rd, Silk KR: State of the art in the pharmacologic treatment of borderline personality disorder. Curr Psychiatry Rep 13(1):69–75, 2011 21140245

Findling RL, Robb A, Bose A: Escitalopram in the treatment of adolescent depression: a randomized, double-blind, placebo-controlled extension trial. J Child Adolesc Psychopharmacol 23(7):468–480, 2013 24041408

Findling RL, Robb A, McNamara NK, et al: Lithium in the acute treatment of bipolar I disorder: a double-blind, placebo-controlled study. Pediatrics 136(5):885–894, 2015 26459650

Geller B, Luby JL, Joshi P, et al: A randomized controlled trial of risperidone, lithium, or divalproex sodium for initial treatment of bipolar I disorder, manic or mixed phase, in children and adolescents. Arch Gen Psychiatry 69(5):515–528, 2012 22213771

Gibbons RD, Brown CH, Hur K, et al: Suicidal thoughts and behavior with antidepressant treatment: reanalysis of the randomized placebo-controlled studies of fluoxetine and venlafaxine. Arch Gen Psychiatry 69(6):580–587, 2012a 22309973

Gibbons RD, Hur K, Brown CH, et al: Benefits from antidepressants: synthesis of 6-week patient-level outcomes from double-blind placebo-controlled randomized trials of fluoxetine and venlafaxine. Arch Gen Psychiatry 69(6):572–579, 2012b 22393205

Glod CA, Lunch A, Flynn E, et al: Open trial of bupropion SR in adolescent major depression. J Child Adolesc Psychiatr Nurs 16(3):123–130, 2003 14603988

Goldsmith L, Moncrieff J: The psychoactive effects of antidepressants and their association with suicidality. Curr Drug Saf 6(2):115–121, 2011 21375477

Golubchik P, Sever J, Zalsman G, et al: Methylphenidate in the treatment of female adolescents with cooccurrence of attention deficit/hyperactivity disorder and borderline personality disorder: a preliminary open-label trial. Int Clin Psychopharmacol 23(4):228–231, 2008 18446088

Goodwin FK, Fireman B, Simon GE, et al: Suicide risk in bipolar disorder during treatment with lithium and divalproex. JAMA 290(11):1467–1473, 2003 13129986

Goodyer I, Dubicka B, Wilkinson P, et al: Selective serotonin reuptake inhibitors (SSRIs) and routine specialist care with and without cognitive behaviour therapy in adolescents with major depression: randomised controlled trial. BMJ 335(7611):142, 2007 17556431

Grunebaum MF, Ellis SP, Duan N, et al: Pilot randomized clinical trial of an SSRI vs bupropion: effects on suicidal behavior, ideation, and mood in major depression. Neuropsychopharmacology 37(3):697–706, 2012 21993207

Hammad TA, Laughren T, Racoosin J: Suicidality in pediatric patients treated with antidepressant drugs. Arch Gen Psychiatry 63(3):332–339, 2006 16520440

Hart SR, Van Eck K, Ballard ED, et al: Subtypes of suicide attempters based on longitudinal childhood profiles of co-occurring depressive, anxious and aggressive behavior symptoms. Psychiatry Res 257(November):150–155, 2017 28755606

Hauser M, Galling B, Correll CU: Suicidal ideation and suicide attempts in children and adolescents with bipolar disorder: a systematic review of prevalence and incidence rates, correlates, and targeted interventions. Bipolar Disord 15(5):507–523, 2013 23829436

Hawton K, Kingsbury S, Steinhardt K, et al: Repetition of deliberate self-harm by adolescents: the role of psychological factors. J Adolesc 22(3):369–378, 1999 10462427

Hawton K, Witt KG, Taylor Salisbury TL, et al: Interventions for self-harm in children and adolescents. Cochrane Database Syst Rev (12):CD012013, 2015 26688129

Hazell P, Mirzaie M: Tricyclic drugs for depression in children and adolescents. Cochrane Database Syst Rev (6):CD002317, 2013 23780719

Hetrick SE, McKenzie JE, Cox GR, et al: Newer generation antidepressants for depressive disorders in children and adolescents. Cochrane Database Syst Rev (6):CD004851, 2012 23152227

Hughes CW, Emslie GJ, Crismon ML, et al; Texas Consensus Conference Panel on Medication Treatment of Childhood Major Depressive Disorder: Texas Children's Medication Algorithm Project: update from Texas Consensus Conference Panel on Medication Treatment of Childhood Major Depressive Disorder. J Am Acad Child Adolesc Psychiatry 46(6):667–686, 2007 17513980

Keller MB, Ryan ND, Strober M: Efficacy of paroxetine in the treatment of adolescent major depression: a randomized, controlled trial. J Am Acad Child Adolesc Psychiatry 40(7):762–772, 2001 11437014

Kelleher I, Lynch F, Harley M, et al: Psychotic symptoms in adolescence index risk for suicidal behavior: findings from 2 population-based case-control clinical interview studies. Arch Gen Psychiatry 69(12):1277–1283, 2012 23108974

Kovacs M: Presentation and course of major depressive disorder during childhood and later years of the life span. J Am Acad Child Adolesc Psychiatry 35(6):705–715, 1996 8682751

Kuba T, Yakushi T, Fukuhara H, et al: Suicide-related events among child and adolescent patients during short-term antidepressant therapy. Psychiatry Clin Neurosci 65(3):239–245, 2011 21507130

Kutcher S, Papatheodorou G, Reiter S, Gardner D: The successful pharmacological treatment of adolescents and young adults with borderline personality disorder: a preliminary open trial of flupenthixol. J Psychiatry Neurosci 20(2):113, 1995 7703220

Lewinsohn PM, Joiner TE Jr, Rodhe P: Evaluation of cognitive diathesis-stress models in predicting major depressive disorder in adolescents. Abstract Psychol 110(2):203–215, 2001 11368074

Libby AM, Orton HD, Valuck RJ: Persisting decline in depression treatment after FDA warnings. Arch Gen Psychiatry 66(6):633–639, 2009 19487628

Lieb K, Völlm B, Rücker G, et al: Pharmacotherapy for borderline personality disorder: Cochrane systematic review of randomised trials. Br J Psychiatry 196(1):4–12, 2010 20044651

Linden S, Bussing R, Kubilis P, et al: Risk of suicidal events with atomoxetine compared to stimulant treatment: a cohort study. Pediatrics 137(5):e20153199, 2016 27244795

Linehan MM: Suicide intervention research: a field in desperate need of development. Suicide Life Threat Behav 38(5):483–485, 2008 19014300

Lu CY, Zhang F, Lakoma MD, et al: Changes in antidepressant use by young people and suicidal behavior after FDA warnings and media coverage: quasi-experimental study. BMJ 348(June):g3596, 2014 24942789

Machell KA, Rallis BA, Esposito-Smythers C: Family environment as a moderator of the association between anxiety and suicidal ideation. J Anxiety Disord 40:1–7, 2016 27035729

Man KKC, Coghill D, Chan EW, et al: Association of risk of suicide attempts with methylphenidate treatment. JAMA Psychiatry 74(10):1048–1055, 2017 28746699

Mann JJ, Emslie G, Baldessarini RJ, et al: ACNP Task Force report on SSRIs and suicidal behavior in youth. Neuropsychopharmacology 31(3):473–492, 2006 16319919

Manor I, Gutnik I, Ben-Dor DH, et al: Possible association between attention deficit hyperactivity disorder and attempted suicide in adolescents—a pilot study. Eur Psychiatry 25(3):146–150, 2010 19699060

March J, Silva S, Petrycki S, et al: Fluoxetine, cognitive-behavioral therapy, and their combination for adolescents with depression: Treatment for Adolescents With Depression Study (TADS) randomized controlled trial. JAMA 292(7):807–820, 2004 15315995

March JS, Klee BJ, Kremer CME: Treatment benefit and the risk of suicidality in multicenter, randomized, controlled trials of sertraline in children and adolescents. J Child Adolesc Psychopharmacol 16(1–2):91–102, 2006 16553531

Marcus RN, McQuade RD, Carson WH, et al: The efficacy and safety of aripiprazole as adjunctive therapy in major depressive disorder: a second multicenter, randomized, double-blind, placebo-controlled study. J Clin Psychopharmacol 28(2):156–165, 2008 18344725

Marttunen M, Henriksson M, Aro H, et al: Suicide among female adolescents: characteristics and comparison with males in the age group 13 to 22 years. J Am Acad Child Adolesc Psychiatry 34(10):1297–1307, 1995 7592267

Melhem NM, Brent DA, Ziegler M, et al: Familial pathways to early onset suicidal behavior: familial and individual antecedents of suicidal behavior. Am J Psychiatry 164(9):1364–1370, 2007 17728421

Miller M, Swanson SA, Azrael D, et al: Antidepressant dose, age, and the risk of deliberate self-harm. JAMA Intern Med 174(6):899–909, 2014 24782035

Mullins N, Perroud N, Uher R, et al: Genetic relationships between suicide attempts, suicidal ideation and major psychiatric disorders: a genome-wide association and polygenic scoring study. Am J Med Genet B Neuropsychiatr Genet 165B(5):428–437, 2014 24964207

Neale G, Smith AJ: Self-harm and suicide associated with benzodiazepine usage. Br J Gen Pract 57(538):407–408, 2007 17504594

Nelson JC, Spyker DA: Morbidity and mortality associated with medications used in the treatment of depression: an analysis of cases reported to U.S. Poison Control Centers, 2000–2014. Am J Psychiatry 174(5):438–450, 2017 28135844

Nemeroff CB, Kalali A, Keller MB, et al: Impact of publicity concerning pediatric suicidality data on physician practice patterns in the United States. Arch Gen Psychiatry 64(4):466–472, 2007 17404123

Niculescu AB, Le-Niculescu H, Levey DF, et al: Precision medicine for suicidality: from universality to subtypes and personalization. Mol Psychiatry 22(9):1250–1273, 2017 28809398

Nock MK, Green JG, Hwang I, et al: Prevalence, correlates, and treatment of lifetime suicidal behavior among adolescents: results from the National Comorbidity Survey Replication Adolescent Supplement. JAMA Psychiatry 70(3):300–310, 2013 23303463

Olfson M, Shaffer D, Marcus SC, et al: Relationship between antidepressant medication treatment and suicide in adolescents. Arch Gen Psychiatry 60(10):978–982, 2003 14557142

Olfson M, Marcus SC, Shaffer D: Antidepressant drug therapy and suicide in severely depressed children and adults: a case-control study. Arch Gen Psychiatry 63(8):865–872, 2006 16894062

Pandey GN, Rizavi HS, Ren X, et al: Proinflammatory cytokines in the prefrontal cortex of teenage suicide victims. J Psychiatr Res 46(1):57–63, 2012 21906753

Patorno E, Bohn RL, Wahl PM, et al: Anticonvulsant medications and the risk of suicide, attempted suicide, or violent death. JAMA 303(14):1401–1409, 2010 20388896

Perlis ML, Grandner MA, Chakravorty S, et al: Suicide and sleep: Is it a bad thing to be awake when reason sleeps? Sleep Med Rev 29:101–107, 2016 26706755

Picouto MD, Villar R, Braquehais MD: The role of serotonin in adolescent suicide: theoretical, methodological, and clinical concerns. Int J Adolesc Med Health 27(2):129–133, 2015 25411983

Pitzianti M, Marciano S, Minnei M, et al: Asynchronicity of organic and psychiatric symptoms in a case of sertraline intoxication. Clin Neuropharmacol 39(5):269–271, 2016 27454389

Podobnik J, Foller Podobnik I, Grgic N, et al: The effect of add-on treatment with quetiapine on measures of depression, aggression, irritability and suicidal tendencies in children and adolescents. Psychopharmacology (Berl) 220(3):639–641, 2012 22173852

Rappaport N, Prince JB, Bostic JQ; Association of Medical School Pediatric Department Chairs, Inc: Lost in the black box: juvenile depression, suicide, and the FDA's black box. J Pediatr 147(6):719–720, 2005 16356415

Ren X, Rizavi HS, Khan MA, et al: Altered Wnt signalling in the teenage suicide brain: focus on glycogen synthase kinase-3β and β-catenin. Int J Neuropsychopharmacol 16(5):945–955, 2013 23110823

Richmond TK, Rosen DS: The treatment of adolescent depression in the era of the black box warning. Curr Opin Pediatr 17(4):466–472, 2005 16012257

Rihmer Z, Akiskal H: Do antidepressants t(h)reat(en) depressives? Toward a clinically judicious formulation of the antidepressant-suicidality FDA advisory in light of declining national suicide statistics from many countries. J Affect Disord 94(1–3):3–13, 2006 16712945

Runyan CW, Becker A, Brandspigel S, et al: Lethal means counseling for parents of youth seeking emergency care for suicidality. West J Emerg Med 17(1):8–14, 2016 26823923

Schneeweiss S, Patrick AR, Solomon DH, et al: Comparative safety of antidepressant agents for children and adolescents regarding suicidal acts. Pediatrics 125(5):876–888, 2010 20385637

Schreffler SM, Marraffa JM, Stork CM, et al: Sodium channel blockade with QRS widening after an escitalopram overdose. Pediatr Emerg Care 29(9):998–1001, 2013 24201980

Sharp C, Ha C, Carbone C, et al: Hypermentalizing in adolescent inpatients: treatment effects and association with borderline traits. J Pers Disord 27(1):3–18, 2013 23342954

Sheridan DC, Lin A, Zane Horowitz B: Suicidal bupropion ingestions in adolescents: increased morbidity compared with other antidepressants. Clin Toxicol (Phila) 56(5):360–364, 2018 28944696

Simeon JG, Dinicola VF, Ferguson HB, Coppiing W: Adolescent depression: a placebo-controlled fluoxetine treatment study and follow-up. Prog Neuropsychopharmacol Biol Psychiatry 14(5):791–795, 1990 2293257

Starcevic V, Janca A: Pharmacotherapy of borderline personality disorder: replacing confusion with prudent pragmatism. Curr Opin Psychiatry 31(1):69–73, 2018 29028643

Storrow AB: Bupropion overdose and seizure. Am J Emerg Med 12(2):183–184, 1994 8161393

Thomas KH, Martin RM, Davies NM, et al: Smoking cessation treatment and risk of depression, suicide, and self harm in the Clinical Practice Research Datalink: prospective cohort study. BMJ 347(October):f5704, 2013 24124105

Tragesser SL, Jones RE, Robinson RJ, et al: Borderline personality disorder features and risk for prescription opioid use disorders. J Pers Disord 27(4):427–441, 2013 23718741

Vita A, De Peri L, Sacchetti E: Antipsychotics, antidepressants, anticonvulsants, and placebo on the symptom dimensions of borderline personality disorder: a meta-analysis of randomized controlled and open-label trials. J Clin Psychopharmacol 31(5):613–624, 2011 21869691

Vitiello B, Ordóñez AE: Pharmacological treatment of children and adolescents with depression. Expert Opin Pharmacother 17(17):2273–2279, 2016 27690663

von Knorring AL, Olsson GI, Thoimsen PH, et al: A randomized, double-blind, placebo-controlled study of citalopram in adolescents with major depressive disorder. J Clin Psychopharmacol 26(3):311–315, 2006 16702897

Wagner KD, Ambrosini P, Rynn M, et al: Efficacy of sertraline in the treatment of children and adolescents with major depressive disorder: two randomized controlled trials. JAMA 290(8):1033–1041, 2003 12941675

Wagner KD, Robb AS, Findling RL, et al: A randomized, placebo-controlled trial of citalopram for the treatment of major depression in children and adolescents. Am J Psychiatry 161(6):1079–1083, 2004 15169696

Wagner KD, Jonas J, Findling RL, et al: A double-blind, randomized, placebo-controlled trial of escitalopram in the treatment of pediatric depression. J Am Acad Child Adolesc Psychiatry 45(3):280–288, 2006 16540812

Weisberg HI, Hayden VC, Pontes VP: Selection criteria and generalizability within the counterfactual framework: explaining the paradox of antidepressant-induced suicidality? Clin Trials 6(2):109–118, 2009 19342462

Wilkinson P, Kelvin R, Roberts C, et al: Clinical and psychosocial predictors of suicide attempts and nonsuicidal self-injury in the Adolescent Depression Antidepressants and Psychotherapy Trial (ADAPT). Am J Psychiatry 168(5):495–501, 2011 21285141

Wöckel L, Goth K, Matic N, et al: Psychopharmacotherapy in adolescents with borderline personality disorder in inpatient and outpatient psychiatric treatment [in German]. Z Kinder Jugendpsychiatr Psychother 38(1):37–49, 2010 20047175

Xu Y, Bai SJ, Lan XH, et al: Randomized controlled trials of serotonin-norepinephrine reuptake inhibitor in treating major depressive disorder in children and adolescents: a meta-analysis of efficacy and acceptability. Braz J Med Biol Res 49(6):pii: S0100-879X2016000600704, 2016 27240293

Yovell Y, Bar G, Mashiah M, et al: Ultra-low-dose buprenorphine as a time-limited treatment for severe suicidal ideation: a randomized controlled trial. Am J Psychiatry 173(5):491–498, 2016 26684923

Zouk H, Tousignant M, Seguin M, et al: Characterization of impulsivity in suicide completers: clinical, behavioral and psychosocial dimensions. J Affect Disord 92(2–3):195–204, 2006 16545465

Zullig KJ, Divin AL, Weiler RM, et al: Adolescent Nonmedical Use of Prescription Pain Relievers, Stimulants, and Depressants, and Suicide Risk. Subst Use Misuse 50(13):1678–1689, 2015 26576505

Index

Page numbers printed in **boldface** type refer to tables and figures.